GRAND ROUNDS

ONE HUNDRED YEARS OF INTERNAL MEDICINE

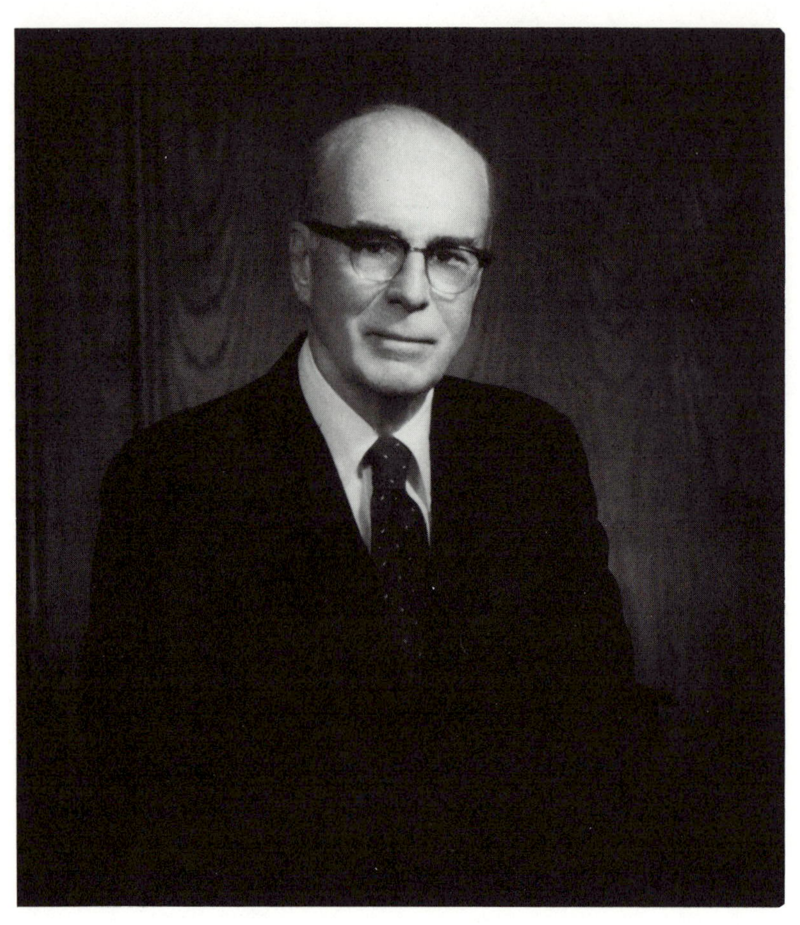

This volume is dedicated to Francis C. Wood, M.D., Professor Emeritus of Medicine at the University of Pennsylvania and Past President of the College of Physicians of Philadelphia. Grand Rounds: One Hundred Years of Internal Medicine *was the second conference of the Francis C. Wood Institute for the History of Medicine at the College of Physicians of Philadelphia.*

GRAND ROUNDS

ONE HUNDRED YEARS OF INTERNAL MEDICINE

RUSSELL C. MAULITZ *and*
DIANA E. LONG *Editors*

upp
UNIVERSITY OF PENNSYLVANIA PRESS *Philadelphia*

Printed in the United States of America

Library of Congress Cataloging-in-Publication Data

Francis Clark Wood Institute for the History of Medicine. Conference (2nd : 1986 : College of Physicians of Philadelphia)
Grand rounds : one hundred years of internal medicine / Russell C. Maulitz and Diana E. Long, editors.
p. cm.
"Second Conference of the Francis C. Wood Institute for the History of Medicine at the College of Physicians of Philadelphia" —P. facing t.p.
"Dedicated to Francis C. Wood"—P. facing t.p.
Includes bibliographies and index.
ISBN 0-8122-8080-6
1. Internal medicine—United States—History—Congresses. 2. Wood, Francis C. (Francis Clark), 1901– —Congresses. I. Maulitz, Russell Charles, 1944– II. Long, Diana E. III. Wood, Francis C. (Francis Clark), 1901– IV. Title.
[DNLM: 1. Internal Medicine—history—United States—congresses. W3 FR818 2nd 1986g / WZ 70 AA1 F8 1986g]
R151.F73 1986
616'.009—dc19
DNLM/DLC
for Library of Congress *87-30237*
CIP

Designed by Adrianne Onderdonk Dudden

CONTENTS

PART II
THE SUBSPECIALTIES OF INTERNAL MEDICINE: CASE STUDIES

PART III
HISTORICAL PROBLEMS IN DIAGNOSIS AND THERAPY

PART IV
A CONCLUDING VIEW

PREFACE

In March 1986 the Francis C. Wood Institute for the History of Medicine of the College of Physicians held its second national conference on the history of internal medicine in the United States in the last hundred years. The conference, like this book, aimed to enrich our historical understanding of American medicine while giving honor to a man who played a large role in the advancement of internal medicine, Francis C. Wood.

Internal medicine has been a dominant force in American medicine during the last century, but only recently have its practitioners and academic observers asked questions about the the emergence of this most general specialty. In a period of shifting boundaries in medical theory and in the medical profession itself, practitioners have begun to search for a clearer view of how the field emerged, defined itself, and evolved in response to new discoveries and institutions. Historians of late nineteenth- and early twentieth-century American medicine, a lively area of research in the 1980s, have also turned to the recent past of internal medicine as an especially telling case history of American medicine in an age of specialization.

Aware of the possibilities of this professional and historical interest in internal medicine, the editors of this volume convened "Grand Rounds: One Hundred Years of Internal Medicine" at the College of Physicians of Philadelphia. Since its founding in 1787, the College has grown into a modern medical academy whose historical collections, museum, and fellowship combine to make it an ideal setting for conferences and research in the history of medicine. Francis Clark Wood played a major role in the creation in 1978 of the Institute named for him. In November 1984 the Institute held its first national conference on the history of the American general hospital. The overall goal of the Institute is to enlarge our understanding of "contemporary medicine in historical perspective."

The two-day conference on the history of internal medicine included papers and discussions of the institutions, intellectual development, and professional concerns of internists and of the subspecialty fields of internal medicine. In Chapter 1 Russell Maulitz describes the themes and contributions of the papers to our understanding of medical science, practice, and institutions in the American context.

Francis C. Wood

The remarkable transformation of American medicine from the 1920s to the present was the setting for the professional life of Francis C. Wood. Born to Protestant missionaries in South Africa and educated at Princeton University in the 1920s, Francis Wood fulfilled a childhood ambition to become a doctor at one of America's newly reformed centers of academic medicine, the University of Pennsylvania. He has spoken of his good fortune to have encountered men who fired his intellectual ambition—E. G. Conklin at Princeton and A. Newton Richards at the University of Pennsylvania. After medical training at Penn, Francis Wood moved into the life of the full-time academic clinician; he developed a private practice, attended medical wards, and taught medical students. In line with scientific expectations of the post-Flexner period in American medical schools' history, he also did laboratory research and joined Charles Wolferth at the newly formed Cardiac Clinic at the University. In this setting, he was able to create and fulfill a specialized research program in cardiology that enriched medical understanding of the heart and provided a new tool of diagnosis and therapy for the clinician: precordial electrocardiographic leads. His individual studies of angina pectoris, coronary occlusion, and myocardial infarction were milestones of cardiology. Taken as a whole, these discoveries exemplify beautifully the strategic development of an overall research program on the function of the heart in health and disease.

From 1928 to 1941 Francis Wood published over fifty papers on a wide range of cardiovascular problems that won him the honor and recognition of the elite medical scientific societies, the Association of American Physicians, and the American Clinical and Climatological Association. His presidential addresses to these societies give us insight into his curiosity and understanding as a scientist and as an observer of the human scene. In this he was "the true internist," defined by his friend O. H. Perry Pepper in 1940 as an "ingenious man in the old sense of that word, when it was properly used to indicate an active intellectual inquiring mind." More particularly, Pepper says in *Annals of Internal Medicine*,

> An internist is a physician fitted by a sound and applicable knowledge of the basic sciences, a continuing training in clinical medicine, a familiarity with fields outside his own, and an intellectual rather than a manual or technical approach, to study, diagnose and treat the diseases of the field of internal medicine to which he strictly limits himself and to integrate with the knowledge of his own field that of the allied specialties. [1940, 13]

Pepper does not discuss the institutional characteristics of the internist's life—a subject of much importance in this book. Francis Wood made his mark as a scientist while he was progressing up the track of "full-time" clinical medicine in the medical school, a member of the first generation committed to this role. He has left some characteristically humorous comments on this organizational innovation in his presidential address to the Association of American Physicians (AAP).

Francis Wood describes in his address to the AAP the diffidence with which he took on his role as leader of the Department of Medicine at the University of Pennsylvania in 1947; this diffidence and the success of his chairmanship add a dimension to our understanding of internal medicine *qua* institution as well as *qua* scientific specialty. Along with a number of his medical colleagues at Penn, Francis Wood left the Cardiac Clinic and his assistant professorship of medicine in 1941 to form the 20th General Hospital in Assam, India. World War II provided an opportunity for the scientific clinician to demonstrate the large-scale effectiveness of the new internal medicine. Francis Wood served first as Assistant Chief of Medicine and then as Chief of Medicine at the 20th General Hospital, which had remarkable success. More than 99 percent of patients treated at the Assam Hospital survived.

Becoming a full professor and chairman of the Department of Medicine in 1947, Francis Wood was able to combine scientific practice with his innate skills as a leader of a complex organization. As the essays in this book illustrate, American medicine was infused with not only large-scale science projects ("Big Science") but Big Money (from the federal government's newly formed medical philanthropies) and Big Institutions (with complex roles) in the postwar period. Departments of medicine were at the center of this transformation. One is impressed, however, with Wood's creativity in working with his medical school community. William Williams, one of his admiring students, speaks of his "endless ingenuity to provide opportunities for young men to develop their academic skills unhampered by service obligations or administrative assignments . . . in the almost complete absence of University funding." Francis Wood found funding from private donors and from the "ethical" drug companies for his students, just as the University was finding it for its new scientific and clinical institutes. The academic medical center at the University of Pennsylvania was fortunate indeed to have Francis Wood as its medical leader.

Recollections from his students and colleagues illustrate his genius at teaching, organizing, and providing a moral model for all his colleagues, the students, house staff, postdoctoral fellows, specialized colleagues, and visitors who made up the community of internal medicine in the 1950s. He was awarded the Distinguished Teacher Award of the American College of Physicians in 1976, thirty-nine years after he was certified in internal medicine and cardiology by that organization.

How did he integrate and lead this complex community? Francis Wood provides the historian with some puzzling answers, which refer back to his personal beliefs. He made sure that his department was a place where "the finest, most intelligent young gentlemen would want to come to work and stay" (*Transactions Association of American Physicians* 79 [1966]: 10). The work of medicine had a shared meaning and value in this environment that united the departmental and institutional family. He made sure that he—and his colleagues—were enjoying themselves.

Francis Wood retired from the chairmanship of the Department of Medicine in 1964. He has long been a leader in the affairs of the College of Physicians of Philadelphia and was its president from 1967 to 1970. His most recent project at the College has been the Francis C. Wood Institute for the History of Medicine at the College of Physicians. Characteristically, he has worked hard in this new role, as a scholarly participant at all our meetings, as an organizational advisor on the advisory committee, and most of all as a friend, making sure that we are all having fun. This new role comes at a time when he has many laurels that could be a resting place: honorary doctorates from Thomas Jefferson University, the University of Pennsylvania, Princeton University, and Trinity College, Dublin.

This book is a token of thanks offered to Francis Wood from his new historical colleagues and friends, looking back on the extraordinary success of a man who integrated and nourished the new field of internal medicine and became one of its best exemplars as a scientist, doctor, and friend.

Diana E. Long

ACKNOWLEDGMENTS

Many individuals and institutions contributed to *Grand Rounds* as a conference and as a book. From the beginning, several departments of the College of Physicians have taken an active part in the work. The Office of Special Events offered hospitality to the conference; the Historical Collections of the Library and the Mütter Museum supported the research for this book; and the Advisory Committee of the Francis C. Wood Institute helped with arrangements. We are especially grateful to Vaughan Simmons, who provided videotape of the conference and of the dinner in honor of Francis C. Wood. That dinner was enlivened by the after-dinner comments of Jonathan Rhoads.

The Henry J. Kaiser Family Foundation provided a planning grant for the conference, which was supported in addition by generous grants from the Benjamin and Mary Siddons Measey Foundation and the Josiah Macy Foundation.

The authors of the essays in this volume were all participants at the conference. In addition, this study benefitted from the involvement of other speakers and chairpersons at the conference: Saul Benison, John Eisenberg, William Felch, Palmer H. Futcher, A. McGehee Harvey, Halsted Holman,

Edward J. Huth, Robert J. T. Joy, James Pittman, Eugene Stead, and Samuel Thier.

Eva Artschwager provided invaluable research assistance for this project. Our special thanks to John Parascandola and Margaret Kaiser for sending us a printout from the National Library of Medicine on their holdings in internal medicine.

LIST OF FIGURES

LIST OF TABLES

GRAND ROUNDS

ONE HUNDRED YEARS OF INTERNAL MEDICINE

PART I

INTRODUCTION: HISTORICAL PERSPECTIVES

1

Grand Rounds: An Introduction to the History of Internal Medicine

RUSSELL C. MAULITZ

To write about the history of internal medicine we have to find a way to think about it. How should we conceptualize the history of a medical specialty that is as broadly based and amorphous as internal medicine?

Many years have passed since George Rosen's brief, classic history of one of the earliest specialties, ophthalmology.[1] The medicine of the eye was, moreover, a relatively straightforward prototype. It allowed Rosen to go a long way toward developing an ideal type or model of a "specialty." That model relied most heavily on the notion that a body of professional work might crystallize around a particular organ system and a particular set of esoteric technical skills. In the case of ophthalmology, then, the introduction of the ophthalmoscope in the mid to late nineteenth century was critical, because it allowed a cohort of doctors to hive off into the well-demarcated practice of a new specialty.

The classic model, unfortunately, may apply most distinctly to that small circle of specialties that reached something like their modern form in the late nineteenth century, fields such as ophthalmology, dermatology, otolaryngology, or pathology. It is much less clear how such a pattern applies to twentieth-century specialties, especially protean ones like internal medicine.[2] No single organ system or single set of skills has provided a clear field for monopolization. Modern internists do too many different things, occupy too many disparate niches, for us to give this diverse group of physicians a straightforward lineage, or even a common ancestor.

Yet internists, having trained together for three or more years, band together in colleges of physicians. So they do see themselves, however tenuously, as having something in common, if only because they all treat "the contents of the skin" and because they agree on the educational drill that defines their neophytes' basic expertise. But what is it, historically, that necessarily links internists together? It is a thorny question. Perhaps the problem we have answering it would be less refractory if we let go of the attempt to find elegant, purposeful, and purely rational explanations to account for the internist's emergence from the ranks of medical generalists. The formation of internal medicine might then be conceived as a series of historical contingencies.

Why, for example, is endocrinology part of internal medicine whereas neurology, for the most part, is not? Maybe it is for the same reason that cardiology became a subspecialty of internal medicine until recently when, in at least a few locales, its practitioners budded off from their colleagues the internists: simply put, a process of negotiation. In this rubric internal medicine is a specialty and its subspecialties are organically part of it because (1) internists behave as if such structures are primary, and (2) their behavior is accepted by other physicians.[3] Earlier, unicausal explanations, based on the inexorable expansion of knowledge and technique, then, seem rather inadequate and beg the questions they are meant to answer.

We are reminded of this complexity, and of the necessity to understand it in broad historical rather than narrow instrumental terms, by many of the case studies in this volume. Gastroenterology, for example, according to several of the criteria of specialty formation—societies, special techniques, journals, and so forth—had emerged as a free-standing specialty by the beginning of the twentieth century. Hence, as Joseph Kirsner demonstrates in his chronicle of the specialty of digestive diseases, gastrointestinal (GI) medicine as an organized domain actually predated internal medicine. In an important sense, gastroenterology was thus a specialty before it was a subspecialty and gained the latter status when, a generation later, it was captured by internal medicine.

In this less unidirectional and more elastic framework, the internist's mandate did not simply grow out of a single population (as did the obstetrician's or pediatrician's), a single instrument (as did the otolaryngologist's), or a single disease (as did the claims of the pulmonologists [tuberculosis] and perhaps the dermatologists [venereal diseases]). Rather, nineteenth-century practitioners of "physick" may have laid the foundations for the internal medicine of the twentieth century through the use of various resources: organizational support patterned, however loosely, on the venerable colleges of physicians of western Europe; professional and ideological support from the new scientific disciplines of the late nineteenth century; and intellectual and economic support from a variety of technological advances, most particularly diagnostic machines and new drug regimens.

The problem, of course, in presenting the history of internal medicine in this less tidy fashion is that it places greater, not smaller, demands on its recruits. It demands much of the medical practitioner who tries to look back at his or her collective history. No simple model, be it George Rosen's, Thomas Kuhn's,[4] or anyone else's, will suffice to explain elegantly the dramatic changes in internal medicine witnessed by mid-twentieth-century participant-observers. With easy explanations left wanting, we can be left with the diluted, celebratory "centennial histories" we are used to seeing from time to time. Another result, albeit a rather more useful one, may be the proverbial narrative of one damn thing after another.

The professional historian, choosing to look at a scientifically demanding twentieth-century medical specialty, and viewing internal medicine in a different set of contexts, faces different sorts of demands. Technical understanding is one of these requirements. If an understanding of the basic science and clinical essentials is lacking, the alternative, no matter how theoretically sophisticated the commentator, can be a one-sided and simplistic neglect of key research sources. One may grasp the fundamentals of institutional history and still disclose a disregard for (or perhaps intimidation by) the key ideas of modern physiology, pathology, clinical medicine, and epidemiology.[5] Needless to say, the institutional history, and the political context within which it is embedded, remain essential to the story as well.

It is therefore understandable that few historians of modern medical specialties have sought to "get inside" their material enough to pay attention to the technical *and* the social dimensions. The resulting schism is a daunting one in both methodological and emotional terms. In the late 1980s, which for both medicine and society is a troubling time of brisk epidemiological and professional change, of AIDS and the doctor glut, the emotional schism has begun to be bridged. Antagonisms have become somewhat muted, and appropriate lip service is being paid to the notion of dialogue between participant-historians and professionals. But attempts to create an actual discourse, especially an engaged discourse centered on the task of connecting medical and historical events, have been for the most part lacking. The effort to find the links between notions of institutional structure and intellectual content has scarcely begun.

Given the state of our "dichotomous discipline,"[6] the planners of the second Wood Institute Conference on the history of medicine found that the idea of bringing students of history together with its makers meant a journey into challenging and slightly unfamiliar terrain. It meant promoting the sort of dialogue seen more often, perhaps, in politics: a leader of government imports a resident historian to start molding the "long view" before the short view has dissipated. Even among statesmen and politicians, though, this is not something that we see happening very often; in medicine it occurs even less often.

In the last few years, by default, a sort of two-pronged historiography of medicine has persisted in lieu of the highly demanded integrative approach. Indeed, little has changed in the nearly ten years since historian Morris Vogel examined the same phenomenon in the essay with which he introduced *The Therapeutic Revolution*, an important medico-historical work from the publisher of the present volume.[7] Vogel noted how nineteenth- and early twentieth-century ideas of progress informed early "teleological" accounts of the march of scientific medicine. Lately, he added, more critical efforts were undertaken to probe the American medical system, with all its weaknesses and contradictions. Frequently those efforts entailed the examination of those parts of the system of health care and science that seemed most controversial—the role of psychiatry, the labeling of disease, the making of health care policy, and the business of educating and professionalizing doctors.[8]

Despite the dichotomous history of recent years, it is nonetheless possible to find among the early chroniclers of twentieth-century scientific medicine a few figures who both narrated medicine's positive progress and were themselves also among its engineers. In an earlier generation of the makers of twentieth-century medicine, some, like George Corner, went from developing its knowledge base to describing its triumphal march.[9] As Paul Beeson and Russell Maulitz point out in this volume, now another, later generation—this time focusing on internal medicine as a specialty—coming to retirement at the end of the twentieth century, follows suit. These men of the 1940s, 1950s, and 1960s are providing us with their own self-portraits, individually and collectively. In so doing they probably signal the end of an extraordinary post-World War II growth spurt.[10]

In view of the foregoing, we sought for *Grand Rounds* two kinds of participants. The first group consisted of more senior participant-observers, makers and shakers who were willing now to look back over the formation of their own subspecialties of internal medicine. Our second group comprised a handful of younger historians, participant-observers of a different sort, who were willing to peer more theoretically at a different cross-section of issues in the development of diagnosis, treatment, and other medical subspecialties. The reader of this volume will have little difficulty distinguishing between the two groups' analyses, and we have not sought to blur the distinctions.

By the same token, in the conference on which the volume is based, there was much lively dialogue and gratifying contention. Some of the ways in which this interaction was fruitful will only be apparent (one hopes) in future publications. Not a little of this back-and-forth colloquy made its way into the revised papers that make up this volume. Both genres will have lasting value, as primary sources in some cases, secondary sources in some, and hopefully a bit of each in still others.

The chapters in *Grand Rounds* are bracketed by two perspectives on internal medicine, viewed, as it were, through opposite ends of the telescope. Paul Beeson and Russell Maulitz view the twentieth-century development of the specialty from the inside looking out, while Rosemary Stevens concludes the volume by taking another look, from the outside, so to speak, looking in. Beeson and Maulitz describe the internal history of the internist's work. They explore in turn each of the three levels at which the internist experienced this work: institutionally, as a constituent of the larger social and cultural system of scientific medicine; professionally, as the individual charged with confronting disease through diagnosis and treatment; and experientially, as a career. They describe some of the early milestones in the rise of a medical research and education establishment, beginning with the Rockefeller and Johns Hopkins institutions and continuing with the development of the full-time professorial system and the growth of organized specialty bodies. They then discuss the implications for the internist of changing disease patterns, from the acute infections of the late nineteenth century to the chronic degenerative processes of an aging population in the late twentieth century. Finally, in more anecdotal and personal terms, Maulitz and Beeson reflect on the changing nature of internal medicine itself, introducing what may count as this volume's essential tension: the internist as generalist versus the internist as subspecialist.

In the third introductory chapter, Bruce Fye examines internal medicine as a body of written knowledge, demonstrating the relations between the literary record and the internist's place in a universe of both practice and science. By emphasizing trends rather than microanalysis of particular publications, he explores how the adoption of a research ethic changed the literature of medicine in the United States. Fye focuses on the journal literature but considers other key forms of publication as well. Finally, he balances the roles of the author, editor, publisher, librarian, and reader, showing that concerns about the quality and quantity of medical publications are at least as old as internal medicine itself.

In the chapters on the subspecialties of internal medicine, five contributors look at several of the subspecies of practitioners and scientists that evolved from the mid-twentieth-century fragmentation of general internal medicine. It is perhaps at this level, that of the subcommunity, that one may most fruitfully seek out the theoretical links between science and practice, and the historical links between clientele and expertise. Not every subspecialty is covered: notably absent are pulmonology, endocrinology, and hematology-oncology. Indeed, we have not attempted to provide a definitive history of internal medicine, but rather a set of case studies and initial explorations. Nor have we tried to impose uniformity on each author's treatment of the subspecialties that are covered: some are mainly chronological while others are mainly thematic. All strive, however, to identify those critical links of which we just spoke—between science and practice, clientele and expertise.

Edward Kass, for example, after first surveying epidemic and sporadic contagions since the founding of the United States, describes the quite recent development of infectious diseases (ID) as a medical subspecialty. Kass describes the protracted course by which individual bits and pieces of the internist's understanding of infection came to be assimilated. Remarkable in this course was the lack of a specific technical procedure, or body of technical procedures, to drive the ID subspecialists into their own separate camp. Yet split off they did, at a remarkably late date (the 1950s and 1960s). In a comprehensive narrative of its organizational and literary apparatus, Kass suggests some of the institutional reasons for this rather recent development.

In contrast, another pioneer, Joseph Kirsner, shows the evolution of gastroenterology from one of the earliest subspecialties. Initially based on rather restricted areas of technical expertise, primarily radiological assessment and intubation of the gut, gastroenterology developed into what is now arguably a "superspecialty," that is, a composite of many clinical and scientific disciplines. Kirsner describes what he calls the branch points in the development of the study of diseases of the digestive system. In doing so he furnishes a useful narrative of the technical achievements of gastroenterologists, as well as an exhaustive account of the organizational development of the field in which he was an early innovator. He also suggests that there was a glaring disjunction between the mastery of craft that justified the specialty in practice and the investigative research paradigms that came to be imported in the era of National Institute of Health (NIH) research sponsorship. In this respect the case of gastroenterology, one of the earliest subspecialties of internal medicine, oddly resembles that of some of the most recent ones. Nephrology is the most conspicuous recent case of a similar phenomenon discussed in these pages.

Thomas Benedek's study of the subspecialty of rheumatic diseases is also a chronological narrative. In rheumatology, the author claims, specialization depended on both technical and cultural factors. He establishes the importance of a consistently large and chronically ill clientele as a basis for the support of rheumatology. Like infectious diseases, the rise of a rheumatic diseases specialty was hampered by the lack of specific diagnostic methodologies and, for a long time, a similar lack of specialized therapy. But around 1950, several new diagnostic, therapeutic, and economic factors intersected and began to change this state of affairs. Benedek examines the convergence of elements as disparate as diagnostic tests for rheumatoid arthritis and lupus erythematosus, the acute and demonstrable effects of cortisone and corticotropin, and the funding of specialized research and education activities through organizations such as the Arthritis and Rheumatism Foundation and the National Institute of Arthritis and Metabolic Diseases.

In his study of the emergence of a subspecialty of renal diseases, Steven Peitzman argues persuasively for another, quite different configuration of practitioners, tools, and expertise. He shows that nephrology began in America when clinical investigators embraced functional diagnosis and chemical investigation. Leaders like Otto Folin and Donald Van Slyke imparted a distinctly physiologic-chemical cast to early renal research, a direction followed by other contributors in an era of close collaboration between clinicians and bench scientists. The rediscovery of acute renal failure in World War II added consultative roles for nascent kidney diseases subspecialists. And, critically, clinicians' and investigators' attempts to confront renal failure fostered the midcentury development of two key technical developments, one diagnostic and one therapeutic: renal biopsy and renal dialysis. These two techniques unquestionably helped denote and delimit the new subspecialty. Yet the old metabolic-physiologic wing sustained its early leadership of societies, publications, certification mechanisms, and medical school divisions.

Finally, Joel Howell examines one of the other early subspecialties of internal medicine, cardiology. Using heart medicine thematically as a case study in the development of organizational relationships, Howell redresses the traditional view, which cardiology has always seemed superficially to support, that the early emergence of subspecialties is technologically driven. He argues that cardiology was historically much more than the now familiar bastion of high technology instrumentation. He shows us a different cardiology, evolving in response to a wide variety of changing circumstances both inside and outside of internal medicine. In some instances those circumstances involved specialty groups and institutions elsewhere in medicine—pediatrics was one key example. In some cases, such as the rise of the social medicine movement and the voluntary health societies, important influences flowed from surprising places that lay outside medicine altogether.

A thematic section, addressing diagnosis and therapeutics, follows the history of the subspecialties. In a contemplative essay, Stephen Kunitz suggests that diagnostic classification is a halfway house between the concreteness of the individual and the abstraction of statistical insight. Internists, Kunitz points out, have emphasized the importance of diagnostic classification to defend the uniqueness of their specialty against those arrayed at opposite poles: family practitioners who assert the importance of their knowledge of the unique individual patient, and researchers concerned with underlying mechanisms of disease. Clinical internists have attempted to hold the middle ground. Kunitz discusses the emerging role of the general internist in terms of the post-World War II erosion of the specialist's ability to occupy simultaneously the roles of master-clinician and laboratory investigator, and he comments on the probabilistic sorts of diagnostic classifications that result. He argues that knowledge is thus used not only to guide practice, but also to defend professional boundaries. In some cases, he speculates, echoing Howell's case study, new knowledge may even be generated to justify the continued development of subspecialties that may have formed originally for very different reasons.

Finally, Harry Marks presents a case study in the history of therapeutics, expanding on the same issue of probabilistic reasoning in internal medicine. But whereas Kunitz is concerned rather generally with the epistemology of the diagnostician, Marks focuses on the particularities of the negotiations between key early arbiters of what constituted therapeutic efficacy—and how to prove it. In his inquiry into the early roots of clinical trials, Marks stresses the role of therapeutic researchers between the two world wars in preparing the ground for the postwar introduction of statistical methods. He shows how a scientific elite within internal medicine began to abandon its confidence in the ability of clinical specialists to produce reliable information about the merits of new treatments. He suggests why this elite might have turned in the postwar period to a greater reliance on statisticians and statistical methods, a reliance which some critics perceived to imperil clinicians' bedside autonomy. The power of therapeutic ideas, asserts Marks, cannot in itself explain their eventual acceptance. Instead, he claims (in concert, one suspects, with Kunitz, Peitzman, and Howell), they must be placed in the larger context of various communities of scientists and practitioners finding themselves at times in competition and at other times in collaboration.

A concluding essay by Rosemary Stevens picks up many of the threads woven through the preceding chapters of *Grand Rounds.* From her vantage point as both a policy analyst and historian of medicine, Stevens points out the contradictions of a specialty trying to be all things—or many different things—to all people. She surveys the development of internal medicine in terms of its various audiences and clienteles, returning to the theme of the general specialist versus the subspecialist. Internal medicine, she concludes, is defined in part by the tensions that both divide and mobilize its spokesmen and practitioners and in part by its institutions. In the final analysis, though, in view of the extraordinary social and cultural role internal medicine will continue to be called upon to play, Stevens ventures a rather favorable prognosis.

Certain common themes suffuse the contributions to *Grand Rounds.* Clearly one we have already mentioned is the disjunction, or at least the lack of any necessary conjunction, between the craft and science elements of either the specialty or its individual subspecialties. Hence, one useful way of understanding the tortuous development of domains like cardiology or gastroenterology, each with "something old, something new," may be to analyze their historical evolution in terms of both technique (craft) and academic paradigm (science), understanding the distinctness, and perhaps at times the interdependence, of the two sorts of criteria for specialty formation.

Another theme pervading the individual accounts in the book is the peculiar centrality of the war experience. There is nothing new about the contention that war has always been the perverse handmaiden of medical progress. It was so at the introduction of gunpowder and long before that. But twentieth-century global war, especially World War II, exerted a remarkable array of quite singular effects on internal medicine, fostering the growth of everything from penicillin production to the internist's status in the medical community.

Finally, an overarching theme is the curious manner in which men and ideas intersect with institutions and larger social roles to produce historical change. In recent years much of that change, driven by technology and economics, has been marked by fragmentation and a crisis of identity associated with it. The late 1980s seems to be an especially felicitous time to examine those new patterns as internal medicine, like Humpty-Dumpty, strives to put itself back together again.

I wish to thank Diana E. Long, Charles Rosenberg, and Rosemary Stevens for helpful suggestions in reviewing the manuscript.

NOTES

1. George Rosen, *The Specialization of Medicine with Particular Reference to Ophthalmology* (New York: Froben, 1944; repr. Arno, 1972).

2. This point is made elegantly by Bonnie Ellen Blustein in "New York Neurologists and the Specialization of American Medicine," *Bull Hist Med* 53 (1979): 170–83.

3. For a variant of this interpretation see Grace De Santis, "Medical Work: Accommodating a Body of Knowledge to Practice," *Sociology of Health and Illness* 2 (1980): 133–50.

4. A brief but useful discussion of this point in connection with a specialty that borders internal medicine is Glenn Gritzer and Arnold Arluke, *The Making of Rehabilitation: A Political Economy of Medical Specialization, 1890–1980* (Berkeley and Los Angeles: University of California Press, 1985), 1–14, especially 2–6. The original referent is to Thomas Kuhn's classic, *The Structure of Scientific Revolutions* (Chicago: University of Chicago Press, 1962; new ed. 1970).

5. S. E. D. Shortt, "Clinical Practice and the Social History of Medicine: A Theoretical Accord," *Bull Hist Med* 55 (1981): 533–42, cf. 534–35 in particular. Shortt provides a useful overview of the schismatic process working itself out through the intellectual and social tumult of the 1960s and 1970s.

6. Shortt, "Clinical Practice and the Social History of Medicine," 536.

7. Morris Vogel, "Introduction," in *The Therapeutic Revolution: Essays in the Social History of American Medicine*, Morris Vogel and Charles Rosenberg, eds. (Philadelphia: University of Pennsylvania Press, 1979), vii–xiii. See also Susan Reverby and David Rosner's useful introductory essay, "Beyond the Great Doctors," in their *Health Care in America: Essays in Social History* (Philadelphia: Temple University Press, 1979), 3–16.

8. It is not possible here to survey the wealth of writings of the past 15–20 years on the "new" history of medicine. But for those looking for recent (as of

1987) guides to this literature, reasonable beginnings include Charles Rosenberg, "Disease and Social Order in America: Perceptions and Expectations," *Milbank Quarterly* 64 (1986) (Suppl. 1): 34–55; Daniel Fox, "The Decline of Historicism: The Case of Compulsory Health Insurance in the United States," *Bull Hist Med* 57 (1983): 596–610; and, for a British perspective, Peter Wright and A. Treacher, *The Problem of Medical Knowledge: Examining the Social Construction of Medicine* (Edinburgh: Edinburgh University Press, 1982).

9. George Corner, *The Hormones in Human Reproduction* (Princeton: Princeton University Press, 1942). Corner, of course, was one of a now-vanishing breed of scientists and physicians who sustained a profound and lifelong interest in history.

10. For a study in this genre of one late-blooming subspecialty see, for example, Maxwell M. Wintrobe, *Hematology, the Blossoming of a Science: A Story of Inspiration and Effort* (Philadelphia: Lea & Febiger, 1985). For broader views of this "golden age of scientific medicine" see A. McGehee Harvey, *Science at the Bedside: Clinical Research in American Medicine, 1905–1945* (Baltimore: Johns Hopkins University Press, 1981), and the essays by Paul Beeson, Leighton Cluff, Robert Petersdorf, et al., collected in the special issue of *Daedalus* (spring 1986) entitled "America's Doctors, Medical Science, Medical Care."

2

The Inner History of Internal Medicine

PAUL B. BEESON and RUSSELL C. MAULITZ

Origins

What is internal medicine? And who is the internist? The terms have never been clearly understood by much of the public. When lay acquaintances are told that we practice internal medicine, they may respond with blank stares. Fully certified internists must pass specialty board examinations, but their patients nonetheless ask them for referrals "to a specialist." When pressed about what he or she does, the internist may wind up lamely saying something to the effect that internal medicine is "not surgery." To the disinterested outside observer, then, the internist's role and scope may understandably remain confused. The varied settings in which internists practice may add to the confusion. Some practice in rural or suburban settings, supplying general adult health care as providers of primary care. Others, often quite similarly trained, may end up practicing highly subspecialized, technology-dependent medicine in urban, tertiary-care settings. So it is not surprising that ad hoc definitions of this most general of specialties may depend on who is being asked to describe it.

In an era of scarce resources, conclusions about the nature of internal medicine (or for that matter any specialty) cease to be mere academic exercises. They take on crucial political importance: will general internal medicine or family practice most efficiently and effectively serve the social good?

Where do we put our resources? Lately questions of this sort have gained in importance—at the very moment when they are most susceptible to distortions imposed by the perspective of the informant.

One way out of the dilemma of self-definition is a historical description. We are defined as much by where we have been as we are by where we wish to go. It is possible to retrieve the past, at least to the extent that our sense of that past is not overly colored by the desire to see it through the prism of today's agenda. American internists are tempted, for example, to trace their corporate ancestry back to the tiny Royal College elites granted monopoly rights by royal warrant beginning in the sixteenth century.[1] Indeed, the American College of Physicians professes a certain filial relationship thereby to the Royal College of Physicians of London (now of England), empowered by Henry VIII in 1518.[2] But in actuality we need look no further back than a hundred years or so to find the internist's origins both in America and abroad, all part of the inner history of internal medicine. To investigate that inner history in this chapter we will examine the development of the internist's world from three perspectives: first, the scientific; second, the clinical; and finally, the personal and professional.

Among the most significant of the changes that followed the Franco-Prussian and American Civil Wars was the segmenting of the medical marketplace academically and clinically. The process of demarcating new medical specialties, first in Germany and soon after in the other industrial nations, was fueled by two powerful engines: new technology (primarily diagnostic, but also therapeutic) and increased professional competition.[3] New, specialized fields like ophthalmology and otolaryngology found professional niches in the worlds of medical knowledge and medical practice.[4] Slightly later, old fields like surgery, which were increasingly recognized as proper specialties, gained in professional power as they erected their edifices on foundations of science.[5]

Against the backdrop of these changes in the late 1870s and early 1880s, the designation "internal medicine" seems to have originated around 1880 in Germany, with the use of the modifying word *innere*. The term was employed to indicate a field of practice in which concepts were based on an emerging understanding of physiology, biochemistry, bacteriology, and pathology, and in which surgical methods were not employed. The expression was intended to connote special knowledge and training rather than dogma, empty hypotheses, and mere observation of outward manifestations of disease.[6]

At that time North America took most of its medical cues from Germany. Over a few decades, after all, thousands of physicians and medical students were flocking to the laboratories and polyclinics of Strasbourg, Berlin, and Vienna. Consequently the expression "internal medicine," reflecting German institutional arrangements, was adopted quickly in America. But the choice of terms, designed to describe this new self-definition of the specialist in internal diseases, was not unanimous and unequivocal. In 1897, for example, in a lecture entitled "Internal Medicine as a Vocation," William Osler could dispute its status as an incipient specialty, lamenting that

> I wish there were another term to designate the wide field of medical practice which remains after the separation of surgery, midwifery and gynecology. Not itself a specialty (though it embraces at least half a dozen), its cultivators cannot be called specialists, but bear without reproach the good old name physician, in contradistinction to general practitioners, surgeons, obstetricians and gynecologists.[7]

Osler, following the British tradition, would have deemphasized the "specialized" aspect of the field. Instead he chose to stress its role as a gateway to other, more limited "specialties"—domains of scientific knowledge or technical expertise now conventionally thought of as *sub*specialties. But Americans, especially those in academic internal medicine, abandoned the word "physician" along with the nineteenth-century naturalist tradition of which Osler was the apotheosis. American internists chose instead to bow to the then dominant German tradition of scientific medicine, emphasizing the internist's coequal status among the other nascent specialties, and coining the new term "internist."[8]

Early Contributions Made by American Physicians

If one looks for American contributions to "internal medicine" before the Civil War, the harvest is a meager one. Although Benjamin Rush, the best-remembered physician of the eighteenth century, was a leading citizen and statesman, he made few noteworthy contributions to medicine. Even more than his contemporaries, Rush relied on heroic methods of treatment such as purging and bleeding, based on received wisdom about what might benefit the patient. Other antebellum physicians made their mark through precision in their accounts of nosography and nosology. William Gerhard of Philadelphia, for example, differentiated typhoid from typhus and emphasized the distinctive intestinal lesions of typhoid. Nathan Smith of New England wrote a masterful clinical description of typhoid fever. Daniel Drake of Cincinnati carried out epidemiological studies of malaria and other fevers of the Mississippi River Valley. An experimental tradition existed primitively if at all, despite William Beaumont's frequently cited series of studies of digestion in a patient with a gastric fistula.[9]

By the middle of the nineteenth century, a new group of proto-internists, their medical sensibilities forged on the European continent rather than in Edinburgh and London, was beginning to emerge. Men such as Austin Flint, Oliver Wendell Holmes, and Jacob DaCosta placed much greater emphasis on pathological anatomy, physical diagnosis, and therapeutic skepticism than their eighteenth-century counterparts.[10] Austin Flint of New Orleans and New York reported careful observations of cardiac auscultation in which he described the murmur produced at the mitral valve in patients with aortic insufficiency. The Civil War provided many members of this group with unparalleled clinical exposure. Jacob DaCosta described "soldier's heart," characterized by palpitation, tachycardia, fatigability, and shortness of breath.[11] From the mid-1880s William Osler began his remarkable series of case descriptions, including his discussion of bacterial endocarditis before the technique of blood culture was available. His studies of blood included a discourse on the blood platelets and lending his name to two diseases, hereditary hemorrhagic telangiectasia and polycythemia rubra vera.[12] In 1886 Reginald Fitz of Boston provided a clear description of the clinical manifestations of acute appendicitis.

In the early years of the twentieth century, several physician investigators engaged in clinical observations critical to the scientific foundations of internal medicine. Walter Reed of the U.S. Army, conducting experiments in Havana, demonstrated the role of the mosquito in the transmission of yellow fever. Edward Trudeau founded the archetypal American sanitarium for tuberculosis at Saranac Lake, where it was shown that lengthy bed rest, fresh air, and sunlight were beneficial. Elliot Joslin of Boston concentrated attention for many years on patients with diabetes mellitus and wrote a celebrated book on the subject. James Herrick of Chicago made two important contributions to internal medicine by describing in 1910 the deformity of erythrocytes in sickle cell disease and in 1912 the clinical manifestations of acute myocardial infarction.[13]

These early observers extended the borders of both diagnosis and therapeutics. In 1910, for example, Nathan Brill of New York described a febrile disorder seen in adult patients who had emigrated from eastern Europe. Brill noted the similarity of this disease to louse-borne typhus fever. Later work substantiated his conjecture, and it is now agreed that this disease is a recrudescence of typhus long after the original attack. George Minot and William Murphy of Boston in 1926 announced the curative effect of a diet rich in liver for the treatment of pernicious anemia, a discovery for which they received a Nobel Prize, shared with George Whipple. Shortly afterward, their colleague William Castle carried out clinical experiments demonstrating the presence in normal gastric secretion of something called "intrinsic factor."[14] He found this to be lacking in the secretions of patients with pernicious anemia. In the 1920s and 1930s two physicians at the Mount Sinai Hospital in New York, George Baehr and Emanuel Libman, described disseminated lupus erythematosus as we know it today.

The last of the individual contributions we note is that of Philip Hench of the Mayo Clinic. In the 1940s Hench observed spontaneous remissions of rheumatoid arthritis during pregnancy and occasionally in the presence of liver disease. He suggested the possibility that some endogenous product must be capable of reducing the intensity of the inflammation. Following this line of reasoning he persuaded his biochemist colleague, Edward Kendall, to let him have some of the newly isolated adrenocortical hormone, cortisone, for trial in the treatment of patients with rheumatoid arthritis. The response was dramatic, laying open the whole field of investigation of inflammatory processes resulting from immunologic reactions. Later Hench, Kendall, and another biochemist, Tadeus Reichstein, received a Nobel Prize for this work.[15]

The Gilded Age: Important Events

As we noted earlier, the idea of internal medicine as a specialty grew in part from the *innere Medizin* of Germany a hundred years ago. The scientific development of internal medicine also gained impetus in the same period, notably through three influential events between 1886 and 1893. In 1886 the Association of American Physicians was formed by a small group of respected practitioners in the eastern part of the United States and Canada. They joined together in hopes of pooling their experiences and exchanging viewpoints about clinical medicine in an atmosphere free from political and organizational controversy. In 1915 Osler referred to the formation of the Association of American Physicians as the "coming of age party of internal medicine in America." It has had, and still retains, great influence on the thinking of teachers of internal medicine in the United States and Canada.[16]

In 1892 the first edition of Osler's textbook *Principles and Practice of Medicine* was published.[17] It was actually one of the last of the major nineteenth-century single-author surveys of medical practice. But it was clearly the first that came to be regarded as an unalloyed classic. Osler sought to integrate the natural history of disease processes, at which he was the past master, with both their pathological anatomy and their therapeutic tractability. As we shall see, he regarded the last as meager indeed.[18] The *Principles and Practice of Medicine*, because of its systematic and authoritative coverage of the entire field, had a remarkable influence on the teaching and practice of medicine. It not only directed world-wide attention to American internal medicine but, among scholarly physicians, also fostered a sort of collective consciousness of their mission and purpose.

In 1893 the Johns Hopkins Medical School admitted its first class. Opened in conjunction with its own teaching hospital, the medical school boasted an outstanding founding faculty, including Franklin Paine Mall in anatomy, William Welch in pathology, William Osler in medicine, and W. S. Halsted in surgery. The course of instruction was set at four years, of which two were mainly devoted to preclinical subjects and two to clinical medicine. (By way of comparison, many of the existing proprietary medical schools offered only two four-month terms of instruction.) Furthermore, a program of intern and residency training, modeled after the German system of postgraduate clinical training, was instituted.

The entire process could be coordinated because the preclinical departments, with their research laboratories, were located close to the hospital. For the first time in America, medical students had free access to a teaching hospital—its wards, its outpatient clinics, and its operating theaters. The new system of training caused the nation's best young students to flock to Baltimore. Later its graduates fanned out to other cities and other medical schools, taking with them the spirit and style of teaching at Hopkins. At the time of his departure for Oxford in 1905, Osler described Hopkins as "not simply a seed farm, but a veritable nursery from which the whole country has been furnished with cuttings, grafts, slips, seedlings."[19]

The Flexner survey of American medical education, carried out by Abraham Flexner in 1908–1909, and reported in 1910, had a mutually reinforcing relationship with the new medical school at Johns Hopkins. Although the reform of medical education had been well under way even before the founding of Hopkins, Flexner used its curriculum and its faculty as his "gold standard" for comparison. Against that standard, scores of so-called medical schools were seen to be so deficient that many of them closed within a few years of the report's publication.[20]

The Rockefeller Institute

The Johns Hopkins medical institution played a part in the formation of the Rockefeller Institute in New York in 1901. The idea for it was suggested to John D. Rockefeller by his advisor in philanthropy, the Reverend Frederick Gates, who had chanced to browse through a copy of the Osler textbook and had been surprised to find how little effective treatment was available for most diseases. Rockefeller then gave a large sum of money for a research institute. Its first director was Simon Flexner, a pathologist and bacteriologist who had studied under Welch at Hopkins. Welch himself served as chairman of the Board of Scientific Directors of the Institute.[21]

The Rockefeller, more than any other organization, attracted international attention to the United States as a place where important medical scientific work was being done. One of its novel features was the establishment of a clinical research center—a small hospital staffed by scientists at the Institute. None of the physicians on the hospital staff engaged in private practice; each devoted his full attention to research. This precedent inaugurated the full-time system in American medicine. The hospital's first director was Rufus Cole, who had trained under Osler in Baltimore. George Corner would depict Cole's plan for the hospital as

> a bold, though relatively simple plan, calling for clinical staff of young men of exceptional ability, able to undertake independent research. They were not to be mere assistants to a physician-in-chief, nor to visiting physicians; on the contrary, each would have full control of a ward where he could study patients suffering with a disease in which he was particularly interested. Each resident would be provided with enough assistants to leave time for research. Facilities for animal experimentation and laboratory work would be at his disposal. Even the interns—junior members of the resident staff, would be allowed time for research. The director would, himself, foster and lead the work of these.[22]

One can hardly overstate the novelty and importance of this part of the new institute. The research hospital became a workplace for a whole generation of clinical scientists who were to lead American medicine during the following decades. Among them were Donald Van Slyke, father of clinical chemistry; Thomas Rivers, pioneer in animal virology; Rene Dubos, microbiologist and ecologist; and Oswald Avery, whose studies of the transformation of pneumococcal types led to the discovery of the role of DNA in genetic processes.

Clinical Investigation Becomes Scientific

By 1880 the notion of clinical investigation as a coherent set of activities had already been articulated by German physicians. Friedrich von Frerichs, in the introduction to the new *Zeitschrift für Klinische Medizin*, advocated the independence of clinical medicine. He contended that the theoretical branches of science threatened to predominate, and that such a tendency could be detrimental to medical progress. Frerichs maintained that the fundamental method for the study of disease must be the bedside collection of information by every means available to modern science. He regarded animal experimentation as indispensable when observation of patients alone failed to provide solutions to the problems involved. But "experimental pathology," he declared, "should not, as sometimes happens, lay claim as an independent science, to the leading role in studying disease. This method is as little suited to this end as was once chemistry, or physics, or morphology. The decisive method of approach is, and always will be the observation of patients."[23]

Frerichs' idea remained controversial, part of a hidden dialectic within scientific medicine that continued into the twentieth century. Support for bringing the laboratory and the bedside closer together came with the 1911 opening of the Hospital of the Rockefeller Institute. World War I, like all wars, had a major impact on disease and medicine. Surgery was propelled as a specialty further than internal medicine, perhaps because the former was organizationally more advanced, but also due to the overwhelming problem of traumatic shock. In the period just after the war, however, in what amounted to a watershed for clinical science, a new cadre of investigators raised internal medicine to such a level that it was ready to coalesce into a fully recognized specialty.

The crucial events of the period between the wars began in 1915 with the crystallization of thyroxine by Edward Kendall, who later elucidated the nature of the hormonal products of the adrenal cortex. The 1920s, a halcyon period for the first generation of career clinical invesigators, saw the introduction of insulin therapy for diabetes and of liver therapy for pernicious anemia.[24] These achievements, both calling for careful clinical and laboratory supervision of treatment, had a profound effect on clinicians' attitudes.

A new breed of careers had been developed—and they had borne fruit. Henceforth the place of the clinical investigator began to be accepted. The establishment in 1924 of the *Journal of Clinical Investigation* (*JCI*) conferred further prestige; today the *JCI* probably remains the most prestigious American publication for clinical research.

Clinical science, embodied in the internist investigator, could soon boast an impressive series of accomplishments. The net result in many cases was a reversal of the traditional notion that basic research enlightens the clinic. The elucidation of clinical problems led to key disclosures in basic science. Physicians, by virtue of their access to human disease, are able to make observations and develop areas for investigation that would never be reached by other avenues. They can study disorders that take years to develop, as well as conditions that cannot be reproduced in animals. They have as background information the pooled observations of hundreds of thousands of doctors caring for millions of people, wherein chance observations disclose rare disorders and unusual reactions. The experimental subject of the clinical investigator can recite past experiences, can describe symptoms and effects of treatment, and may ultimately provide clues to the still vaguely comprehended relationship between mind and body.[25]

Clinical methods developed to study the function of the human heart, kidney, and lungs produced physiological information that could hardly have been obtained by other means. The study of patients with chronic diseases of the kidneys and lungs, for example, deepened understanding of the mechanisms by which water and electrolyte balance is regulated.[26] Diseased organs revealed previously unexpected clues to their normal function, a notable example being insights into endocrine function. The chance observation that administration of drugs developed to produce diuresis caused lowering of the blood pressure in hypertensive patients, and the linking of this with sodium excretion broadened knowledge of the etiology of high blood pressure. Biopsy techniques used in the study of diseases of the gastrointestinal tract, liver, and kidney permitted application of biochemical and immunological methods in examination of fresh tissues and furnished insight into the pathogenesis of many chronic diseases. The opportunity to maintain anephric patients on chronic dialysis disclosed information about the kidney's role in erythropoiesis, calcium metabolism, and parathyroid function.

In hematology the yield of clinical investigations was especially noteworthy because of the relative ease of sampling blood and bone marrow constituents, enabling biochemical and immunological techniques to be used easily. Enzymatic defects in erythrocytes and polymorphonuclear cells were identified, and correlated with clinical syndromes. The whole area of immune deficiency syndromes, either congenital or acquired, was also derived from clinical observation.[27]

The Full-Time System

Full-time academic posts in clinical subjects were an essential corollary of clinical investigation. They were less conspicuous but probably equally essential as preconditions for the formation of internal medicine as a distinct specialty. One of the first accounts of the beginnings of the clinical full-time system was that provided by Abraham Flexner.[28] Through his connection with the General Education Board of the Rockefeller Foundation, Flexner did much to further the full-time system in the clinical departments of American medical schools. In 1913 funds were made available to the Johns Hopkins University to support full-time clinicians in the departments of medicine, surgery, and pediatrics. By 1925 Flexner was able to count at least thirty full-time clinical chairs, many of them with their own research staffs, in the United States, Canada, and England. In the United States, he noted, the medical schools could "command their entire time for the care of patients, for the instruction of students, and for research." He emphasized the importance of the full-time academic clinician's freedom from the routine necessities of private practice. The new man could deal with patients wherever they offered educational or research value, remaining "free . . . to devote himself in what is for him the most effective fashion to the care of patients, the training of his pupils, and the increase of knowledge."[29]

Flexner's clear-headed assessment of the potential difficulties, as well as the advantages, of the full-time system was remarkably prescient. He foresaw the obstacles and trade-offs that would arise not only in relation to the academic setting, but also to the field of internal medicine writ large. The new field would not succeed, he argued, unless internists

> are enabled to devote their time and energy to painstaking study and experimentation, wide reading in many languages, discursive conversation, and leisurely reflection. . . . For the physician deals with the most complicated of mechanisms—the human body; he must be master of a vast and rapidly increasing volume of knowledge, into which streams from a thousand sources—foreign and domestic—continuously pour; must—spare himself as he will—spend himself in human ways, as no physicist, astronomer or philologian need; must administer an elabo-

> rate and costly organization which will function effectively only if constantly tended; finally, he must teach and somehow supervise the teaching of others. Under these circumstances, full-time itself is sadly inadequate to the opportunities for service—human, educational, and scientific—afforded by a medical clinic. [30]

Unlike his brother Simon, Flexner was not a physician but rather one of the first professional educational consultants. In the ensuing sixty years no one has stated the situation better than this remarkable observer. And the same two questions remain controversial: the proper balance among internists' closely held values of service, education, and research; and the proper balance between a great deal of knowledge about a narrow part of the field, and a shallower knowledge base covering a larger expanse.

The 1930s: Internists Organize

The explosion of knowledge and hopes for combating disease that pervaded the 1920s led to an array of institutional and organizational steps both within and outside of internal medicine in the 1930s. The most important of those occurring outside the internist's own private world was the triumph of the hospital, which was, after all, the internist's clinical laboratory. With the increased emphasis on acute nonsurgical care brought about partly by improved methods of treating acute medical illness, and with the continued growth of the full-time system in the medical schools' clinical departments, the internist became a central figure in directing ward activities. That held true not only for patient care but for the education of the clinical clerkship students as well. From the 1930s until at least the 1970s, and arguably until the present, the locus of medical education moved from ambulatory and some surgical settings to hospital wards, where internists played a central role in directing and teaching patient care.[31]

The 1930s was a time of metamorphosis for internal medicine, a critical decade of transformation. There was a new perception of the importance of chronic degenerative diseases and a sense of urgent need for new knowledge about basic biological processes. Major growth and expansion lay ahead during the war and, especially, the postwar years.[32] But clearly internal medicine was ready for a process of internal differentiation, a process already under way but now reified through the certification system created in 1936. At the end of that year the American Board of Internal Medicine gave its first examination in the specialty, and four years later, under the same aegis, four subspecialties inaugurated their own examinations.[33] Aware of the explosion of knowledge, in 1938 the American College of Physicians undertook a series of postgraduate courses that has continued for nearly fifty years.[34]

Lay perceptions of triumph and progress paralleled professional perceptions of an exploding knowledge base. Daniel Fox has recently documented the change in popular perceptions of the physician and of medical science that, having begun in the 1920s, reached its high water mark in the 1930s. Novels, paintings, plays, photographs, and many of the new talking motion pictures all celebrated the medical profession, portraying recent strides in scientific medicine with bold strokes and high drama. Now the internist could join his better organized and, as a specialist, more prominent surgical counterpart on the pedestal of science. Together they could bask, despite the economic depression, in the new medical optimism.[35]

The 1930s was a remarkable and heady time to be entering medicine. Change was in the air. On the surface, perhaps, that was hard to see in internal medicine itself. Practice was still mainly private. Science was still something that clinicians, except at a few places such as the Rockefeller, did in stolen moments. And academic departments were still small enclaves largely composed of rather privileged individuals. But, as we have indicated, lay and professional observers alike knew that, a generation after medical education had been reformed, clinical dividends were not just around the corner but in fact already evident. This seemed especially clear to young internists just entering the field. Their immediate seniors, men of the Meltzer-Dock-Cohn generation of the 1910s and 1920s, however, saw the opening of the era as a double-edged sword. Robert Loeb, president of the American Society for Clinical Investigation, cautioned that

> keeping pace with the spirit of abandon which characterized the florid twenties, clinical investigation ran riot, recognizing no bounds, philosophical, intellectual, technical or financial. With apparently unlimited financial resources, the business man's concept of mass production tended to creep into academic medical circles.

This situation created the false hope that "the mysteries of medical science must bow before the concerted onslaught and bow promptly." The interwar "boomlet," too brief for departments to scale up significantly (but compelling enough to give Loeb and his colleagues cause for concern about its direction) ended with the stock market crash and the Depression. In 1936 Loeb could argue that

> we are now confronted with the inevitable and healthy task of taking account of stock and separating the wheat from the chaff. . . . [W]hat we desire to save above all else is a backlog of solid and profitable research . . . defined as a product of thoughtful and critical curiosity supported by ingenuity in experimentation. . . . Another approach . . . the *research project* . . . attempts to force progress through regimentation of workers [and] is usually initiated by energetic and misguided promoters inspired by the effectiveness of mass production in big business.[36]

Such warnings about Big Science and Big Medicine were interesting in part because they were sounded again and again in the new era that was about to begin. In the 1930s, however, rhetoric of this sort did not bring irresolution. Internal medicine had been infused by the idea that progress was soon in coming. Within internal medicine progress seemed to hinge on three key S's: science, specialism, and scale—scaling up. It took the new young leaders but a few years to bring them all into play, for the outbreak of another war forced the issue and made certain that there would be no turning back.

World War II

With the advent of World War II, medical research and technology were channeled into fields of military pertinence. While some projects had to be put on hold, others became more pressing, and this time internists were ready to take advantage of the military challenge in an organized fashion. American clinicians were active, for example, in developing better methods of blood storage through blood banking. Several viral vaccines were manufactured on a large scale for the protection of personnel going into parts of the world where problems such as yellow fever, sandfly fever, and dengue were to be expected. Drugs for prophylaxis and treatment of malaria were prepared. When Howard Florey and colleagues in Britain showed that penicillin could bring about dramatic improvement in the types of infection that commonly complicated war injuries, American commercial laboratories succeeded in developing large-scale methods of producing penicillin. The need to extend the World War I level understanding of traumatic shock gave impetus to pioneering work by Dickinson Richards and André Cournand, who used the technique of right-heart catheterization. For these studies they, along with Werner Forssman, were awarded the Nobel Prize.[37]

From the standpoint of organized internal medicine, scientific advances like these were unquestionably important in upgrading the internist's professional status. Also essential to this advancement was the array of administrative arrangements developed in the military to meet the perceived need for specialized, high quality care in nonsurgical areas. Even as late as the 1930s, the peacetime Army had recognized no need for a consultant service. Indeed, the military command continued well into the war years grappling with the problem of how to integrate nonsurgical specialists into their operations. Obstacles abounded. Service command surgeons, for example, did not immediately welcome the idea of consultant internists. There was a sizeable moment of administrative inertia. Between 1942 and 1944 frequent reorganizations resulted as medical consultants sought to overcome these obstacles and to create a standardized system of specialists and subspecialists. Indeed, as late as 1942 no such classification system had been put into place.

Between mid-1942 and late 1943, however, surgeons and internists rallied together to lobby both civilian and military constituencies about the need for some means to get the right expertise out to the right place at the right time. The Surgeon General was caught between consultants in the medical department and higher Army authority. It was left to a few key individuals to press for the implementation of specialist evaluations, or written assessments of physicians according to their level of specialized expertise. Importantly, such evaluations had been prepared even before the war by the Committee on Medicine of the National Research Council. Finally, in October 1943, the Army accepted and promulgated a system for classifying medical officers into four categories, A through D, based on their demonstrated professional qualifications.[38]

The effect of the A-B-C-D system, accompanied by differential salary scales, cannot be overestimated. For the consultants it provided for the all-important double product: demonstrable expertise coupled with distinctive socioeconomic status, both conferred in a manner that was conspicuous and standardized. The result, "thanks to the developments in medical therapeutics since the early 1920's," noted one insider, was that "the internist had become the most effective therapist extant."[39] In part, such statements must be understood in the context of the traditional friendly rivalry between surgeons and internists. Nonetheless, this war had done for the latter group what earlier ones did for the former. And when the consultants—originally products, after all, of civilian medicine—returned to it, they retained the new, hierarchical system. It was a system wherein "more specialized" on some objective scale, and not only a scale of demonstrated ability but also of rewards, now seemed to connote "better."[40]

The Boom in Biomedical Research After 1950

Although World War II brought a temporary halt to many programs of laboratory and clinical investigations, it had an even more important effect. It demonstrated that major scientific goals could be attained by spending large sums of money and by focusing attention on defined objectives. As a consequence, shortly after the fighting ended, governments and private foundations began to make large contributions to medical research. At the same time pharmaceutical manufacturers world-wide began to invest unprecedented sums of money in research and development of new drugs and biological products. Noting the advances already made in biochemistry, radioisotope development, and new instrumentation, the large drug firms realized that the time was ripe for major new investment in medical research.

Beginning in the 1950s, then, from public as well as private sources, American medical school faculty members found themselves being offered undreamed of sums of money to develop extensive tools for biomedical investigation. At the same time they began to be offered many new effective therapeutic agents turned out by the pharmaceutical industry. The combination—interesting, potentially soluble problems and the wherewithal to address them—was a heady one. For participants in this expansion it was an exciting period, welcoming new and effective forms of therapy, building research laboratories, and recruiting young medical scientists into careers as clinical investigators. One paused now and then to ask oneself what else to ask for.[41]

The surge in biomedical research was not confined to the United States. Changes in the scale of funding rippled from nation to nation as each increased its investment in health-related research and services. Rapid travel and swift means of disseminating new knowledge combined to make medical research genuinely a shared world commodity. American workers played an important part in producing new information, but they also borrowed heavily from findings of biomedical scientists working elsewhere.

The amount of money allocated to biomedical research in the United States indicates the scale of this increased expenditure. In the decade 1940–49, the total sum spent on medical research and development was $763 million. In 1950–59 this rose to $3.2 billion; in 1960–69 to $18.4 billion and in

1970–79 to $46.5 billion. During the four-year span 1980–83 the cost amounted to $36 billion.[42]

Changes in the scale of malleable problems for investigation, and of research dollars with which to tackle them, were paralleled by changes in the numbers of personnel. In 1950 all the departments of medicine in United States medical schools were staffed by fewer than 1,000 salaried faculty; at present the number is probably in the vicinity of 12,000. Add to that many thousands of postdoctoral research fellows and research technicians. The resulting "growth spurt" makes pointless any comparison with research before 1949.

In the post-World War II period one area of discovery not only ranked in importance with the nineteenth-century golden age of bacteriology, but was in important ways analogous to it historically: the new understanding of genetics and molecular biology. Oswald Avery's demonstration of the role of DNA in the transformation of the pneumococcus organisms led, ultimately, to the Watson-Crick model of the structure of DNA, the unraveling of the genetic code, discoveries about the function of RNA, cloning, recombinant DNA techniques, restriction endonucleases, regulatory genes, oncogenes, and immunogenetics. It became possible to speak in meaningful fashion of "molecular diseases" after the publication of Linus Pauling's work on sickle-cell hemoglobin. Pauling would later recall that when

> Dr. William B. Castle . . . mentioned that the red cells of patients with [sickle-cell anemia] are deformed (sickled) in the venous circulation but resume their original shape in the arterial circulation, the idea occurred to me that sickle-cell anemia was a molecular disease, involving an abnormality of the hemoglobin molecules that I postulated to be present in the red cells of these patients would have two mutually complementary regions on their surfaces, such as to cause them to aggregate into long columns, which would be attracted to one another by van der Waals forces, causing the formation of a needle-like crystal which, as it grew longer and longer, would cause the red cell to be deformed and would thus lead to the manifestations of the disease.[43]

It thus became possible, in the years just after World War II, for a person with an understanding of physics and chemistry to take advantage of specific clinical observations and to follow their characterization of the underlying disorder down to the molecular level. After 1945 many more specific molecular abnormalities were identified.[44] It seems likely that in the decades that lie immediately ahead, practitioners of internal medicine will have rational approaches to the correction of several molecular diseases. This critical next step will help close the circle of learning about the chronic and malignant disorders that have largely supplanted the infectious disorders of the early twentieth century. Yet this cycle of diagnosis and treatment seems part of a larger historical cycle. It is not dissimilar from the efforts, one hundred years ago, first to establish the etiology of infectious diseases and later to mitigate their impact through specific preventive and chemotherapeutic measures. In each case diagnostic advances led in time to therapeutic applications.[45]

Nearly equal in importance to molecular biology, and probably converging with it, was the field of immunology. Though it traces its roots back to Edward Jenner and Louis Pasteur, modern immunological investigation began in earnest only after World War II. Since the 1940s investigators recognized the role of lymphocytes in graft rejection, paving the way for later characterization of lymphocyte populations and immunoglobulin structure. Clinical medicine benefited from a growing understanding of the immense importance of the immune system, not only in the defense against microbial invaders, but also possibly in the surveillance against some neoplastic diseases, and certainly in the pathogenesis of autoimmune disorders.[46]

Finally, after World War II three additional areas of investigation began to offer the prospect of fundamental new knowledge: the study of cascade mechanisms, the study of basic neurobiology, and improved methods of clinical trial design. In neuroscience the twentieth-century physician witnessed the discovery of the hypophyseal peptide hormones, the different neurotransmitters as well as the enzymes that regulate their actions, and the whole concept of the central nervous system as an endocrine organ, elaborating not only hormones but such entities as the endorphins. Meticulous work, aided by new technology, made it possible to describe the components of cascading mechanisms, as evidenced in blood coagulation, complement activation, and interactions in inflammatory processes, for example the role of kinins and prostaglandins. And, as Harry Marks explains later in this volume, epidemiologists brought together the new clinical science with the arcane methods of statisticians to begin a revolution in the evaluation of medical intervention. That revolution is now robustly bearing its fruit.

Disease: The Internist's Patients

During the twentieth century there have been unprecedented changes in the *kinds* of illness that comprised the work of practitioners of internal medicine. For centuries, infectious disorders were the leading causes of morbidity and mortality: the common contagious diseases, tuberculosis, syphilis, dysentery, pneumonia, malaria, yellow fever, erysipelas, suppurative diseases, and meningitis. Even before the etiological role of microbes in infective processes was recognized, it began to be possible to institute measures to lessen their injurious effects through vaccines, proper safeguarding of food and water, sewage disposal, control of insect vectors, and other similar means. Beginning with the advent of sulfonamides in the 1930s, internists have had the resources to treat many life-threatening processes. As a consequence we have witnessed a striking increase in life expectancy. A century ago a newborn infant would survive for an average of 40 years; now the life expectancy at birth is close to 75 years.

This is not to suggest that therapeutics and increased life expectancy are a simple cause and effect mechanism. Many factors converged to lengthen life. But if one looks further, there is a curious and much less obvious historical relationship between disease itself and the diagnostic tools and categories devised to uncover and classify it. Some of the most intriguing examples of this relationship stem from the first half of the twentieth century, when acute infectious diseases came to be recognized in increasingly fine diagnostic detail, yet remained both pervasive and difficult to treat.[47] In that transitional period, infectious disorders were, for a while, discerned in every nook and cranny. Illnesses from as widely disparate causes as nutritional and psychiatric disturbances were ascribed in many instances to microbial etiologies.[48]

A remarkable example of what might be called the heroic era of microbiology, in its relation to nosology and nosography, was the doctrine of focal infection. The idea had its beginning in a set of 1915 lectures (published the following year) by Frank Billings of Chicago, an eminent practitioner and past president of the American Medical Association. He reported that he had noted clinical improvement in patients with nephritis and arthritis, following the removal of "foci of infection" in other parts of the body—for example, in the periodontal tissues, the tonsils, nasal sinuses, appendix, gall bladder, and uterus. The bacteriologist at the Mayo Clinic, Edward Rosenow, proceeded to find specific strains of streptococci in "foci of infection" and claimed, in the classic fashion dictated by Koch's postulates, to have reproduced the human disease by injecting the organisms into healthy animals. The laboratory model for Billings' clinical ideas lent credibility to the doctrine of focal infection.

The concept was adopted with enthusiasm in many parts of the world. During the next quarter century millions of unneeded surgical and dental procedures were carried out in efforts to eradicate "foci of infection." A standard textbook recommendation for the treatment of any disease of unknown etiology was to search for and remove any possible focus of infection. In addition a brisk business in producing autogenous vaccines developed. Eventually, bacteriologists reported their inability to confirm the supposed associations and the animal experiments. In 1940 a critical review by Hobart Reimann and W. Paul Havens challenged the concept.[49] Thereafter the wholesale attack on tonsils, teeth, sinuses, and other nonessential parts abated. In the mid-1940s Russell Cecil, primarily a rheumatologist, remarked ruefully that his luster began to dim when the focal infection theory was exploded.

In retrospect, Frank Billings' characterization of focal infection may seem misguided. Yet it is not clear that the late twentieth-century internist is any more exempt from shaky diagnostic entities. What is clear is that, since Billings' day, the practice of internal medicine has changed from coping with entities like typhoid fever, tuberculosis, and syphilis—and focal infection—to dealing with the chronic and degenerative processes that tend to increase in importance as the body ages, notably atherosclerotic heart disease, cancer, and rheumatic and neurologic disorders. (A number of the chapters in this volume illustrate the manner in which this shift to chronic diseases has altered the character of the patient population and thereby the internist's practice.)[50] It is tempting to postulate that a "stable" subspecialty of internal medicine is one that succeeds in navigating the transition from acute to chronic disorders.[51]

Diagnosis in Internal Medicine

To the practitioner of internal medicine, diagnosis has always been regarded as an end in itself, in contrast to our surgical colleagues, for whom diagnosis is a way station to the performance of a procedure. The term "diagnostician" was often employed by lay people as a compliment to indicate a physician who possessed unusual competence and wisdom. Perhaps the high value we have placed on diagnosis has its origin in the fact that until recently we possessed so little effective treatment. The role of the internist's predecessors had been to decide about the diagnosis and to estimate prognosis. In a few cases he might be called on to guide palliative treatment as well. That situation changed slowly over the course of the nineteenth century. In the early nineteenth century, the advent of pathological anatomy and the "anatomico-clinical method" led to the development of simple procedures of physical diagnosis.[52] Later in the nineteenth century physicians began to appreciate that helpful information could be obtained from the chemical laboratory. After 1880–90, the microbiological laboratory became another arrow in the diagnostician's quiver, as physicians began to make specific diagnoses by identifying etiologic agents of infectious diseases. Around the turn of the century immunological methods of diagnosis such as the Wasserman reaction and the Widal test further expanded the horizon of the diagnostician.[53]

Roentgen's discovery of the X ray was turned to practical advantage with spectacular speed, first for problems of trauma, but soon afterward in the domain of internal medicine. Within ten years of Roentgen's announcement, a number of physicians, including George Dock in Ann Arbor, were demonstrating pulmonary and cardiac disease by means of what were then called skiagrams. Soon the use of contrast media was introduced to examine particular organ systems: the gastrointestinal tract, the urinary and biliary tracts, and the fluid compartments of the central nervous system. The internist became dependent on colleagues with special skills in order to employ diagnostic methods more complex than palpation, percussion, and auscultation.[54]

In the field of hematology, diagnosis was improved by both pathologists and practicing physicians, because the blood and bone marrow were so well suited to morphologic study by ordinary microscopy. Alongside hematology the field of clinical chemistry steadily grew in importance, and American workers, notably Donald Van Slyke and Otto Folin, played key roles. Clinical chemistry got a special fillip when insulin treatment for diabetes came into use because it called for repeated estimations of the blood sugar and of acid-base balance of the blood. Various colorimetric and gasometric methods of analysis were devised, followed by the flame photometer for blood sodium and potassium determinations; the technique of electrophoresis provided new ways of following metabolic processes or detecting abnormal constituents. From about 1930 to 1950 a two-volume work by John Peters, an internist, and Donald Van Slyke, was the authoritative reference for methods of clinical chemistry and interpretation of the findings.[55]

New techniques were also brought to the bedside. Between 1920 and 1940, for example, electrocardiography became essential to the field of cardiology. In the same period basal metabolic rate determinations were widely employed in the diagnosis of thyroid abnormalities, although this was later outmoded and the patient was again abstracted from the diagnostic process once chemical techniques for measuring circulating thyroid hormones were devised. Methods to determine levels of various enzymes in the blood proved useful, especially in hepatic diseases, where the custom of performing a "battery of function tests" became popular. In the last few decades, technological developments such as radioimmunoassay, immunoelectrophoresis, and immunofluorescence further refined the diagnostician's ability to monitor the most fastidious processes and obscure derangements of organ function.

Since World War II anatomical diagnosis also developed to a point that surely surpassed Roentgen's wildest dreams. Ultrasound, computed tomography, isotopic scanning, and magnetic resonance imaging have brought anatomical diagnosis to a new level. It is interesting, when thinking of the power of the new diagnostic imaging techniques, to recall that one of Osler's lecture topics was the differential diagnosis of abdominal tumors. At that time radiologic and even more revealing procedures had not been devised, so he must have been speaking about the differentiation of lesions large enough to be palpable. We remember a time when the physician making teaching ward rounds sought to be first to feel the tip of the spleen or to detect a heart murmur. Those skills are still badges of a medical education, but have certainly lost some of their direct importance in guiding the medical work-up. Perhaps a more important skill now lies in knowing which test to perform, guided by increasingly precise and explicit methods of medical decision analysis. History taking is still of prime value, but the relative importance of the stethoscope and the rest of the physical examination, especially in cardiac and pulmonary disease, or the reflex hammer in neurology, has diminished substantially.

Therapeutics in Internal Medicine

The notion of therapeutics is one that is just beginning to find its historians.[56] The term derived from the Greek concept of *θεραπεία*, for "healing," but underwent a number of shifts in meaning and emphasis before it reached the modern and quite recent connotation of "specific treatment" now taken for granted. Therapeutics in the early American setting, like that seen in Europe and elsewhere, was characterized by two cardinal features: it was principally empirical, and, of all the aspects of a physician's practice, it had the most immediate impact on the patient's sense of well-being.[57] Various herbal preparations had been used since earliest recorded history, and remained mainstays of American nineteenth-century practice. Until recently the study of botany was a required part of medical education. And indeed, some botanical agents provided effective forms of treatment. A partial list is impressive: morphine, cocaine, colchicine, ipecac, quinine, salicin, digitalis, coumadin, and vincristine. Generally only crude preparations were used, but beginning in the nineteenth century, with the advent of organic chemistry, the active materials began to be extracted and synthesized by pharmaceutical companies.

Empirical herbal treatments were augmented, especially in the eighteenth century, by attempts to restore the proper balance of the putative "humors," the basis of the practices of bleeding, purging, sweating, and blistering. By the middle of the nineteenth century, however, skepticism had begun to make inroads on this sort of heroic therapeutics. Jacob Bigelow of Boston, in his 1835 "Discourse on Self-Limited Diseases," argued that many diseases ran their courses and were not influenced favorably by any therapy then available. This essay was said to have caused physicians to question the custom of treating sick patients so harmfully and to have given rise to a more supportive, less aggressive, kind of treatment. He declared that some diseases had their own "definite and necessary career" that deviated little regardless of the physician's ministrations. Self-limited diseases, in his view, had their own cadence and rhythm; they would "be completed in a certain time; which time and processes may vary with the constitution and condition of the patient, and may tend to death or to recovery, but are not known to be shortened, or greatly changed, by medical treatment."[58]

Heroic notions of bleeding and purging were not, however, easily forsaken. As late as 1892, for example, William Osler could still discuss the treatment of pneumonia in these terms:

> In many cases the question comes up at the onset as to the propriety of venesection. . . . During the first five decades of this century the profession bled too much, but during the last decades we have certainly bled too little. Pneumonia is one of the diseases in which a timely venesection may save life. To be of service it should be done early. In a full-blooded, healthy man with a high fever and bounding pulse, the abstraction of from 20 to 30 ounces of blood is in every way beneficial, relieving the pain and dyspnea, reducing the temperature and allaying the cerebral symptoms, so violent in some instances.

Osler has often been described as a therapeutic nihilist and as we already noted, the idea of creating the Rockefeller Institute flowed in part from his acknowledgment of the futility of most medical treatments. Nevertheless, in light of today's rigorous standards for acceptance of an effective treatment, some of his recommendations give us insight into the best-informed view of therapeutics a century ago. In pneumonia, for example, he noted that "though some hold that alcohol in this condition is not indicated, I believe that it is in many instances the only remedy capable of tiding the patient over the most dangerous period." He espoused the use of strychnine and hypodermic injections of ether as cardiostimulants and recommended as adjuncts the administration of ammoniacal spirits, camphor, and musk. On diabetes mellitus, Osler wrote that "opium alone stands the test of experience as a remedy capable of limiting the progress of the disease. Diabetic patients seem to have a special tolerance for this drug." And, mentioned without comment, in the section on intestinal obstruction, was this intriguing glimpse of nineteenth-century practice:

> Jonathan Hutchison recommends that the patient be placed under an anesthetic, the abdomen thoroughly kneaded, and a copious enema given while in the inverted position. Then, with the aid of three or four strong men, the patient is to be thoroughly shaken, first with the abdomen held downward, and subsequently in the inverted position.

Here is the thinking of the most influential practitioner and teacher of internal medicine that the western world has known—a man of great erudition whose memory is celebrated by scores of "Osler Clubs" in different parts of world, and whose writings and sayings are still being reissued. Current criteria for determining therapeutic efficacy have changed to a point where Osler's approach would likely be labeled "anecdotal."[59] But a perusal of his first edition provides a telling view of the therapy available a century ago. Like the Reverend Gates one is struck by how little there was to be offered in treatment. Osler indeed merited the appellation of therapeutic nihilist. The book is full of expressions such as "no treatment," "unsatisfactory," "not satisfactory," "extremely unsatisfactory," "an incurable disease," "symptomatic," "no remedy is known," "medicinal treatment is of little avail," "treatment can only be palliative," and "no known treatment."

Osler was, of course, able to recommend some agents that were effective. Among them were opium in various forms, antipyrine, phenacetin, salicylates; subcutaneous infusion of saline in cholera, quinine for malaria; chloral hydrate as a sedative, colchicum for gout, cod liver oil for rickets, lemon or lime juice for scurvy; calomel for constipation, bicarbonate of soda or bismuth for gastritis and other disorders of the intestine; venesection for acute pulmonary edema, nitroglycerin for angina pectoris, digitalis for heart failure; iron for secondary anemia, and bromides for epilepsy. In the matter of preventive measures against infection, he listed vaccines for smallpox and rabies.

But the main thrust of medical treatment in Osler's time was reflected in an array of general supportive measures, beginning with good nursing care. Bed rest and absolute quiet or rest of an affected part were often mentioned. Other general measures included nutritious diet, fresh air, and sunlight. Osler emphasized the importance of keeping the bowels open. There was also much about use of heat or cold, either locally or in the form of baths or spongings. Steam inhalations were recommended for respiratory inflammation; liniments and gargles were used. He frequently recommended lavage of the stomach. For painful conditions in the chest and abdomen, he used adhesive strapping of the chest, or turpentine stupes to the abdomen. He suggested a change of climate in some instances, or travel, or time spent at a spa.

During the early decades of the twentieth century progress was made in the development of agents useful in immunization and, in a very few cases, in specific treatment of active disease. After diphtheria antiserum proved successful, many attempts were made to produce other antisera, including, of course, tetanus. Less certainly successful were antisera for treatment of meningococcal meningitis and scarlet fever. In chemotherapy the one significant achievement was the 1909 development of arsenical compounds for use in syphilis and trypanosomiasis. Arsenic, as Fowler's solution, and potassium iodide continued to enjoy great popularity for a wide variety of diseases. But there is little reason to believe that they had much effect, except in syphilis.

Indeed, even up to World War I, specific therapeutics lagged behind the diagnostic techniques that we have already discussed. It is intriguing, but perfectly understandable, that not only the *substance,* but the very *idea* of specific therapeutics was quite distinct from—and more vague than—that taken as a given in the present antibiotic era. In 1910, for example, in surveying the "progress of therapeutics during the past twenty years," it was still possible for a prominent therapeutist and nutritionist, the gastroenterologist A. L. Benedict, to devote more space to "diagnostic therapeutics"—three pages—than he did (one brief paragraph) to the heart or (another paragraph) diabetes mellitus. Much of the excitement in 1910 was focused on tuberculin, iodides, X rays, and methylene blue, products that pharmaceutical firms and chemists conjured up for the internist, not as therapeutist, but as diagnostician.[60]

But the period between the wars brought new circumstances, beginning in the 1920s with two major therapeutic discoveries, the liver diet for pernicious anemia and insulin for diabetes mellitus. In the mid-1930s, when the discovery of the sulfonamide drugs was announced, practicing physicians were stunned by reports that dreaded diseases such as streptococcal septicemia and meningococcal meningitis could be halted and cured simply by giving tablets containing a relatively simple chemical compound. Succeeding years brought penicillin, streptomycin, and a long series of other effective antimicrobial agents. It was a yeasty time for those who had a special interest in infectious disease.

The major pharmaceutical manufacturers saw, from the experience with penicillin and other antibiotics, that large investments in research and development could produce large profits. This work was unsuited to academic departments, due to long latent periods between discovery and marketing, the expense of safety trials, and the need for secrecy before new drugs could be patented. Nevertheless, for the pharmaceutical industry such gambles were good business, hence the large investments in commercial research and development, from which came whole families of effective drugs for use in a wide assortment of disease states. Industrial research yielded many valuable and effective agents: synthetic endocrine preparations, oral diuretics, antihypertensive agents, anticoagulants, histamine inhibitors, prostaglandin inhibitors, antineoplastic agents, vasoactive drugs, antiarrhythmic drugs, the phenothiazines, immunosuppressive compounds, new sedatives and tranquilizers, levodopa, and others. The flood of new compounds to be tested in clinical settings, together with the acceptance of clinical investigation as a branch of science, created a demand for a more scientific and more objective study of drug effects—in essence, the new science of clinical pharmacology.[61]

All this concentration on therapy by medicinal agents has produced substantial benefits. We have moved into a period wherein crude herbal extracts were replaced by compounds of standardized, well-defined composition. Anecdotal evidence, as seen above with Osler's enemas, and which was so commonly trusted at the beginning of this century, came to be considered highly questionable. Several years ago, one of us (P. B.) made a study, disease by disease, of the efficacy of medical treatment, as reflected in a comparison of the first edition of the *Cecil Textbook of Medicine* (1928) with the 15th edition (1976).[62] The findings were encouraging. In 1928, there were effective treatments or preventative measures for 5 to 10 percent of 360 diseases—for example, quinine for malaria and toxoid to prevent tetanus. By 1976 the proportion had risen to 50 to 55 percent, and the progress continues.

Advances between 1928 and 1976 were not limited to the field of infectious diseases; instead they spanned every branch of internal medicine. A patient today has a far better chance of receiving effective treatment, with early return to normal living, than in 1930. The chemotherapy of infections now spans not only the acute septic processes but also the more chronic and nevertheless highly lethal diseases. Half a century ago, a young adult with cavitary tuberculosis had about a 50-50 chance of dying of that disease within five years. A young physician in the second quarter of this century encountered frequent examples of late manifestations of syphilis in the heart, aorta, central nervous system, and other organs. Tertiary syphilis is now so rare that many doctors in midcareer have never seen examples. The polio season in August and September used to be a cause for dread. Smallpox was not as common, but became wholly eradicated. Other, noninfectious chronic processes have proved more obdurate. Yet it is not unthinkable that, in decades to come, people currently in the profession may witness a curative treatment for schizophrenia or a way of arresting the progress of Alzheimer's disease.

Infectious disease may be the most dramatically changed area of internal medicine, but it is not unique. We now have effective treatment (chemotherapy and radiotherapy) for several malignant tumors, for example, choriocarcinoma, childhood sarcoma, testicular cancer, Burkitt's lymphoma, and Hodgkin's disease. Bone marrow transplants save the lives of some people with aplastic anemia, leukemia, and other hematopoietic neoplasms. Diagnostic techniques such as endoscopy and mammography make it possible to find cancers at a stage when they can be removed surgically. The availability of steroids and immunosuppressive agents has greatly altered the prognosis in systemic lupus erythematosus, inflammatory bowel disease, pemphigus, rheumatoid arthritis, polymyalgia rheumatica, pulmonary sarcoidosis, and idiopathic thrombocytopenic purpura.

Our ability to control hypertension is undoubtedly a factor contributing to the declining incidence and mortality of cerebrovascular disease and congestive heart failure. And that terrible disorder, malignant hypertension, has almost disappeared. Many diseases of the endocrine system can be accurately diagnosed and treated by replacement therapy, surgery, or chemotherapy. We can cope with cardiac arrhythmias far more effectively. In neurology there is effective treatment for myasthenia gravis, and substantial palliation can be achieved in some cases of parkinsonism. Schizophrenia and epilepsy are controlled far better now than half a century ago. The treatment of gout is greatly improved. There is no question that the technological methods of life support used in intensive care units make the difference between survival and death in many instances.

In several kinds of disease medical treatments have largely, or totally, supplanted surgery. Fifty years ago surgery for some forms of pulmonary tuberculosis was a major activity: thoracoplasty, resection of diseased lung, permanent collapse by plombage, and rest of affected lung by phrenic nerve interruption. Suppurative processes—abscess and empyema—are now often *prevented* by antimicrobial drugs used in the early stages of infection; similarly, in diseases such as parotitis, osteomyelitis, and mastoiditis, surgical measures are less often needed. A few decades ago one of the desperate measures used to mitigate severe hypertension was thoracolumbar sympathectomy, a procedure now totally abandoned. In the management of peptic ulcer the first line of defense in treatment is use of the H2 receptor antagonist drugs, surgical procedures being necessary only in complicated cases. In Graves' disease subtotal thyroidectomy is only one of the options to be considered, along with radioiodine or antithyroid drugs. Finally, the increasing importance of cytotoxic drugs and biological products used in the treatment of neoplastic diseases is also noteworthy.

The Literature of Internal Medicine: After Osler

The literature of internal medicine is discussed elsewhere in this volume, but a few points bear making in connection with any survey of a century of internal medicine.[63] The Osler textbook held sway among English language books on internal medicine from the first edition (1892) until well into the twentieth century, always as a single-author text. Osler was succeeded by Thomas McCrae as author, for the ninth through the 12th editions, and Henry Christian took responsibility for the last (13th) single-author edition, which appeared in 1938. In 1928, however, a new breed of textbook appeared. It was at the peak of the halcyon years of innovation in clinical investigation between the wars. In the opening paragraph of his new medical textbook, Russell Cecil of New York described how the

> rapid growth of medical science during the last few years has made it almost impossible for a single individual to master the entire field. In internal medicine, as other branches of human knowledge, the age of specialism has of necessity arrived, and some of our ablest practitioners even devote themselves in great measure to one disease. In order that physicians and students of medicine might have the benefit of an authoritative and up-to-date treatise on every medical subject, it seemed

> desirable to prepare a textbook of medicine in which each disease, or group of diseases, would be discussed by a writer particularly interested in that subject. This book represents an effort to carry out such a plan. In all there are one hundred and thirty contributors, each of whom is a student or investigator of the subject upon which he has written.

Although Cecil used the term "specialism" he did not speak of his 130 contributors as specialists, but rather as "writer[s] particularly interested in that subject." In the 1930s and 1940s, the Cecil textbook became the most widely used text, while single-author textbooks on internal medicine lost favor. Later other multiauthor books appeared, notably Tinsley Harrison's text, the *Scientific American* series, and the textbook edited by Jay Stein. The Osler tradition has been brought back, without abandoning the idea of multiple authorship, by members of the Department of Medicine at Johns Hopkins, with A. McGehee Harvey as editor.

Meanwhile, with the proliferation of medical subspecialties, monographs and texts dealing with each subspecialty have appeared in large numbers. Elsewhere in this essay we cite a few examples of the content of a modern textbook of cardiology to illustrate the extent of specialization in a single field. One can find large textbooks dealing exclusively with gastroenterology, hematology, oncology, rheumatology, infectious diseases, or pulmonary diseases. Some of them are as large as standard textbooks of internal medicine—2,000 to 2,500 pages written by fifty to one hundred contributors.

New subspecialty societies have flourished, and are rivaling the major clinical meetings in internal medicine in terms of numbers of papers presented and numbers of persons in attendance.[64] Most of the specialty societies sponsor publication of a journal, so that in major medical libraries one now sees scores of periodicals dealing with various fields within the domain of internal medicine. No doubt this surge in subspecialty publications has also contributed, as a community of readers is fragmented into smaller ones, to the centrifugal influences that we pointed out earlier. A countervailing influence, perhaps, will be the recent spate of textbook publications in general internal medicine. These are not the traditional (and still worthwhile) mega-textbooks, but a new species of texts geared to ambulatory care, consultative medicine, and the needs of the academic general internist.

Specialized Practice in Internal Medicine

It was easier for readers to be generalists when writers were generalists. Although a few clinicians concentrated their attention during the latter half of the nineteenth century on certain kinds of diseases, for example, neurology and dermatology, or tuberculosis, most of the leading physicians at that time were true generalists. For instance, when the famous German professor Friedrich von Mueller visited North America early in this century, he gave clinics on such varied topics as blood diseases, disseminated sclerosis, and pneumonia. Similarly, when William Osler lectured on internal medicine in the first decade of this century, he covered subjects as diverse as infective endocarditis, typhoid fever, pneumonia, tuberculosis, cerebrospinal fever, pancreatitis, intracranial masses, and abdominal tumors.

The range of the elite internist in the earliest years of the twentieth century may be glimpsed in a unique document at the University of Michigan. George Dock was professor of medicine at that medical school during the first decade of this century; his preserved stenographic notes, taken from ward teaching rounds, are a window on the early internist's inpatient practice. He met students twice weekly for clinical discussions based on patients in the hospital. The subjects included virtually everything in the domain of internal medicine: gastrointestinal disease, kidney disease, neurologic disease, diabetes, tuberculosis, neoplastic disease, typhoid fever, and pneumonia, among others. Dock's goal was to cover most subjects in internal medicine in the course of two years.[65]

To a great extent this kind of authoritative generalism was still the fashion when one of us (P. B.) took up the study of medicine. He can remember clinics by Jonathan Meakins of McGill on bronchiectasis, coronary artery disease, fever of unexplained origin, lymphosarcoma, and Bright's disease. In the late 1930s and 1940s he began attending the meetings of the Association of American Physicians in Atlantic City. It was common for some leading figures of the time such as Henry Christian or Emanuel Libman to rise repeatedly to discuss papers dealing with a wide variety of subjects. Nowadays at that society's meetings it is unusual for any member of the audience to comment on more than one paper during a session. By the end of World War II a tendency was developing to recognize special expertise among the various members of an academic department. Nevertheless, all members of that department were expected to be able to function as generalists and to serve as teachers on medical wards without special selection of the cases to be encountered.[66]

After 1950, with the rapid infusion of large amounts of money into medical research and medical education, there was a huge increase in the manpower of departments of medicine. These people, whose salaries were partly or wholly derived from research grants, were expected to spend a large proportion of their time in research. They found it expedient to narrow their focus to diseases of one organ system or to one kind of pathologic process. They became subspecialists, and many were uncomfortable attempting to teach about all facets of the growing knowledge base of internal medicine.

We have not been able to obtain precise figures on the number of full-time salaried faculty members in departments of medicine in the United States medical schools in about 1947. We estimate that for each American school the number generally ranged between six and twelve. Today the range would be from about fifty to four hundred, with an average of about one hundred per department. Lawrence Young has provided figures on the growth of the Department of Medicine at the University of Rochester during the 1960s and 1970s. His predecessor, William McCann, was the only full professor between 1939 and 1957, during which period the total number of salaried department members rose from eight to fourteen. Young held the same position from 1957 to 1974, and during his tenure the number of salaried senior faculty members grew from fourteen to one hundred, and the number of full professors from one to twenty-three.

With so many crowding in to deal with the same number of patients, and without a very great increase in the number of students, it was inevitable that faculty members would tend to "stake out" certain areas, and that those boundaries would be respected by other members of their departments. As early as 1955 Harold Himsworth said this:

> The present situation has arisen because medical knowledge has grown to such an extent that it is no longer, and never again will be, within the capacity of any individual man to master more than a small fraction of it. To decry this is not only to ignore facts; it is to deny the very means that have made our recent progress possible. Specialization is a natural phenomenon. It is comparable in human affairs to differentiation of function in biology.[67]

In academic departments subspecialists needed to attract colleagues to help with patient care and teaching and to collaborate in research. They wanted to have trainees to assist in consultations around the hospital and to participate in the research. Thus it soon developed that an academic department of medicine was organized in subspecialty divisions. The heads of those divisions took responsibility for applying for their own research funding and for recruiting junior faculty and research fellows.

The growing complexity of diagnostic and therapeutic procedures occupied the full attention of research fellows in academic departments. After they had completed a period of training many went out into private practice. They then persuaded the administrators of private hospitals to provide the special equipment they had learned to use in diagnosis and treatment. Thus, academic subspecialty divisions soon produced a large cadre of physicians who had been trained to focus attention on narrow fields within internal medicine. The result was that subspecialty practice flowered in the United States. Now we have come to a situation where there may be more subspecialists than seems desirable.

Among the factors that nurtured subspecialty practice were (1) chronic disease, (2) good basic science correlations, (3) complex diagnostic technology carried out by the subspecialist, (4) lack of a simple curative treatment, but numerous palliative measures, (5) a large volume of current literature dealing with these scientific, diagnostic, and palliative aspects of the disease picture, (6) the "attractiveness" of the field, (7) third-party payment for office procedures or for short-stay hospital care.[68]

To illustrate this in cardiology, one might cite some of the chapter and topic headings in Eugene Braunwald's textbook of cardiovascular medicine.[69] This 2,000-page work has forty-six contributors. In the diagnostic section, after discussing history and physical examination, there are sections on phonocardiography, carotid pulse tracings, apex cardiography, echophonocardiography (all of which are intended to improve on the traditional method of auscultation). Then comes catheterization, coronary arteriography, and radioisotope examination of the cardiovascular system. In this book sixty pages are devoted to the management of heart failure, most of which deals with the use of digitalis preparations; it is bolstered by 569 references. Management of arrhythmias runs to thirty pages, and includes discussions of seven different classes of drugs, as well as electrical methods. Pacemakers are dealt with in a chapter with just under four hundred references. Therapy of hypertension occupies thirty-six pages, covering dietary measures, diuretics, adrenergic blocking drugs, vasodilators, and renin-angiotensin inhibitors. The chapter on management of acute myocardial infarction discusses mobile coronary care units, hospital coronary care units, use of anticoagulants and fibrinolytic agents, treatment and prophylaxis of arrhythmias and hemodynamic disturbances, and measures designed to limit infarct size.

We have provided enough examples here to show the enormous scope of modern cardiology. It is no surprise, then, that cardiologists seldom seem to read articles on general internal medicine, and fail to attend general medical meetings, at home or away from home, unless the topic for discussion lies in the domain of cardiology. Although cardiology is our largest subspecialty in terms of practitioners, it is not unique in complexity.

The result of all this is that academic departments of medicine have become loose amalgamations of clans each more or less independent of the next. This arrangement has in many cases propagated itself into the outside world, because for better or worse the organization of the clans has become the model for practice patterns. Opinions differ about whether the model is most efficacious and economical, but only recently have health systems scientists begun rigorously testing the model that was previously accepted as a given. In academic medicine, the independence of subspecialty groups has been fostered by the greater role that personally generated funds—either in the form of research grants or fees for patient care—have played in providing faculty support. In the late 1940s, when support for faculty salaries first became available from sources outside the university, the question was sometimes raised whether a faculty member whose salary came partially or predominantly from "outside" sources would soon become more or less a "visitor" at the university. Certainly as time has passed, the requirements of granting agencies or of remunerative clinical work have led to increased tension between obligations to maintain funding and university faculty responsibilities.[70]

The Future Prospects of Internal Medicine

A century ago internal medicine was regarded as a branch of practice which, though broad in scope, could be mastered by a single individual. Now we must ask ourselves whether there can continue to be a field of practice of such breadth. Will it be fragmented gradually into independent specialties, as has taken place with so many of the branches of surgery? To be sure, the field of internal medicine seems fairly stable right now: general periodicals such as the *New England Journal of Medicine* and the *Annals of Internal Medicine* continue to thrive. The American College of Physicians continues successfully to offer programs of interest to the general internist. Most medical schools have departments or divisions bearing the name "general internal medicine," and one finds it on letterheads or lists of doctors in group practices, even in the Yellow Pages of telephone directories. But threatening the durability of general medicine as a major field of professional practice is the rise of hyperspecialism. Neurology and dermatology already constitute separate departments in many medical schools. Indeed, it is unlikely that most dermatologists or neurologists today would or could describe themselves as internists.

Is it not likely then, that the same kind of budding off will take place in several other branches of internal medicine? We have already quoted Himsworth's thought-provoking words: "Specialization is a natural phenomenon . . . comparable in human affairs to differentiation of function in biology." We also take note of the firm links that exist between certain medical specialties and other branches of professional work. Some cardiologists, for example, collaborate with surgeons more closely than with other internists. Oncologists must plan their therapy in close liaison with surgeons and radiologists. Clinical pharmacologists often have appointments in departments of pharmacology.

We pointed out earlier that single-author textbooks of internal medicine are a phenomenon of the past, and also that widely competent physicians are rare among medical school teachers. Nowadays when we want authoritative information we go to specialists or consult books and periodicals dealing with restricted fields. Other evidence of this trend is found in the vigor of the many specialist societies. Subspecialist practitioners are more likely to travel to meetings in which the discussion pertains only to their chosen field. Even the Association of American Physicians, from which so much of the progress in American internal medicine was first reported, is currently asking opinions of its members whether subspecialty sessions should replace the general sessions at its meetings. The American College of Physicians has already moved in that direction.

Of course we will always need special knowledge and skills and can all take pride in the advances that made it necessary to create these narrower fields of interest. But many symptoms that bring people to the doctor do not automatically fall into one or another of the specialty fields—headache, for example, or low back pain, fever, fatigability, anorexia, weight loss, edema, dyspnea, syncope, jaundice, dementia, and many others. The general internist is best qualified to assess such manifestations and, often, to manage them. In addition, the fact is that many physicians prefer not to limit their work to a narrow spectrum of disorders. Those practitioners who have completed residency training and have been certified by the American Board of Internal Medicine are usually competent to deal with many major illnesses that could be claimed by specialists—for example, cardiac decompensation, hypertension, fluid and electrolyte disorders, cerebrovascular disease, diabetes mellitus, peptic ulcer, cirrhosis of the liver, rheumatoid arthritis, epilepsy, pernicious anemia, and many of the infectious diseases.

Walsh McDermott has presented a strong argument that our health care system needs a plentiful supply of good doctors who can deal with most medical events, but who will know when there is need for help by a specialist. His list of the characteristics of general medical care includes wide responsibility, the "first contact" or primary care positioning of the generalist, a substantial expectation of continued patient observation when it is needed, a largely ambulatory population, and a guiding role in managing referrals and tests.[71]

Another factor to be taken into consideration for the future is the aging of the population. Older patients often have disabilities related to more than one organ system. In these individuals, care by more than one doctor can lead to serious confusion. Also, medical care of the elderly less often requires the use of aggressive diagnostic and therapeutic measures; instead the need is for long-term supervision, preventive medicine, and measures to retard the rate of progress of the decrements that come with aging.

However, it is no simple matter to redress what seems to have grown into an imbalance between specialism and generalism. Although most heads of departments of internal medicine concede that it would be desirable to produce more generalist and fewer specialist physicians, nevertheless they know the real obstacles that must be overcome to bring this about.[72] General internal medicine does not flower exuberantly in modern medical academia. In that setting professional success, signified by promotion and pay, carries the requisite that new knowledge be produced. This is somewhat easier for the faculty member whose clinical interests are narrow, especially when some basic science, or some special technique, can be employed in the investigative work. Teachers who serve as generalist physicians, although they perform valuable service as role models and as providers of patient care, experience difficulty in exhibiting scholarly productivity.

The centrifugal effect of all this power-to-the-subspecialties, particularly in but not exclusive to the academic setting, has also had an odd effect on the struggling new (actually old, but newly revived) upstart, general internal medicine. To grasp power, it has paradoxically been forced to prove itself as a sort of subspecialty in its own right. Its proponents have felt compelled to arm themselves with their own arcane "technologies." So far these tools have mainly consisted of "high tech" mathematical modeling and statistical techniques and economic analysis of health services; they have also included, albeit to a much more limited extent, "low tech" fields such as medical ethics and medical history.

The paradox lies in the fact that few, if any, of these technologies, although they may promote the academic survival of general internal medicine, have been demonstrated as truly essential in the training of internists equipped to provide high quality primary care in the community. The general internist remains caught between opposite roles, between the family practitioner and the subspecialist, toiling mightily to gain something of the virtues of each while evading its vices. Whether such narrow straits can be navigated successfully remains an open question. One measure designed to further the success of the venture has been the formation of a special society, General Medicine. The organization now also sponsors a medical journal. Its members realize that they face handicaps when it comes to published evidence of scholarly productivity.[73]

Despite its trials and tribulations, general internal medicine should be—and will be—maintained as a large and important kind of medical practice. There are grounds for arguing that it should in fact regain some of its former strength and influence. We share the view of many, namely that we have produced an imbalance in our field, with too many specialists and not enough generalists. We believe that the quality of medical care will be served best if we can find ways to limit the proportion of physicians engaged in specialty practice and ensure an adequate number of generalists.

We wish to thank John Eisenberg, Janet Golden, David Rytand, and Rosemary Stevens for their helpful suggestions in the course of revising the manuscript of this article.

NOTES

1. Harold Himsworth, "The Integration of Medicine: The Endeavour of Thomas Linacre and its Present Significance," *Brit Med J* 2 (1955) : 217–31.

2. For studies emphasizing this continuity see, for example, R. H. Kampmeier, "The American College of Physicians: Past and Present," *J Roy Coll Physicians Lond* 2 (1973) : 237–49. On the London College there is a large literature. A useful brief introduction to its early history is Theodore Brown, "The College of Physicians and the Acceptance of Iatromechanism in England, 1665–1695," *Bull Hist Med* 44 (1970) : 12–30; the exhaustive "house history" remains Sir George Clark, *A History of the Royal College of Physicians of London*, 3 vol. (Oxford: Clarendon, 1964, 1966, and 1972).

3. On German scientific medicine, its institutional development and clinical context see *Institutes and Ideas*, William Coleman and F. L. Holmes, eds. (Berkeley and Los Angeles: University of California Press, 1987), especially Timothy Lenoir's chapter on the relationship of physiology and internal medicine under Carl Wunderlich, "Science for the Clinic: Carl Ludwig and the Institutional Revolution in German Science." On the clinical specialties per se see Hans-Heinz Eulner, *Die Entwicklung der Spezialfächer an den Universitäten des deutschen Sprachgebietes* (Stuttgart: F. Enke, 1970). It provides a finely detailed survey of the explosion of specialties which, in the critical final decades of the nineteenth century, occurred in the German-speaking academic domains of Central Europe.

4. Cf. George Rosen, *The Specialization of Medicine* (New York: Froben, 1944). Also useful, for a broader economic picture of the early twentieth-century American specialist, is George Rosen, *The Structure of American Medical Practice, 1875–1941* (Philadelphia: University of Pennsylvania Press, 1983), especially 19–32 and (on institutional aspects) 43–51.

5. See Theodore Billroth, *The Medical Sciences in the German Universities* (New York: Macmillan, 1924), and George Crile, "The Progress of Surgery During the Past Quarter of a Century," *Int Clin* 4 (1915) : 249–55.

6. Arthur L. Bloomfield, "Origin of the Term 'Internal Medicine'," *JAMA* 169 (1959) : 168–69. See also Edward Atwater, "Internal medicine," in *The Education of the American Physician*, Ronald Numbers, ed. (Berkeley and Los Angeles: University of California Press, 1980), 145.

7. William Osler, *Aequanimitas: With Other Addresses to Medical Students, Nurses and Practitioners of Medicine*, ed. 3 (New York: McGraw-Hill, 1923), chapter 8.

8. The contrast between the German and English systems of clinical training is discussed in a number of places, although no single work concentrates explicitly on this intriguing subject, and no author provides a comparative view of internal medicine per se in the two contexts. An important recent point of departure is Kenneth Ludmerer, *Learning to Heal: The Development of American Medical Education* (New York: Basic Books, 1985), 47–71. Ludmerer underscores the point others have made, that the *choice* of the German model over the English was just that, not happenstance or the result of "drift," but a conscious choice, mediated in considerable measure by John Shaw Billings. In support of this Ludmerer supplies useful references to the published and unpublished documents of Billings.

9. Shryock remains the best introductory source for the eighteenth and early nineteenth centuries. On Gerhard see Dale C. Smith, "Gerhard's Distinction Between Typhoid and Typhus and its Reception in America, 1833–1860," *Bull Hist Med* 54 (1980) : 368–85.

10. On American physicians in Paris see Russell M. Jones, *The Parisian Education of an American Surgeon: Letters of John Mason Warren* (Philadelphia: American Philosophical Society, 1978), and John Warner, *The Therapeutic Perspective: Medical Practice, Knowledge, and Identity in America, 1820–1885* (Cambridge, MA: Harvard University Press, 1986).

11. Among the key "trigger diseases" in cardiology were rheumatic fever and, as discussed here, soldier's heart. On the importance of the former, see Chapter 8 by Joel Howell in this volume; on the latter in another national context, see his "'Soldier's Heart': The Redefinition of Heart Disease and Speciality Formation in Early Twentieth-Century Great Britain," in *The Emergence of Modern Cardiology, Medical History*, W. F. Bynum, C. Lawrence, and V. Nutton, eds., Suppl. No. 5 (London: Wellcome Institute for the History of Medicine, 1985), 34–52. On the third obviously central syndrome in cardiology, the paradigmatic aspect of which is more problematic vis-à-vis the formation of cardiology, see J. O. Leibowitz, *The History of Coronary Heart Disease* (London: Wellcome Institute for the History of Medicine, 1970).

12. See A. M. Harvey and V. A. McKusick, eds., *Osler's Textbook Revisited* (New York: Appleton-Century-Crofts, 1967).

13. Herrick's early paper attracted little attention, but his second communication on the subject, in 1919, gained immediate acceptance, and thereafter the clinical syndrome began to be recognized throughout the world. See Joel Howell, "Early

Perceptions of the Electrocardiogram: From Arrhythmia to Infarction," *Bull Hist Med* 58 (1984) : 83–98.

14. The pernicious anemia story is well told in Maxwell Wintrobe, *Hematology, the Blossoming of a Science: A Story of Inspiration and Effort* (Philadelphia: Lea & Febiger, 1985), 215–38.

15. On the steroid hormones in relation to arthritis and other disorders see the chapter by Thomas Benedek in this volume. On Kendall's broader importance, see Clark Sawin, "Defining Thyroid Hormone: Its Nature and Control" (in press).

16. William Osler, "The Coming of Age of Internal Medicine in America," *Int Clin* 4 (1915) : 1–5.

17. William Osler, *Principles and Practice of Medicine* (New York: Appleton, 1982).

18. For a survey of nineteenth-century textbooks of medicine in relation to their incorporation of scientific data, see Russell Maulitz, " 'The Whole Company of Pathology': Pathology as Idea and as Work in American Medical Life," in *History of Pathology*, Teizo Ogawa, ed. (Tokyo: Taniguchi Foundation, 1986), 139–61. On Osler's relative therapeutic nihilism see "Therapeutics in Internal Medicine," below.

19. Osler, *Aequanimitas*, chapter 19. Over the years a virtual cottage industry has grown up to survey the history of the Johns Hopkins medical institutions. The most recent work treating the subject, which has the signal virtue of both providing a reliable guide to further literature and appropriately placing the history of the Baltimore institutions in their larger context, is Ludmerer, *Learning to Heal*, especially 47–71 and 102–22.

20. See Ludmerer, *Learning to Heal*, and Gert H. Brieger, "The Flexner Report: Revised or Revisited?" *Medical Heritage*, 1 (1985) : 25–34.

21. The standard work on the subject remains that of George Corner, *A History of the Rockefeller Institute, 1901–1953: Origins and Growth* (New York: Rockefeller Institute Press, 1964).

22. Corner, *History of the Rockefeller Institute*, 93.

23. On insulin see Michael Bliss, *The Discovery of Insulin* (Chicago: University of Chicago Press, 1982). On pernicious anemia see Wintrobe, *Hematology*. On the idea of clinical investigation see Russell Maulitz, "Pathologists, Clinicians, and the Role of Pathophysiology," in *Physiology in the American Context, 1850–1940*, Gerald Geison, ed. (Bethesda: American Physiological Society, 1987).

24. Knud Faber, *Nosography in Modern Internal Medicine* (New York: Hoeber, 1923).

25. An excellent and readable introduction to this principle is Judith Swazey and Karen Reeds, *Today's Medicine, Tomorrow's Science: Essays on Paths of Discovery in the Biomedical Sciences* (Washington: U.S. Public Health Service, 1978).

26. See Steven Peitzman's essay on the evolution of nephrology, Chapter 7 in this volume.

27. Likewise the occurrence of hypertension or thromboembolic disease in users of contraceptive pills opened new vistas for study. On hematologic investigation see Wintrobe, *Hematology*.

28. The most recent account is Ludmerer's succinct exposition in *Learning to Heal*, 207–17 and passim.

29. Abraham Flexner, *Medical Education* (New York: MacMillan, 1925), 49–58.

30. Flexner, *Medical Education*.

31. See Edward C. Atwater, "Internal Medicine," in *The Education of the*

American Physician, Ronald Numbers, ed. (Berkeley and Los Angeles: University of California Press, 1980), 143–74.

32. We refer to expansion (obviously related one to the other) of both cadres: academic internists in departments of medicine and graduating medical school classes set to go out and practice. See Robert G. Petersdorf, "The Evolution of Departments of Medicine," *N Engl J Med* 303 (1980): 489–96.

33. See Joel D. Howell, "Specialties and the American Board of Internal Medicine: A Historical Perspective," paper presented at the 50th Anniversary meeting of the ABIM, 17 June 1986.

34. Kampmeier, "The American College of Physicians," 245.

35. Daniel M. Fox, "Acrimony and Realignment: The United States, 1932–1940," in *Health Policies, Health Politics: The British and American Experience, 1911–1965,* Daniel M. Fox, ed. (Princeton: Princeton University Press, 1986), 70–79.

36. Robert Loeb, "Comments on Clinical Investigation," *Science,* 83 (1936): 423, quoted by Edwin D. Kilbourne, "The Emergence of the Physician–Basic Scientist," *Daedalus* 115 (1986): 51. Of course Loeb's ambivalence and his nervousness about false expectations resonate deeply with current debates over the efficacy and the potential of the "war on cancer" begun in the 1970s.

37. The best general resource on internal medicine in World War II remains the valuable and rather neglected source, W. Paul Havens, ed., *Internal Medicine in World War II,* vol. 1 of the series edited by John B. Coates, Jr., under the general title *Activities of Medical Consultants* (Washington: Dept. of the Army, Government Printing Office, 1961). Several of the authors of individual chapters (e.g., William S. Middleton, Herman Blumgart) went on themselves to become important internist-educators and internist-investigators in the postwar period. And some of them, notably Hugh J. Morgan on the medical consultants division of the Surgeon General's office, were remarkably candid about the administrative and political difficulties encountered in developing and deploying specialist services during wartime.

38. Hugh J. Morgan, "Medical Consultants Division, Office of the Surgeon General," 1–70, in Havens, *Internal Medicine in World War II.* It should be noted that, when consultant positions were first assigned to the Army, through the Office of the Surgeon General, they were allocated not only in internal medicine but also in surgery and in neuropsychiatry. The consultants were ultimately responsible for directing the activities of that portion of the 1,300 or so medical officers of the regular Army in these three divisions, but (interestingly enough) not in the divisions of preventive medicine, veterinary medicine, dentistry, nursing, planning and training, hospitalization, or medical supply. See Henry M. Thomas, Jr., "Southwest Pacific Area," in Havens, *Internal Medicine in World War II,* 566.

39. Havens, *Internal Medicine in World War II,* 70.

40. This was the senior author's observation and is confirmed by virtually every civilian internist involved in the war effort. Eugene A. Stead of Emory and Duke Universities, for example, discusses the point explicitly in the transcript of the oral history memoir (interviewed by R. C. M.) 16 May 1985.

41. For a contrasting view of the chairman's role at the end of the twentieth century, specifically in relation to matters of scale—expansion versus contraction—see Robert G. Petersdorf, "Medical Schools and Research: Is the Tail Wagging the Dog?" *Daedalus* 115 (1986): 99–118.

42. James Wyngaarden, personal communication, 1985.

43. Linus Pauling, quoted in Horace Judson, *The Eighth Day of Creation*, (New York: Simon and Schuster, 1979), 301–2.

44. D. J. Weatherall, *The New Genetics and Clinical Practice* (London: Nuffield Provincial Hospitals Trust, 1982), and G. J. V. Nossal, *Reshaping Life: Key Issues in Genetic Engineering* (Cambridge: Cambridge University Press, 1985).

45. This process of diagnostic specificity leading to therapeutic specifics occurred at each key level: cognitive, understanding the pathophysiology of a process; professional, leading investigators from one pursuit to the other within individual careers; and institutional, developing major, funded therapeutic initiatives out of cognitive and professional resources. For an example of this approach in connection with early bacteriology and serology, see Timothy Lenoir on Paul Ehrlich and serotherapy in "Binding Science: the Science-Technology Continuum and the Growth of Knowledge in Late Nineteenth Century Germany," *Minerva* (in press).

46. The history of modern immunology, especially that of the past fifty years, remains a major lacuna in the historiography of twentieth-century scientific medicine.

47. See Edward Kass's paper on infectious diseases, Chapter 4 in this volume.

48. For a classic example cf. K. Codell Carter, "The Germ Theory, Beriberi, and the Deficiency Theory of Disease," *Med Hist* 21 (1977) : 119–36.

49. Hobart Reimann and W. Paul Havens, "Focal Infection and Systemic Disease: A Critical Appraisal," *JAMA* 114 (1940) : 1–6.

50. See especially the chapters by Joel Howell, Steven Peitzman, Edward Kass, and Thomas Benedek in this volume.

51. This notion is exemplified by endocrinology, in which acute presentations such as addisonian crisis and thyroid storm are now infrequent; or rheumatology (viz. Chapter 6 by Benedek below); or pulmonary diseases, on which we do not present a specific chapter, but in which the acute and subacute presentations of tuberculosis have given way in large part to the "bread and butter" management of obstructive lung disease. A counter-example is given in this volume by Joel Howell, who demonstrates the move cardiology took in the opposite direction, from chronic care of rheumatic fever to acute care of ischemic and valvular heart disease.

52. For an account of these developments see the second author's recent monograph: Russell C. Maulitz, *Morbid Appearances: the Anatomy of Pathology in the Early Nineteenth Century* (Cambridge and New York: Cambridge University Press, 1987).

53. On the Wasserman test as an example of how immunological diagnosis could change concepts of disease, see Ludwik Fleck, *The Genesis and Development of a Scientific Fact* (Chicago: University of Chicago Press, 1979).

54. For a study of the introduction of X ray apparatus based on examination of patient records in a local clinical setting, see Joel Howell, "Machines and Medicine: Technology Transforms the American Hospital," in *Hospitals/Communities: A Contemporary Institution in Historical Perspective*, Janet Golden and Diana Long, eds. (Ithaca, NY: Cornell University Press, in press).

55. John Peters and Donald Van Slyke, *Quantitative Clinical Chemistry*, 2 vols. (Baltimore: Williams & Wilkins, 1931–32).

56. A useful introduction to this literature is Warner, *The Therapeutic Perspective*.

57. See Charles Rosenberg's title essay in his and Morris Vogels's *The Therapeutic Revolution: Essays in the Social History of American Medicine* (Philadelphia: University of Pennsylvania, 1978), 47–48.

58. Jacob Bigelow, *Discourse of Self-Limited Disease* (Boston: Nathan Hale, 1835).

59. For an appraisal of some key events in the development of clinical trials as a means of effacing the anecdotal nature of therapeutic evidence, see Chapter 10 by Harry Marks in this volume.

60. A. L. Benedict, "The Progress of Therapeutics During the Past Twenty Years," *Int Clin* 2 (1910): 11–31, cf. especially 14–16.

61. Alvan Feinstein has summarized the historical development of the randomized clinical trial in *Clinical Epidemiology* (Philadelphia: Saunders, 1985), 683–90; see also Harry Marks' chapter in this volume (Chapter 10).

62. Paul Beeson, "Changes in Medical Therapy During the Past Half Century," *Medicine* 50 (1980): 79–99.

63. A fuller survey of this topic is provided by Bruce Fye in Chapter 3 of this volume.

64. L. H. Smith, Jr., "Presidential Address," *Trans Assoc Am Physicians* 89 (1976): 1–9.

65. We are grateful to Professor Horace Davenport, of the University of Michigan, for permission to examine these notes. A portion have been published as H. Davenport, ed., *Doctor Dock: Teaching and Learning Medicine at the Turn of the Century* (New Brunswick and London: Rutgers University Press, 1987).

66. On the shifts in emphasis and audience at the "Atlantic City meetings," as well as an informative perspective on the "end of an era" notion, see Gordon N. Gill, "The End of the Physician-Scientist?" in *American Scholar* (summer 1984): 353–68.

67. Himsworth, "The Integration of Medicine."

68. Paul Beeson, "The Natural History of Medical Subspecialties," *Ann Intern Med* 93 (1980): 624–26.

69. Eugene Braunwald, *Heart Disease: A Textbook of Cardiovascular Medicine* (Philadelphia: W. B. Saunders, 1980).

70. This tension forms the theme of several of the essays in the special issue of *Daedalus*, "America's Doctors, Medical Science, Medical Care" (spring 1986), in which the senior author touches on "The changing role model and the shift in power." For a percipient modern view by a pioneer of the general medicine movement, see John Eisenberg, "Sculpture of a New Academic Discipline: Four Faces of Academic General Internal Medicine," *Am J Med* 78 (1985): 283–92.

71. Walsh McDermott, "Education and General Medical Care," *Ann Intern Med* 96 (1982): 512–17.

72. R. H. Friedman and J. T. Pozen, "The Academic Viability of General Internal Medicine," *Ann Intern Med* 103 (1985): 439–44.

73. Robert Fletcher, "Faculty Training and Fellowships in Research in General Medicine," *J Gen Int Med* 1 (1986) (Suppl.): S50–S55. See also Eisenberg, "Sculpture of a New Academic Discipline," 283–92.

3

The Literature of Internal Medicine

W. BRUCE FYE

The advance of medical knowledge and the style of medical practice depend to a large degree on the literature of medicine. Discoveries must be made known to others if they are to have any significant effect on medical science or practice. Similarly, the attitudes of physicians on the social aspects of medical practice have been shaped by their reading of textbooks, articles, and editorials for generations. The central role of the medical literature in the emergence of modern medicine is often overlooked. In this chapter I will trace the development of the literature of medicine over the past century. Although European influences will be mentioned, the emphasis will be on the evolution of medical writing and publishing in America. I focus on the late nineteenth century because in that era the field of internal medicine (and many other medical specialties) originated, along with a literature specifically devoted to physicians concerned with nonsurgical diseases. The same forces that shaped the specialty of internal medicine contributed to the changing character of the American medical literature during the past century.

The literature of internal medicine, like the literature of any medical specialty, serves several purposes. The fundamental purpose of medical writing and publishing is the transmission of knowledge. The character of the medical literature in a given era depends on the goals of the authors and editors who produce it, the nature of its content, the technology of printing, and many other factors. Moreover, the literature of medicine, like all literature, is shaped by the social and intellectual climate in which it appears. This cultural context determines such things as the level of sophistication of the author and reader, the writing style, and such practical matters as the cost and form of the publication. The content of medical writing is dependent on the medical knowledge of the time as well as the accepted approaches to expanding and presenting this knowledge.

Although medical authors have undoubtedly always believed that their writings had intrinsic merit, before the nineteenth century the medical literature contained little more than speculation and case reports based on random observation. Until the pathophysiology and natural history of diseases were better understood, and objective laboratory techniques and statistics were introduced and refined, it was difficult to differentiate beneficial from useless or even harmful interventions. We now recognize this and expect medical researchers to devote considerable effort to the design of their studies and to the analysis of their results prior to publication. These expectations are not necessarily being met, however. It has been suggested recently that the quality of study design of clinical research papers published in three general medical journals over the past thirty years has not improved despite growing sophistication in the design of research and in biostatistics.[1]

Beginning around 1850, the French physiologist Claude Bernard and several German biomedical scientists redefined how new medical knowledge should be acquired and old theories tested. The Europeans forcefully declared that medicine was a science and that experimental techniques were necessary to expand one's understanding of the body in health and disease. They were correct: new knowledge regarding the structure and function of living organisms began to pour from European laboratories. At the same time, greater insight into the nature and clinical course of disease was resulting from the careful study of patients in European clinics and hospitals. Instruments of precision were used in the laboratory, and ultimately at the bedside, to supplement the techniques of physical diagnosis introduced or refined earlier in the century. Operative procedures became more daring and sophisticated as anesthesia and aseptic surgery were introduced and accepted. The discoveries of Louis Pasteur, Robert Koch, and other pioneering microbiologists were watched with anticipation by the medical world and educated lay population. Specific cures for infectious diseases were predicted, but in their absence sanitary reforms and public health measures were introduced to reduce the likelihood of disease transmission.[2]

Through the medical literature, nineteenth-century American physicians were apprised of these dramatic advances in medical science and practice. Moreover, they were told that these developments were due, in large part, to the unique structure and philosophy of the European, especially German, system of medical education. Indeed, thousands of American practitioners witnessed these changes firsthand during trips abroad for postgraduate training.[3] If America was to compete in the arena of medical science, reforms in medical education were required, and the research ethic that permeated the German medical faculties had to be adopted by American medical schools.[4] Specialization in medical practice was encouraged by a growing number of reformers who believed this would result in an acceleration of medical discovery and improve patient care. The model for specialization in medicine already existed in Europe, and in the context of a general trend toward specialization in many aspects of postbellum American society it is not surprising that a growing number of physicians encouraged and participated in this movement.[5]

During the closing decades of the nineteenth century, the movement to reform American medicine gathered momentum. The small band of reformers was composed of a coalition of basic medical scientists, educators, medical editors, and scientifically oriented medical practitioners. This last group, which included such well-known physicians as William Osler, Nicholas Senn, Abraham Jacobi, and Weir Mitchell, played a crucial role: they were largely responsible for gaining the support of America's medical practitioners for the reform movement. In rhetoric heard with increasing frequency and conviction during the closing years of the century, the reformers argued that Americans could make meaningful contributions to medical knowledge if American medical education were endowed with salaries for full-time faculty members committed to research.[6] By the turn of the century, the reformers attracted the attention of philanthropists and soon found their cause championed by the American Medical Association and the Carnegie and Rockefeller foundations. The predictions of the reformers proved accurate. America became the leading producer of biomedical knowledge during the twentieth century as the full-time faculty system and the research ethic were adopted by medical schools throughout the country.[7]

This revolution in the structure and philosophy of medical education had a significant effect on the nature of the medical literature. Several trends that began a century ago continue to affect medicine and its literature. The reform of American medical education led to a better educated medical profession. Higher standards of preliminary education resulted in more sophistication in science and improved foreign language skills among medical matriculants. The appearance and dramatic expansion of the full-time faculty system resulted in a large body of medical scientists imbued with the research ethic and eager to publish the results of their investigations.

There has been a steady trend toward specialization in response to intellectual and economic forces in American society. A century ago it was claimed that "specialism, in the mind of the medical student, is always associated with pecuniary success."[8] Although the economics of specialization continue to encourage specialty practice, and the growing complexity of medical research mandates a narrow focus, there are many other factors that lead a high percentage of medical graduates to specialize. Moreover, medical specialization has given way to subspecialization. In internal medicine, this trend began a half century ago, but gained momentum in the 1960s.[9] It originated, as Paul Beeson has outlined, in academic departments of internal medicine.[10] With the appearance of subspecialty disciplines following World War II, the demand for subspecialty societies and journals grew as well.

Recently, in response to concerns that specialization and technology have gotten out of hand, there has been a resurgence of interest in the concept of the family physician. When A. McGehee Harvey and his colleagues at Johns Hopkins revived Osler's *Principles and Practice of Medicine* their goal was to "produce a book which is built around the patient rather than the disease."[11] Such concerns are not new; James B. Herrick observed half a century ago, "medicine shows more concern than formerly to regard the patient as a human being; medicine is rubbing elbows with sociology . . . physicians and the public are considering, more seriously than ever, questions as to the social and economic relations of the doctor, the patient and the state."[12]

Medical Authors

To assess the literature of internal medicine, it is useful to consider the goals of medical writing and publishing. Although the fundamental purpose of the medical literature is the dissemination of information, each author, editor, publisher, librarian, and reader has his own set of expectations and needs. The changing concerns and goals of each of these groups have helped to shape the character of the literature of medicine over the past century. Just as an author needs an outlet for his literary creation, an editor needs manuscripts to review and revise, and a publisher needs material to print and distribute. The balance of power between the partners in the world of medical publishing has shifted over the past 150 years. When it was founded in 1828 the *American Journal of the Medical Sciences* paid its authors for their contributions. The journal's editor Isaac Hays explained, "in respectfully inviting contributions . . . the publishers . . . repeat the assurance, that all articles that may be inserted, will be liberally paid for."[13] Daniel Drake, the energetic medical teacher, author, and editor offered authors a fee of $1.00 per page for publications that appeared in his *Western Journal of the Medical and Physical Sciences.*

Some leaders of nineteenth-century medicine believed that even greater financial incentives were needed to induce America's physicians to contribute to the medical literature. The eminent surgeon and prolific author Samuel D. Gross declared in 1876,

> the compensation of medical authors is seldom flattering. . . . First editions, even of works of great value, rarely afford any compensation to their authors. . . . The contributors to our medical journals, even the ablest of them, are seldom adequately paid, a dollar a page, doled out in greenbacks, being the ordinary compensation. This is simply disreputable, and is, perhaps, one reason why so much of the periodical medical literature of the country is so indifferent. Self-respect should induce our better class of writers to demand higher rates of compensation, both for their own sake and for that of our literature.[14]

John Shaw Billings expanded on this theme a quarter of a century later in a letter to G. Stanley Hall, who had solicited a manuscript from the Army surgeon. Billings stated:

> Such a paper as you want, if carefully prepared is worth from two to five hundred dollars. We are trying to induce the best of our young men to invest the time and money requisite to make themselves expert original investigators and workers—with the idea that they can support themselves and their families by means of the information which they can give. On the other hand energetic philanthropists and journalists—Hospital and School Trustees—are trying to pump out this information for nothing,—they feel liberal—and think others should be also. I do not approve of skilled lawyers and physicians giving away advice gratis merely because they themselves can afford to do so—because they are taking the bread out of the mouths of younger men by so doing. . . . It seems to me that leaders of thought in your position should try to establish the custom that brain work should be paid for, and should not compete gratuitously with those whose sole means of support and hope of doing future work lies in their obtaining remunerative employment.[15]

Things have changed! Not only do the more prestigious medical journals no longer pay for manuscripts, they charge for them. Citing the economics of medical publishing, some medical journals now require authors to pay a manuscript submission fee, a page charge, or both. This turn of events is due, in large part, to the development of modern academic medicine. Aspiring academic physicans need outlets for their publications and are willing to pay a premium to have their work appear in prestigious journals. As Samuel Shapiro has recently observed, "the investigator is under considerable pressure to publish. Advancement of a career may depend to a large degree on a continually thickening pile of reprints. The publication of even a 'marginal' finding may be tempting since it can be used, with the aid of some political skill, to enhance status and to acquire a grant."[16] Some journals have fared well in their quest for high quality manuscripts; others have not. Once one of America's most highly regarded medical journals, the *Bulletin of the Johns Hopkins Hospital,* recently ceased publication. Explaining his decision to end the *Johns Hopkins Medical Journal* in 1982, Richard Ross observed that, in recent decades, most faculty members had decided to "publish their best material in specialty journals which have a high degree of visibility."[17]

Visibility and prestige, as noted by Ross, have come to influence authors far more than monetary considerations in most cases. The incentives for publishing changed as America's system of medical education evolved from a part-time to a full-time occupation. When the American Medical Association was founded in 1847, there were thirty-three regular medical schools, but fewer than 200 faculty members to instruct the nation's 4,000 medical students.[18] Virtually all of the professors were practitioners who devoted a few hours a week to their lectures. There was only one professor for each major branch of instruction, so academic advancement was nonexistent. Moreover, medical school appointments were usually awarded on the basis of social and political factors, rather than the candidate's proved or potential ability in research or scientific writing.[19] Still, the medical teachers of a century ago were responsible for a significant share of the medical literature. After reviewing the literary output of American physicians in 1876, the respected Louisville physician and medical educator Lunsford Yandell observed: "teachers have both greater leisure and greater facilities than others of the profession for making books, as they are also more likely to find sale for them; and they write text-books rather than monographs, because students demand them."[20]

The small part-time medical faculty of the nineteenth century has evolved into a huge body of full-time medical teachers and researchers. Currently, there are almost 60,000 full-time faculty members in America's medical schools, a number nearly equal to the number of students. Internal medicine and its subspecialties account for one-fifth of the full-time faculty members at the present time.[21] As was true a century ago when Yandell made his observations on the medical literature, medical school faculty members still produce a major proportion of the medical books and journal articles. The incentives for publishing have increased, which has resulted in several notable trends in the medical literature. Today, medical faculty members whose careers depend on publication are not likely to discard a manuscript once it has been completed, despite one or more rejections by editors. The manuscript will probably be submitted to another journal, lower in prestige perhaps, but more in need of material. Julius Comroe, an astute observer of medical science, recently claimed,

> I believe that almost every [medical] scientist working today can get his work published, somewhere, once he decides to 'write it up'; maybe it will be in the Bulletin of the Podunk County Medical Society rather than in the journal with international prestige or readership, or maybe it will be published only as an abstract. The main determinant of what is or is not published therefore seems to be the scientist, for it is he who decides to become or not to become an author.[22]

Concern about the quality of medical publications is not new. In a centennial review of American medical literature, Billings observed, "many articles intended to be practical, are very far from being such, although the authors would probably be surprised and indignant to hear them termed otherwise. . . . Their productions read curiously, and are to be classed with old women's advice, amusing generally; practically suggestive sometimes; clear, scientific, and conclusive, never."[23] In another assessment of America's medical literature at the time of the centennial, Samuel Gross explained that most physician-authors had little leisure time to devote to writing. After listing the few Americans who devoted themselves primarily to teaching and writing, among them Charles Caldwell, Robley Dunglison, John Draper, and George Wood, Gross went on to claim, "it is very different, with a man actively engaged in practice, and dependent for his livelihood upon the number of daily visits he makes. Such a man, if he aspires to elaborate authorship, must work early and late, long, indeed, before ordinary mortals rise in the morning, and long after they have retired at night, or he will accomplish very little."[24]

If one compares the literature of medicine published a century ago with that of today, one of the most striking changes is what Victor Strasburger has termed "author inflation."[25] Single-author papers were the standard a century ago when most medical writers were active practitioners. Solo office-based practice was the norm, and collaboration with colleagues was unusual. But medical research became more complex, requiring increasingly sophisticated apparatus and the participation of trained assistants. Experiment replaced observation and collaboration became more common. As Durack notes in an entertaining article on "The Weight of Medical Knowledge," more than 98 percent of the articles published in the *Boston Medical and Surgical Journal* a century ago were written by a single author. Today, by contrast, fewer than 5 percent of the papers in the journal's successor, the *New England Journal of Medicine*, were written by one individual. By 1980 the average number of authors per article in this journal was nearly five.[26]

The German Model

There was a model for the development of a more sophisticated American medical literature a century ago. George Shrady, the indefatigable medical reformer and editor of the *Medical Record*, accurately depicted the German literature of a century ago and anticipated the content and character of current American medical journals when he claimed:

> The German-speaking race is abundantly supplied with medical journals of every conceivable kind, and they reflect very well the character of the German medical mind. The number of special medical journals is particularly great. . . . They are filled with heavy original articles, most of which are so laboriously scientific and minutely technical that they would appear to the American mind extremely dull. Interspersed with these, however, there are not rarely the rich original contributions to medical science which makes [*sic*] Germany so famous. A characteristic of German periodical literature is that it is almost all written by the Professors or their assistants, or by some of the various instructors at the universities. One hears almost nothing from the general practitioner who is so prominent a person in American medical journalism.[27]

Shrady's unintended prophecy reflects how much the German philosophy and structure of medical education influenced American reformers at the turn of the century. They, in turn, shaped our present system of educating physicians and expanding medical knowledge.

Medical Journals

The medical journal is the subject of much of this essay due to its central role in the literature of medicine. During the nineteenth century, the medical periodical evolved as the primary means of conveying medical information. The primacy of the medical journal has been acknowledged for more than a century. John Shaw Billings declared in 1876, "It is not in text-books or systematic treatises on special subjects that the greater part of the original contributions to the literature of medicine have been made public during the last century. Since the year 1800 medical journalism has become the principal means of recording and communicating the observations and ideas of those engaged in the practice of medicine, and has exercised a strong influence for the advancement of medical science and education."[28]

America's first medical journal, the *Medical Repository,* appeared in 1797. Patterned after the Edinburgh *Annals of Medicine,* it was edited by two prominent New York practitioners, Samuel L. Mitchell and Edward Miller. The venture was successful; demand was such that the earlier volumes of the journal were reprinted. Additional medical journals were soon founded in Philadelphia, Baltimore, and Boston. These early American medical journals contained some case reports by American physicians and surgeons, but were composed mainly of reprints of British contributions. Nathaniel Chapman, editor of the *Philadelphia Journal of the Medical and Physical Sciences,* reproduced a quotation from British preacher and essayist Sydney Smith on the title page of this new journal when it appeared in 1820. Whether Chapman cared to believe it or not, Smith was exaggerating only slightly when he claimed, "in the four corners of the globe, who reads an American book? or goes to an American play? or looks at an American picture or statue? What does the world yet owe to American Physicians or Surgeons?" Indeed, Anglo-American hostility continued to varying degrees in the medical literature throughout the nineteenth century.[29]

A century ago, Harvard's poet-anatomist Oliver Wendell Holmes described the ascent of the medical journal:

> Now there has come a great change in our time over the form in which living thought presents itself. The first printed books—the incunabula—were enclosed in boards of solid oak, with brazen clasps and corners; the boards by and by were replaced by pasteboard covers with calf and sheepskin; then cloth came in and took the place of leather; then the pasteboard was covered with paper instead of cloth; and at this day the quarterly, the monthly, and the daily journal, naked as it came from the womb of the press, hold the larger part of the fresh reading we live upon. We must have the latest thought in its latest expression; the page must be newly turned like the morning bannock; the pamphlet must be newly opened like the ante-prandial oyster. Thus a library, to meet the need of our time, must take, and must spread out in a convenient form,

a great array of periodicals. Our active practitioners read these by preference over almost everything else. Our specialists, more particularly, depend on the month's product, on the yearly crop of new facts, new suggestions, new contrivances, as much as the farmer on the annual yield of his acres.[30]

Why did journals become so popular in mid-nineteenth-century America? Daniel Drake attributed the proliferation of medical journals to the unique cultural climate of America. While it is true that antebellum Americans sought to educate the masses and established institutions and publishing houses to achieve these goals, the medical journal also grew in prominence in Europe and Great Britain in the context of very different social conditions. Local medical journals were especially prevalent in America. The regionalism of Americans contributed to this, but Daniel Drake also attributed the growth of the periodical literature of medicine to the opening of dozens of new medical schools.[31] Billings agreed, although he cautioned, "our medical journals vary so much in character, style, and purpose, that it is hardly possible to make any assertion with regard to the mass which shall be at the same time broad and true."[32] Billings distinguished three categories of medical journals: those without any institutional affiliation, whose contributions were drawn from many sources and regions; those whose contributors were mainly affiliated with a medical school or hospital, but which were "not specifically devoted to its interests"; and finally, "those which are mainly devoted to advocating the interests of a school, and the attacking [of] rival institutions."[33] By the end of the nineteenth century there were scores of general medical journals published in America. Most cities with medical schools—and there were nearly 150 regular medical schools a century ago—had local or regional medical journals.[34]

One of the perceived merits of the medical journal is its ability to get information to the reader in a timely fashion. Technological advances in transportation and printing made possible the rapid publication and dissemination of medical knowledge a century ago. Today, newer electronic forms of information transfer such as television and computers are encroaching on the traditional position of medical journals as the primary means of rapid dissemination of new knowledge.[35] This has led to concern among medical editors and has resulted in some controversial rules regarding journal publishing. The *New England Journal of Medicine* has established a strict policy precluding the release of material to the lay press prior to its formal publication in the journal. Arnold Relman, the journal's editor, explained that this "news embargo" was introduced to serve "the best interests of the public and the medical profession," but he admitted that another purpose was "to protect the newsworthiness of the *Journal*."[36]

Concern about the currency of medical information is not new. The prominent Boston physician and pioneer of public health Henry Ingersoll Bowditch declared in 1867, "modern science does not let any book remain long useful."[37] Bowditch's Harvard colleague Oliver Wendell Holmes touched on this theme in an 1881 assessment of the medical literature:

> I have spoken of the importance and predominance of periodical literature . . . but the almost exclusive reading of it is not without its dangers. The journals contain much that is crude and unsound . . . yet I have known a practitioner—perhaps more than one—who was as much under the dominant influence of the last article he had read in his favorite medical journal as a milliner under the sway of the last fashion-plate. The difference between green and seasoned knowledge is very great, and such practitioners never hold long enough to any of their knowledge to have it get seasoned.[38]

It is impossible to satisfy all the individuals involved in the creation, publication, and consumption of medical papers. Premature publication of the results of medical research may result in censure, particularly if there is the potential for unjustified optimism among the public that practical benefits to human beings might result from the discovery. A recent example of this was the news conference held by French researchers in which they presented the results of preliminary studies on the therapy of the acquired immune deficiency syndrome (AIDS) with immunosuppressive therapy.[39] The primary concern in this case was the lack of peer review prior to the announcement of the researchers' results. Peer review necessitates a time lag between manuscript submission and ultimate publication, and this lag has been criticized by some observers of the medical literature. The reviewing process has become more difficult, however, as specialization proceeds and research methodologies become increasingly complex.[40]

The format of medical journals has changed surprisingly little over the past century. Indeed, in 1977 Franz Ingelfinger acknowledged that the "basic character" of the *New England Journal of Medicine* had been maintained for half a century, and that this "reflected the high value that the *Journal*'s editors have placed on maintaining traditions that have gradually developed since the first issue . . . appeared in 1812."[41] Most nineteenth-century medical journals contained case reports, review articles, original articles, transcriptions of lectures, medical society transactions, correspondence, editorials, and book reviews.

Case reports were the predominant form of American medical publication until recently. Their value has long been the subject of debate. Writing a century ago, Billings revealed his ambivalence toward them. The great bibliographer claimed that carefully prepared case reports "are most useful and valuable, and are the best contributions to a journal which the majority of physicians can make, although [they are] by no means the highest class of medical literature."[42] Nevertheless, in the same article he protested, "we have reached that stage of development, when it is in no way desirable that we should be informed that one dislocated shoulder was reduced, one leg amputated, and two hare-lips operated upon, not even if the usual text-book explanations are added, so as to make up the five or six pages of the report of a college clinic."[43] Although case reports are the mainstay of some current medical journals, many prestigious journals discourage them, and some routinely reject them.

Review articles continue to appear regularly in the medical literature. In contrast to the situation in the nineteenth century, current review articles reflect the important contributions Americans have made to medical knowledge. During most of the nineteenth century, American publications drew heavily on the British and European literature. Oliver Wendell Holmes claimed in 1848, "the great forte of American Medical scholarship has hitherto consisted in 'editing' the works of British authors. . . . Sometimes the additions by the 'American Editor' have been real and important, oftener nominal and insignificant."[44] Although some Americans were reluctant to admit it, an editor of the *Boston Medical and Surgical Journal* accurately portrayed the situation in the middle of the last century: "The fact is, that it is only until very recently that scarcely any medical works of real merit or originality, have been produced by American authors; and if physicians kept pace at all with medical science, they were obliged to consult foreign works."[45]

Original articles in medical journals are based on clinical or scientific investigations that have yielded results considered worthy of publication. It is in the area of original investigation that the American medical literature has changed most dramatically in recent years. Medical educator Victor Vaughan complained a century ago, "little attention is given in this country to original investigation." He believed that medical editors contributed to the problem by refusing to publish this type of contribution: "Editors claim that such articles 'will not take' with readers. They want something for the 'busy practitioner.' Is not this 'busy practitioner' a much abused person? Does he not at times, at least, have a faint desire for some true advance in knowledge?"[46] Vaughan argued that the practice of refusing to publish papers based on scientific research discouraged American physicians from pursuing original investigation. Another major factor that retarded research in nineteenth-century America was the lack of financial support for this activity. There were virtually no full-time medical teachers in America and there was little incentive for medical research. Physicians subsidized their research from their practice income, but this was far from optimal. Although idealists argued that physicians should "labor less for money and more for science," a stable source of funding for research was necessary before Americans made sustained and significant contributions to medical knowledge.[47]

Medical lectures by prominent practitioner-teachers were often published in local or regional medical journals a century ago. They appeared in a serialized fashion and were occasionally reprinted in a single volume following their journal appearance. This practice has virtually disappeared, although some current introductory textbooks are reworked lectures that have been published. Similarly, medical society transactions were often published in nineteenth-century American medical journals. These were usually composed of case reports but occasionally included important papers based on original scientific or clinical research. Indeed, local and regional medical societies were once a major forum for the presentation of new medical knowledge. For example, leading physicians frequently presented important scientific papers before the New York Academy of Medicine, the College of Physicians of Philadelphia, and the Medical and Chirurgical Society of Maryland. The same was true of lesser known state and local societies.

The development of specialization, improvements in transportation, and the dramatic growth of academic medicine led to a shift in focus of most local societies, however. They are now mainly concerned with social and political issues as they relate to medical practice. Scientific presentations are less prominent because there is less prestige associated with the presentation of papers before a regional medical society than before a national specialty organization. The same generalization applies to publication; most contemporary authors prefer to have their work appear in a national rather than a local journal. If the author is a practitioner rather than a full-time academic physician, however, he might choose a state medical journal hoping to encourage referrals through enhancement of his image locally.

As subspecialization became more formalized through board certification, and as specialty meetings drew internists who subspecialized away from the traditional parent discipline of internal medicine, new journals appeared, creating more perceptible interspecialty boundaries. In cardiology, progressive sub-subspecialization has proceeded actively, giving rise to individuals identified as electrocardiographers, echocardiographers, electrophysiologists, and interventional angiographers. The epidemiology of cardiac disease permits this degree of subspecialization; it is economically as well as intellectually feasible.

Just as new specialties continue to develop, some old ones disappear. Effective chemotherapy of mycobacteria led to a dramatic decline in the incidence of tuberculosis, and it is no longer possible for a physician to specialize in the diagnosis and treatment of this infectious disease. The literature of medicine reflects these changes. There are journals devoted to electrocardiography, echocardiography, and cardiac catheterization as well as to general cardiology. The decline of tuberculosis is reflected in the rapid sequential changes in title of one medical journal over a seven-year period. From its inception in 1917 until the early 1950s, the *American Review of Tuberculosis* had a stable title. With the advent of chemotherapy for tuberculosis, however, the name changed three times in seven years. The sequence of titles reveals the efforts of the editorial board and the American Trudeau Society to redraw their territory as tuberculosis rapidly declined in importance (*Table 3.1*). The sponsoring society also changed its name from the American Trudeau Society: Medical Section of the National Tuberculosis Association to the American Thoracic Society: Medical Section of the American Lung Association, to avoid being left without a disease. The other journal of pulmonary disease, *Diseases of the Chest*, changed its name to *Chest* in 1970 because the "journal has become a forum for clinical investigations in areas far removed from those envisioned at the time *Diseases of the Chest* became the official journal of the American College of Chest Physicians. The era of empirical treatment of mycobacterial infections has been superseded by an era of emphasis on pathogenesis and management of disease entities such as emphysema, bronchitis, and atherosclerotic involvement of the myocardium and the peripheral vessels."[48]

Many medical subspecialties sponsor journals devoted to the scientific and clinical aspects of the specific subspecialty. Often, the societies use their sanctioned journals as official organs to transmit policy to their readers. Occasionally, overt changes in society-journal affiliations occur that underscore this special relationship. When the American Heart Association inaugurated *Circulation* in 1950, the *American Heart Journal* lost its position as the official organ of this large organization. The new journal was created, in part, to acknowledge the growing volume of, and interest in, basic research on the circulatory system. Ultimately, another journal, *Circulation Research*, was founded for the publication of even more basic research papers. The *Ameri-*

TABLE 3.1.
SEQUENCE OF TITLE CHANGES FOR
THE AMERICAN REVIEW OF TUBERCULOSIS

Year	Title
1952	*The American Review of Tuberculosis*
1954	*The American Review of Tuberculosis: A Journal of Pulmonary Diseases*
1955	*The American Review of Tuberculosis and Pulmonary Diseases*
1959	*The American Review of Respiratory Diseases*

can Journal of Medicine was founded in 1946, in the words of its editor Alexander Gutman, "to add to the available media for publication of the results of sound clinical investigation."[49] More recently, the American College of Cardiology ended its formal affiliation with the *American Journal of Cardiology* and inaugurated a new journal, the *Journal of the American College of Cardiology*. In the words of the editor, "for the first time, the College owns its own journal and controls its editorial and business policies."[50]

Letters to the editor have been a feature of many American medical journals since the early nineteenth century. The content of these letters has remained surprisingly constant for generations. Many nineteenth-century medical journals contained letters to the editor that shared many similarities with recent letters. In some journals letters undergo the same review process as submitted articles. It has been found that letters published in specialty journals serve as a peer review mechanism, since they often relate to material already published in the journal.[51]

Medical Editors

Editorials have consistently been a prominent part of medical journalism. Editors have long sought to shape their readers' opinions. Their editorials provide valuable insight into the social and political concerns of the profession as well as helping to place clinical or scientific papers in perspective. Editors of medical journals have had substantial influence on the development of American medicine over the past century. Commenting on the situation in this country during the nineteenth century, historian James Cassedy claimed, "whatever their motivations and longevity, the physician-editors collectively occupied one of the best possible positions for influencing and bringing about professional change in the American medical community."[52] In Billings' opinion, "the motive for the existence of the minor journals is not for direct profit, but as an indirect advertisement for certain individuals, or—and this is more common—the desire to have a place in which the editor can speak his mind and attack his adversaries without restraint."[53]

Today's medical editors retain their ability to influence attitudes and behavior, although they are less independent than their predecessors. George Shrady asserted in 1870, "the general want of success of Medical Journalism in this country is . . . a fact." He attributed the demise of many American medical journals to their failure to achieve independence. Instead, they sacrificed "their self-respect to cliquism, base puffery, to petty intrigues, and to the dictation of different medical schools." Another cause for the attrition of many medical journals according to Shrady was their failure to attract "the requisite quantity and quality of contributions."[54] Editors continue to play a critical role in eliciting contributions for their journal. William Bean has written, "any editor realizes that a journal will never be any better than the papers that the editor and the advisory board receive and process; it can be a lot worse. But to get good material it is necessary to get good writers, good physicians, and good investigators to submit papers."[55]

Debates over editorial control, a controversial issue for decades, have intensified. Editors have come under fire for restricting the flow of information (the "Ingelfinger rule" issue), being insensitive to authors in their boiler plate rejection letters, lacking consistency in what they accept and what they reject, and favoring manuscripts submitted by better known investigators or from more prestigious institutions.[56] Editors must have thick skins, because they are regularly faulted for their decisions and policies. This has probably always been true. In 1876 Yandell claimed, "editors in too many cases devote only such odds and ends of their time to their publications as they can spare from more profitable engagements. Deriving hardly any pecuniary emolument from their journals, they are compelled to look to other employment for subsistence. Nearly all their time and thoughts are engrossed by other duties, and their editorial functions are necessarily performed in a hurried and slovenly manner."[57] Most editors of medical journals continue to have a wide variety of obligations and do not devote their entire time to their journal responsibilities. Professional staffs now assist with many aspects of production, however. Moreover, as medicine has become more subspecialized, and publications often reflect narrow fields and sophisticated scientific approaches, editors have come to rely on editorial boards and referees to screen manuscripts.

Book reviews are included in most medical journals. Many physicians and librarians depend on reviews to help them select titles for addition to their personal or institutional collections. Commenting on the value of book reviews, medical librarian Patricia Morton observed, "the great number of medical books published, their similar titles, their inconsistent quality, their higher prices, the greater reliance by physicians on libraries to supply books, and tight library budgets, all combine to make book selection a more arduous process than ever for medical librarians."[58]

The most prominent journals of internal medicine have been in existence for a long time: the *New England Journal of Medicine*, the *Lancet*, and the *American Journal of the Medical Sciences* have been published for more than 150 years; the *Annals of Internal Medicine*, the *Archives of Internal Medicine* and *Medicine* for more than half a century; and the *American Journal of Medicine* for forty years.[59] Over time, however, the market share of these journals fluctuates. Journals do not survive if they cannot attract and maintain a sufficient number of subscribers. Once widely read, the *Medical News* and the *Medical Record* no longer exist, and the venerable *American Journal of the Medical Sciences* has lost the status it once had as America's premier medical periodical. Few of the medical journals published in the nineteenth century survived the lifetime of their founding editors. Dozens of new titles appeared annually, and nearly as many ceased publication. According to Billings, the number of subscribers for the majority of America's medical journals was less than 1,000 a century ago.[60] Edwin Gaillard bragged that the 7 January 1882 issue of his *American Medical Weekly* was sent to 60,000 physicians. This entrepreneurial physician-editor claimed this was the "largest issue that has ever been made of any medical publication in this country or in Europe."[61] This blanket mailing was to inaugurate the new weekly format of his publication which could be purchased for $2.00 per year in the form of cash, money order, or postage stamps. It would be sent free to subscribers who purchased their medical texts through the journal rather than directly from the publisher. Special offers still may be found; Yorke Medical Publishers have actively promoted the *American Journal of Medicine* in recent years by methods that have included unsolicited free issues and discount subscriptions.

Editors and publishers cannot usually depend on the income from subscriptions alone to subsidize the cost of production of medical journals. Although advertising has always been an important source of revenue for medical journals, editors have routinely claimed independence from their advertisers. Gaillard, editor and publisher of the *American Medical Weekly*, explained in 1882, "as is well known, the editor of this journal never inserts editorial notices as part of an advertising contract, never has done so, and never will, but it is a pleasure to call attention to the advertisements in this number. They represent the oldest and best Houses in this country, and they will be read with profit by all who need what is thus advertised. Every one of these Houses, without exception, is declared to be entitled to entire confidence and respect."[62]

It is interesting to review the ads in medical journals because they demonstrate how ephemeral specific medicines and treatment approaches have been. This is apparent even in medical journals from the 1960s, but is quite dramatic if the ads of a century ago are considered. The 10 February 1881 of the *Boston Medical and Surgical Journal* contained advertisements for several medicinal agents, including Lactopeptine, Quinine, Vaseline, mineral water, maltine, hypophosphites, saccharated pepsin, fluid beef extract, and wine of iron with beef extract. Physicians were assured that one company's vaccine virus was obtained from healthy country children who were not syphilitic. In addition, there were advertisements for mustard paper, pessaries, nipples, soluble medicated urethral bougies, prostatic bougies, intrauterine pencils, clinical thermometers, and various forms of electrotherapy apparatus.

Although the cost of medical journals can be subsidized to varying degrees by advertisements, this is not generally the case with books. The cost of medical books has been a source of concern for generations. A British practitioner complained in 1803, "the enormous price of books is an evil calling loudly for redress. . . . My little library might have been twice its magnitude, if half of its prime value had not been sunk in the quality of type and paper. . . . To remedy these evils, I humbly beg leave to recommend that all writers on subjects connected with medicine and surgery should publish on coarse paper with a plain type."[63] Concern regarding the economic aspects of medical publishing persists. Some journals are assured of a substantial circulation by virtue of their selection as the official organ of a society. Members of the society receive the publication as part of their dues. Physicians have not been alone in their concern about the cost of the medical literature. Librarians have had to confront the economics of medical book publishing in the context of budgetary restrictions, continued rapid growth in the number of titles published, and the appearance of a controversial dual pricing policy for institutional subscribers to journals.[64]

Readers

So much for the writers and medical editors. What about the readers, who are presumably the fundamental reason for the existence of a medical literature? Medical students are infused with a sense of duty with regard to the medical literature: to subscribe is mandatory, to read desirable, to absorb and recite on demand ideal. In 1850 Henry Grant encouraged new Yale medical graduates to read journals: "I am well aware that you can not wade through all the trash that is written in these book-making days—neither would I wish it; but in addition to one or more standard authors on each subject, I would advise a liberal subscription to some of the leading medical reviews of the day."[65] Two decades later Shrady claimed, "probably not one physician in ten really imagines that he has any use for a medical journal, at least we can safely assert that not more than that proportion are supporters of our periodical literature."[66] Elsewhere, he wrote, "the physicians of America are not, as a whole, a reading and studious class. . . . The great majority of practitioners are non-subscribers to any journal, and manifest an appalling indifference to the benefits which would otherwise accrue to them."[67] It has often been claimed that physicians do not read enough. Perhaps motivated in part by postbellum regionalism, a Philadelphia writer exclaimed a century ago, "Whether they are too busy, or too illiterate . . . it seems a fact . . . that scarcely one-half of the 26,000 physicians practicing in the Western and Southwestern states take a medical journal of any kind."[68]

Today, it seems likely that physicians read only a small fraction of the literature they purchase. The so-called throw-aways fare less well, often being discarded without even a glance at the table of contents. Pressed by time constraints and growing specialization, few contemporary physicians read broadly; most read on subjects of special interest or relevance to them in their practice or research. Writing in 1881, Billings declared, "there is a vast amount of . . . effete and worthless material in the literature of medicine, and it is increasing rapidly."[69] Forty-five years ago Wilburt Davison of Duke wrote, "no physician can read all of the current literature in his specialty and retain his reason."[70] Concern about how to cope with the enormous amount of medical publishing persists, yet few solutions have been put forth. Computers and related technological developments promise to revolutionize how medical knowledge is transmitted, stored, and recalled, but the challenge to the individual absorbing and retaining this knowledge remains.

The educational attainments of physicians have changed dramatically over the past century. The standards of admission and competition for medical school acceptance in recent decades are in stark contrast to the situation in this country a century ago.[71] Until the opening of the Johns Hopkins School of Medicine in 1893, no American medical school required a collegiate degree for matriculation. There were many poorly educated physicians, some of whom were nearly illiterate if contemporary accounts are to be believed.

Nevertheless, the elite physicians of a century ago were often highly cultured. Many of the leaders of American medicine at the turn of the century spent one or more years of postgraduate study abroad. They subscribed to German medical journals and were familiar with the older literature of medicine. They were the elite of the profession, however, and most physicians were relatively unsophisticated readers who had little insight into, or appreciation of, the increasingly technical and specialized medical publications appearing from the European presses.

A century ago, American physicians demanded a literature that was practical, while their European counterparts were writing and reading scientific articles and books. In 1853 one concerned editor bemoaned the lack of interest among American physicians in what he called "heavy" medical journals, "in which articles of fifty pages or more in length could have insertion . . . but however ably conducted, such a work would certainly languish and die in a single year. . . . Journals of medicine must conform to the spirit of the age, or languish. Articles in them are required to be comprehensive, without being tedious."[72] The loss of language skills and the growing acceptance of English as the primary language of medicine and science has led to a dramatic reduction in the dependence of American physicians on contributions published in foreign languages.

Medical Textbooks

Although journals have been the most important vehicle for the publication of medical information for more than a century, they have not been the only form in which physicians and biomedical scientists have reported their observations. Students of medicine continue to rely almost exclusively on textbooks, for example, as they attempt to learn the language and facts of medical science and practice. This has been true for more than a century, and the purpose and character of this type of publication has changed little during this period. The author of a textbook seeks to synthesize accepted medical knowledge and present this information in an orderly, concise and straightforward fashion. Writing in 1876, Billings characterized textbooks as "for the most part compilations, but their importance is by no means to be underestimated, for the practice of the majority of physicians of this country to-day is based on [them]."[73]

A few American physicians wrote textbooks of medicine during the first half of the nineteenth century, but they drew heavily on British works. Although the medical textbooks written by Americans James Thacher (1817) and John Eberle (1838) were popular in their time, they contained little original material. Revealing his cultural nationalism, Samuel D. Gross reported in 1856 that the Jefferson faculty recently agreed to stop recommending European textbooks to their students. The Philadelphia surgeon observed, "we have seen that there is no need of borrowing from Great Britain as text-books for our medical schools; we have shown that many of our writers are men of great talent and erudition, yielding a ready and prolific pen."[74] Despite this declaration, European and English textbooks continued to be widely used in America during the second half of the nineteenth century.

Some hopeful signs were appearing, however. Austin Flint, a peripatetic medical teacher and prominent practitioner, published his popular *Treatise on the Principles and Practice of Medicine* in 1866. Flint came under the influence of the French school of medicine through his teachers at Harvard Medical School. As a practitioner he kept careful records of the cases he saw and read extensively. His textbook reflected his familiarity with the contemporary medical literature and his extensive clinical experience. It was the content as much as the arrangement of Flint's textbook, however, that made it a noteworthy contribution to the American medical literature. Flint synthesized accepted knowledge and recent observations and presented his conclusions in a lucid style that appealed to contemporary American practitioners and students of medicine. Gross considered Flint's textbook "by far the most original treatise on the principles and practice of medicine ever published in this country, an opinion in which I am supported by the entire profession."[75]

Flint's textbook remained popular and went through six editions before he died in 1886. As knowledge was rapidly expanding in the closing years of the nineteenth century, and more medical schools opened, the demand for medical textbooks grew steadily. Nathan Smith Davis of Chicago and Alfred L. Loomis of New York published comprehensive textbooks of medicine in 1884. Like Flint, these authors confined their subjects to what would soon come to be termed internal medicine. The specialties of obstetrics, surgery, ophthalmology, and otolaryngology, among others, were already established and had their own book and journal literature. The medical textbooks of the era contained sections devoted to diseases of the respiratory tract, digestive system, cardiovascular system, kidneys, nervous system, and contagious diseases, the main cause of morbidity and mortality a century ago. Although contemporary understanding of the pathophysiology of most diseases was imperfect, and diagnostic tests were limited to the microscopic examination of body fluids, the authors often included substantial sections on the etiology and differential diagnosis of the conditions they discussed. There were few efficacious remedies, and conservative approaches to therapy had replaced the heroic approaches of the physicians of the earlier generation, but medical authors were quite willing to elaborate complex regimens to deal with the ailments they discussed.

The most influential medical textbook published in America in the nineteenth century was the work of the Canadian-born physician William Osler. His *Principles and Practice of Medicine* appeared in 1892 and was immediately acknowledged as the leading English language textbook of internal medicine. A decade earlier, Osler "remarked upon the paucity of American text-books of medicine" and found the works which appeared in the mid-1880s from the pens of American physicians generally unsatisfactory.[76] Osler was a master of clinicopathologic correlation. His familiarity with the classic and contemporary medical literature, enormous clinical experience, and literary style enabled him to produce a textbook of unprecedented popularity. A great proponent of the medical literature, Osler remarked in 1901, "to study the phenomena of disease without books is to sail an uncharted sea, while to study books without patients is not to go to sea at all."[77]

Osler adapted the European approach to his textbook, and there are many similarities between his volume and Adolf Strümpell's *Text-book of Medicine* which appeared a few years earlier.[78] Osler's textbook was notable for the inclusion of a historical summary for many subjects he discussed. With this exception, Osler's work was organized on the pattern of Strümpell's work. For each disease he included sections on etiology, morbid anatomy, symptoms, diagnosis, prognosis, and treatment. This arrangement has been followed in most subsequent American medical textbooks.[79] It was not the arrangement, however, or even the subjects covered in his book, that made Osler's textbook so noteworthy. A contemporary reviewer placed the book in perspective: "Everywhere throughout the work one feels the delightful personality of the man. Every page contains evidences of original observation and is marked by an enlightened conservatism."[80]

Monographs

As medicine became progressively more specialized throughout the nineteenth century, the scope of textbooks became more limited. Monographs were also published that dealt with a single subject or closely related group of subjects. American physicians wrote important treatises on subjects such as smallpox and vaccination (Benjamin Waterhouse, 1800), hydrophobia (James Thacher, 1812), typhoid fever (Nathan Smith, 1824), pulmonary tuberculosis (Samuel Morton, 1834), pneumonia (René La Roche, 1854), and heart disease (Austin Flint, 1859), to list but a few. The demand for monographs among America's physicians in the last years of the nineteenth century is reflected in the success of the William Wood publishing company's "Library of Standard Medical Authors." Over eight years, one hundred titles appeared in the series, which was sold by subscription to thousands of American physicians. Many of the titles were reprints of British works or translations of European monographs; a few were original American contributions. The scope of the series was broad, but many volumes were devoted to subjects dealing with the diagnosis and treatment of medical ailments. Included among the titles was a classic of geriatrics, *Clinical Lectures on the Diseases of Old Age,* by the French neurologist Jean Martin Charcot. Americans contributed original medical works on rheumatism (Morris Longstreth, 1882), climatology (A. N. Bell, 1885), therapeutics (Robert Edes, 1883), malaria (George Sternberg, 1884), cholera (Edmund Wendt, 1885), and venereal diseases (Edward Keyes, 1880). The number of medical monographs published in American grew steadily during the early decades of the twentieth century. Although it was rare for a physician to devote himself to a subspecialty of medicine until the middle third of the century, there were numerous works devoted to the diagnosis and treatment of diseases of specific organ systems.[81]

"Systems" of Medicine

Energetic editors and authors have attempted to collect medical knowledge in multivolume encyclopedias or "systems" of medicine for generations. When the Paris School was assuming its position of leadership in the world of medicine in the early nineteenth century, a group of physicians and surgeons collaborated in the publication of the monumental sixty-volume *Dictionnaire des Sciences Médicales* between 1812 and 1822. The English translation of Hugo von Ziemssen's *Cyclopaedia of the Practice of Medicine* was published in New York between 1874 and 1881 in twenty volumes. Billings described this as "the most extensive work, native or foreign, which has ever been issued in the United States."[82] The American editor of Ziemssen's *Cyclopaedia,* Albert Buck of New York, claimed,

> For some time past, physicians . . . have felt the need of a work, or series of works, which should furnish a complete picture of the present state of medical knowledge in the departments of etiology, pathology, and treatment. The ordinary text-books do not supply this want, and the busy practitioner cannot afford to spend either time or money upon the scores of monographs which are constantly being published. A series of treatises, however, written by men who are skilled in the different departments of medicine . . . would meet in great measure this demand.[83]

Buck remained committed to the concept of medical encyclopedias and edited the massive eight-volume *Reference Handbook of the Medical Sciences* in 1885. This work comprised articles written by America's leading physicians. Other notable multivolume systems of medicine were edited by William Pepper in 1885 and William Osler in 1907. Although they survive, multivolume encyclopedias of medicine are far less popular than they were a generation ago.

In 1927 Russell Cecil extended the philosophy of the multiauthor medical encyclopedia to a single volume textbook. Recalling the planning of this medical textbook, Cecil observed, "after all, what is a medical textbook but a condensed system of medicine?"[84] In the preface to his volume, Cecil declared, "the rapid growth of medical science during the last few years has made it almost impossible for a single individual to master the entire field. In internal medicine, as in other branches of human knowledge, the age of specialism has of necessity arrived."[85] Cecil's textbook included contributions by 130 authors, "each of whom is a student or investigator of the subject upon which he has written."[86] The first edition received, in Cecil's words, "only a moderately warm welcome from the medical profession."[87] Nevertheless, in little more than a decade it was the standard textbook in many of the leading American medical schools. This was due, in part, to the broad representation of medical school faculty members among the book's more than one hundred contributors.

Medical Bibliography

Anyone seeking information on a medical topic recognizes the critical importance of sophisticated indexes of the literature of scientific and clinical medicine. In 1876 Billings observed that few American authors made use of bibliographic research despite the existence of important medical libraries in many of America's major cities. This led the Army surgeon and bibliophile to develop the *Index Medicus,* which he believed would help physicians gain access to the large and rapidly growing medical literature of the world.[88] Three years later in the introduction to the first volume of the *Index Medicus,* Billings declared,

> Few words are required to demonstrate the utility of the projected serial. In its pages the practitioner will find the titles of parallels for his anomalous cases, accounts of new remedies, and the latest methods in therapeutics. The teacher will observe what is being written or taught by the masters of his art in all countries. The author will be enabled to add the latest views and cases to his forthcoming work, or to discover where he has been anticipated by other writers, and the publishers of medical books and periodicals must necessarily profit by the publicity given to their productions.[89]

Index Medicus was "perfectly indispensable to true workers," according to Francis Brown of Boston, who made this claim in 1881.[90] The same year Oliver Wendell Holmes observed that "indexing is the special need of our time in medical literature."[91]

In addition to the *Index Medicus,* in which he indexed the contemporary periodical literature of medicine, Billings inaugurated the *Index Catalogue of the Library of the Surgeon General's Office,* in which old as well as new monographs, pamphlets, and offprints were listed by author and subject. These two new bibliographical tools were immediately acknowledged to be invaluable by the medical and scientific communities of the entire world. Upon the occasion of the dedication of the new building of the Boston Medical Library, S. Weir Mitchell observed, "I often remember with regret the great waste of time in my younger days when there were no great libraries, and when John Billings had not indexed the medical thought of all the centuries. The enormous labor then involved in any mere literary research as to facts no one can imagine today. A great library . . . well managed, practically lengthens life by saving time."[92]

The literature of medicine continues to evolve in response to diverse scientific and cultural forces. Despite this there are many features of the medical literature that have remained remarkably stable for decades. New technologies promise to alter the mechanics of information transfer, storage, and recall. Social pressures may well alter the balance between basic research, specialization, and primary care. The literature of medicine will be affected by all of these influences. Authors will continue to write, editors to edit, and publishers to publish for the foreseeable future, but they will have to continue to adapt, as did the editors of the *American Review of Tuber-*

culosis a quarter of a century ago, if they wish to be successful in attaining their goals.

NOTES

1. Robert H. Fletcher and Suzanne W. Fletcher, "Clinical Research in General Medical Journals," *N Engl J Med* 301 (1979) : 180–83.

2. For background on these themes see John Harley Warner, "Science in Medicine," *Osiris* 1 (1985) : 37–58; Ronald L. Numbers and John Harley Warner, "The Maturation of American Medical Science," in *Science & Health in America: Readings in the History of Medicine and Public Health,* Judith Walzer Leavitt and Ronald L. Numbers, eds., ed. 2 (Madison: University of Wisconsin Press, 1985), 113–25; Morris J. Vogel and Charles E. Rosenberg, eds., *The Therapeutic Revolution: Essays in the Social History of American Medicine* (Philadelphia: University of Pennsylvania Press, 1979); Stanley Joel Reiser, *Medicine and the Reign of Technology* (Cambridge: Cambridge University Press, 1978); and Richard H. Shryock, *American Medical Research: Past and Present* (New York: Commonwealth Fund, 1947).

3. Thomas Neville Bonner, *American Doctors and German Universities: A Chapter in International Intellectual Relations: 1870–1914* (Lincoln: University of Nebraska, 1963).

4. W. Bruce Fye, *The Development of American Physiology: Scientific Medicine in the Nineteenth Century* (Baltimore: Johns Hopkins University Press, 1987).

5. For background on the development of specialization in medicine, see George Rosen, *The Specialization of Medicine with Particular Reference to Ophthalmology* (New York: Froben Press, 1944); Rosemary Stevens, "Egalitarianism in Medicine and the Challenge of Specialism, 1860–1900," in *American Medicine and the Public Interest* (New Haven: Yale University Press, 1971), 34–54; and Edward C. Sequin, "The Cultivation of Specialties in Medicine," *Arch Med* 4 (1880) : 280–93.

6. Fye, *Development of American Physiology.* See also James Bordley III and A. McGehee Harvey, *Two Centuries of American Medicine: 1776–1976* (Philadelphia: W. B. Saunders, 1976); Kenneth M. Ludmerer, *Learning to Heal: The Development of American Medical Education* (New York: Basic Books, 1985); and Paul Starr, *The Social Transformation of American Medicine* (New York: Basic Books, 1982).

7. See Joseph Ben-David, "Scientific Productivity and Academic Organization in Nineteenth Century Medicine," *Am Soc Rev* 25 (1960) : 828–43, and Numbers and Warner, "Maturation of American Medical Science."

8. [George Shrady], "Specialism and General Practice," *Med Rec* 11 (1876) : 631–32.

9. Alvin S. Tarlov, "Consequences of the Rising Number of Physicians and of the Growth of Subspecialization in Internal Medicine," in *Academic Medicine: Present and Future,* John Z. Bowers and Edith E. King, eds. (North Tarrytown, NY: Rockefeller Archive Center, 1982), 106–21. See also Robert G. Petersdorf, "Internal Medicine 1976: Consequences of Subspecialization and Technology," *Ann Intern Med* 84 (1976) : 92–4.

10. Paul B. Beeson, "The Natural History of Medical Subspecialties," *Ann Intern Med* 93 (1980) : 624–26.

11. Foreword, in A. McGehee Harvey, Leighton E. Cluff, Richard J. Johns, et al., eds., *The Principles and Practice of Medicine*, ed. 17 (New York: Appleton-Century-Crofts, 1968), xxiii.

12. James B. Herrick, "Changes in Internal Medicine Since 1900," *JAMA* 105 (1935) : 1312–15.

13. [Isaac Hays], "Advertisement," *Am J Med Sci* 1 (1827) : vii.

14. Samuel D. Gross, *History of American Medical Literature from 1776 to the Present Time* (1876; repr. New York: Burt Franklin, 1972).

15. John Shaw Billings to G. Stanley Hall (c. 1895), John Shaw Billings Papers, Rare Books and Manuscripts Division, New York Public Library, New York.

16. Samuel Shapiro, "The Decision to Publish: Ethical Dilemmas," *J Chronic Dis* 38 (1985) : 365–72. See also Michael R. Rosen and Brian F. Hoffman, "The Cost of Scientific Communication: The Scientist as Ad-Man," *Circ Res* 40 (1977) : 1–2.

17. Richard S. Ross, "Memorandum to the Advisory Board of the Medical Faculty" (21 June 1982), *Johns Hopkins Med J* 151 (1982) : 264–65.

18. *Proceedings of the National Medical Conventions, Held in New York, May, 1846, and in Philadelphia, May, 1847* (Philadelphia: American Medical Association, 1847).

19. W. Bruce Fye, "S. Weir Mitchell, Philadelphia's 'Lost' Physiologist," *Bull Hist Med* 57 (1983) : 188–202.

20. Lunsford Pitts Yandell, "Address on American Medical Literature," in *Transactions of the International Medical Congress of Philadelphia 1876*, John Ashhurst, Jr., ed. (Philadelphia, 1877), 223–64.

21. Anne E. Crowley, Sylvia I. Etzel, and Edward S. Petersen, "Undergraduate Medical Education," *JAMA* 254 (1985) : 1565–72.

22. Julius Comroe, "Publish and/or Perish," *Am Rev Respir Dis* 113 (1976) : 561–65. See also Rand B. Krumland, Edward E. Will, and G. Anthony Gorry, "Scientific Publications of a Medical School Faculty," *J Med Educ* 54 (1979) : 876–84.

23. John S. Billings, "Literature and Institutions," *Am J Med Sci* 72 (1876) : 439–80.

24. Gross, *History of American Medical Literature*.

25. Victor Strasburger, Jr., "Righting Medical Writing," *JAMA* 254 (1985) : 1789–90.

26. David T. Durack, "The Weight of Medical Knowledge," *N Eng J Med* 298 (1978) : 773–75.

27. [George F. Shrady], "German Medical Journals," *Med Rec* 26 (1884) : 71–72.

28. Billings, "Literature and Institutions." See also James H. Cassedy, "The Flourishing and Character of Early American Medical Journalism, 1797–1860," *J Hist Med Allied Sci* 38 (1983) : 135–50; Norman Shaftel, "The Evolution of American Medical Literature," *Int Rec Med* (July 1958) : 431–54; and Victor Robinson, ed., "Medical Journalism Number: Origin of Medical Journalism in America," *Med Life* 36 (1929) : 553–606.

29. James Eckman, "Anglo-American Hostility in American Medical Literature of the Nineteenth Century," *Bull Hist Med* 9 (1941) : 31–71.

30. Oliver Wendell Holmes, "Dedicatory Address," in *Dedication of the New Building and Hall of the Boston Medical Library Association* (Cambridge: Riverside Press, 1881), 1–21.

31. Cassedy, "Early American Medical Journalism."

32. Billings, "Literature and Institutions."

33. Billings, "Literature and Institutions."

34. *Medical Education and the Regulation of the Practice of Medicine in the United States and Canada*, rev. ed. (Chicago: W. T. Keener, 1884).

35. Harold M. Schoolman, "The Impact of Electronic Computers and Other Technologies on Information Resources for the Physician," *Bull NY Acad Med* 61 (1985) : 283–89. See also Mary E. Corning and Martin M. Cummings, "Biomedical Communications," in *Advances in American Medicine: Essays at the Bicentennial*, John Z. Bowers and Elizabeth F. Purcell, eds., 2 vols. (New York: Josiah Macy, Jr., Foundation, 1976), 2 : 722–73, and Theodore Berland, "The Challenge of Medical Writing in America," *Perspect Biol Med* 26 (1983) : 587–94.

36. Arnold S. Relman, "An Open Letter to the News Media," *N Engl J Med* 300 (1979) : 554–55.

37. Henry Ingersoll Bowditch to Olivia Bowditch, 14 October 1867. Vincent Y. Bowditch, ed., *Life and Correspondence of Henry Ingersoll Bowditch*, 2 vols. (Boston: Houghton, Mifflin, 1902), 2 : 146.

38. Holmes, "Dedicatory Address."

39. Robert Walgate, "Politics of Premature French Claim of Cure," *Nature* 317 (1985) : 3.

40. See Della Mundy, "Time Needed for Publication of Journal Articles," *Ann Intern Med* 101 (1984) : 61–62, and Julius Comroe, "Publisher's Dawdle: An Incurable Disease," *Am Rev Respir Dis* 115 (1977) : 131–34.

41. Franz J. Ingelfinger, "The New England Journal of Medicine: Editor's Report, 1967–1977," *N Engl J Med* 296 (1977) : 1530–35.

42. Billings, "Literature and Institutions."

43. Billings, "Literature and Institutions."

44. Oliver Wendell Holmes, Enoch Hale, G. C. Shattuck, Jr., et al., "Report of the Committee on Medical Literature," *Trans AMA* 1 (1848) : 249–88.

45. "Editing Foreign Medical Works by American Physicians," *Boston Med Surg J* 56 (1857) : 115–20.

46. [Victor Vaughan], "Original Investigation," *Physician and Surgeon* 5 (1883) : 13–14.

47. [George Shrady], "Medical Authorship," *Med Rec* 2 (1867) : 445–46.

48. Alfred Soffer, "Why a New Journal Title?" *Chest* 57 (1970) : 1–2.

49. Alexander B. Gutman, "The Objective of the American Journal of Medicine," *Am J Med* 1 (1946) : 1–2.

50. Simon Dack, "The Journal of the American College of Cardiology: Editor's Perspective," *J Am Coll Cardiol* 1 (1983) : 3–4.

51. David H. Spodick and Robert J. Goldberg, "The Editor's Correspondence: Analysis of Patterns in Selected Specialty and General Journals," *Am J Cardiol* 52 (1983) : 1290–92.

52. Cassedy, "Early American Medical Journalism."

53. Billings, "Literature and Institutions."

54. [George Shrady], "American Medical Journalism," *Med Rec* 5 (1870) : 349–50.

55. William B. Bean, "My Sampler of Editors," *N Engl J Med* 303 (1980) : 229–33.

56. These issues are considered by Lawrence D. Grouse, "The Ingelfinger Rule," *JAMA* 245 (1981) : 375–76, and Strasburger, "Righting Medical Writing."

57. Yandell, "American Medical Literature."

58. Patricia Morton, "Medical Book Reviewing," *Bull Med Libr Assoc* 71 (1983) : 202–6.

59. See Joseph Garland, "The New England Journal of Medicine, 1812–1968," *J Hist Med Allied Sci* 24 (1969) : 125–39; Edward C. Streeter, "The Boston Medical and Surgical Journal: Beginnings and Development," *N Engl J Med* 198 (1928) : 24–26; Leslie T. Morton, "British Medical Periodicals: 1868–1968," *Practitioner* 201 (1968) : 224–30; Lester S. King, "Medical Journalism, 1847–1883," *JAMA* 250 (1983) : 744–48; Edward Bell Krumbhaar, "Early Days of the AJMS," *Med Life* 36 (1929) : 239–56; and Edward J. Huth, "Annals of Internal Medicine: The First 50 Years," *Ann Intern Med* 87 (1977) : 103–10.

60. Billings, "Literature and Institutions."

61. Edwin S. Gaillard, "Sixty Thousand Copies!!" *Am Med Weekly* 14 (1882) : 27–28.

62. Edwin S. Gaillard, "The Advertisers," *Am Med Weekly* 14 (1882) : 28.

63. John Wilson, "[Letter] on the Medical Library," *Med Phys J* 10 (1803) : 334–39.

64. See Michael R. Kronenfeld and Sarah H. Gable, "Real Inflation of Journal Prices: Medical Journals, U.S. Journals, and Brandon List Journals," *Bull Med Libr Assoc* 71 (1983) : 375–79, and Dick R. Miller and Joseph E. Jensen, "Dual Pricing of Health Sciences Periodicals: A Survey," *Bull Med Libr Assoc* 68 (1980) : 336–47.

65. Henry A. Grant, *The Annual Address to the Candidates for the Degree of Doctor of Medicine in the Medical Institution of Yale College* (New Haven: William H. Stanley, 1850). Joseph Garland, former editor of the *New England Journal of Medicine*, addressed this theme more recently. See Joseph Garland, "Medical Journals in the Continuing Education of the Student and Physician," in *Training of the Physician* (Boston: [Boston City Hospital], 1964), 94–96.

66. [George Shrady], "American Medical Journalism."

67. [George Shrady], "Medical Journalism," *Med Rec* 1 (1866) : 453–54.

68. "Physicians Who Do Not Read," *Coll Clin Rec* 3 (1883) : 39.

69. John S. Billings, "Our Medical Literature" (1881), reprinted in *Selected Papers of John Shaw Billings*, Frank B. Rogers, comp. ([Chicago]: Medical Library Association, 1965), 116–38.

70. Wilburt C. Davison, "Reflections on the Medical Book and Journal Situation," *Bull Hist Med* 11 (1942) : 182–200.

71. Overviews of the history of American medical education are Ronald L. Numbers, ed., *The Education of American Physicians: Historical Essays* (Berkeley and Los Angeles: University of California Press, 1980), and Ludmerer, *Learning to Heal*.

72. "Heavy Medical Journals," *Boston Med Surg J* 48 (1853) : 43–44. See also F. Gaskell, "Medical Literature," in *Medicine and Science in the 1860s*, F. N. L. Poynter, ed. (London: Wellcome Institute, 1968), 289–309.

73. Billings, "Literature and Institutions."

74. Samuel D. Gross, "Report on the Causes Which Impede the Progress of American Medical Literature," *Trans AMA* 9 (1865) : 337–62.

75. Gross, "Causes Which Impede American Medical Literature."

76. William Osler, "Reviews. Art. XVI. Recent Works on Practice," *Am J Med Sci* 89 (1885) : 175–81.

77. William Osler, "Books and Men," *Boston Med Surg J* 144 (1901) : 60–61.

78. Adolf Strümpell, *A Text-Book of Medicine for Students and Practitioners*, Herman F. Vickery and Philip C. Knapp, trans., Frederick C. Shattuck, ed. (New York: D. Appleton & Co., 1887).

79. A. McGehee Harvey and Victor A. McKusick, eds., *Osler's Textbook Revisited* (New York: Appleton-Century-Crofts, 1967).

80. "Reviews" *Med News* 60 (1892) : 442.

81. Medical monographs have traditionally been the most sought after items by medical bibliophiles. For surveys of medical book collecting see John L. Thornton, *Medical Books, Libraries and Collectors: A Study of Bibliography and the Book Trade in Relation to the Medical Sciences,* ed. 2 (London: Andre Deutsch, 1966); W. Bruce Fye, "Collecting Medical Books: Practical and Theoretical Considerations with an Annotated Bibliography," *Trans Stud Coll Physicians Phila* 1 (1979) : 305–23; idem, "A Primer on Medical Books," *AB Bookmans Weekly* 67 (1981) : 3658–96; and idem, "Collecting Medical Books: Challenges and Opportunities in the Eighties," *Bull NY Acad Med* 61 (1985) : 250–65.

82. Billings, "Literature and Institutions."

83. Albert H. Buck, "Preface to the American Edition," in *Cyclopaedia of the Practice of Medicine,* H. von Ziemssen, ed., 20 vols. (New York: William Wood & Co., 1874), 1 : iii.

84. Russell L. Cecil, "The Editing of a Modern Medical Textbook," in *Medicine and Writing,* Russell L. Cecil, Morris Fishbein, John F. Fulton, et al., eds. (New York: M.D. Publications, 1956), 1–7.

85. Russell L. Cecil, ed., *A Text-Book of Medicine by American Authors* (Philadelphia: W. B. Saunders, 1927).

86. Cecil, *Text-Book of Medicine.*

87. Cecil, "Editing of a Modern Medical Textbook."

88. Billings, "Literature and Institutions."

89. John S. Billings, "Prospectus," *Index Medicus* 1 (1879) : 1–2. See also Leonard Karel, "Selection of Journals for *Index Medicus:* A Historical Review," *Bull Med Libr Assoc* 55 (1967) : 259–78, and John B. Blake, ed., *Centenary of Index Medicus: 1879–1979* (Bethesda: National Library of Medicine, 1980).

90. Francis Brown, "Indexes to Medical Literature," *Boston Med Surg J* 104 (1881) : 318–20.

91. Holmes, "Dedicatory Address."

92. S. Weir Mitchell, "Letter [for the dedication of the new building of the Boston Medical Library]," *Boston Med Surg J* 144 (1901) : 65.

PART II

THE SUBSPECIALTIES OF INTERNAL MEDICINE: CASE STUDIES

4

History of the Subspecialty of Infectious Diseases in the United States

EDWARD H. KASS

The history of infectious diseases is, perhaps more than in any other field of medicine, inextricably intertwined with the history of medicine in general. It takes little analysis to recognize the enormous impact of fevers and of transmissible diseases on social organization, culture, religion, wars and virtually every aspect of daily life. To discuss the history of infectious diseases even in outline would require an extensive treatise, beyond the scope of this summary. Therefore, I shall take a truncated approach, with particular emphasis on recent developments. I shall also say relatively little about contributors to the field who are still alive; this is not in order to suggest a means for achieving immortality in this field, but because evaluation of contemporaries is difficult, often offends sensibilities, and is, in any event, lacking in the perspective that comes from time.

For convenience, the history of infectious disease can be divided into three broad phases. In the earliest phase a large share of ordinary medical practice was concerned with infections, as we now recognize them. There was no need for infectious disease specialists—every physician was necessarily an infectious disease specialist—and the number of specific preventive and therapeutic methods was small (e.g., quinine for fevers, variolation or vaccination for smallpox). In consequence, clinical and investigational emphasis was on the recognition of the clinical syndromes and natural history of different infections.

The United States during the colonial and postcolonial periods offered no exception to this natural historical sequence: Jamestown was settled in 1607, the year that William Harvey became a Fellow of the Royal College of Physicians. Those colonial settlers who were recognized as doctors often were also farmers, teachers, and sometimes, like Cotton Mather and John Wilson, clergymen as well.

The second phase of the history of infectious diseases can be considered to have begun in the early nineteenth century, with its attendant advances in prosperity and public health. These advances led, by the end of that century, to the discovery of microbial causes of disease and to the appearance of many specific vaccines and antisera with their well-known consequences.

As mortality rates fell, the public became increasingly aware that disease, mostly infectious, was not a necessary and preordained lot in life, and that health, which was improving, could be further improved by individual and community actions. This awareness was translated into an increasing desire for medical care, even though in retrospect such care, apart from offering important but not life-saving emotional support, did little to improve the lot of the patient, and was sometimes harmful. The public desire for the same medical care received by the wealthy, the sense that doctors had brought about the improving health, and the striking advances in diagnosis, chemistry, physiology, and pathology led to increased social prestige for members of the medical profession, and to increased numbers of societies, regulatory bodies, medical schools, hospitals—the process of professionalization of medicine as a recognizable self-governing force in society.

The third phase of the history of infectious disease was possible only when the incidence, mortality, and societal consequences of infections had become so small that detailed knowledge of them was no longer fundamental to every practitioner of medicine, except for the commonest infections. The advent of specific chemotherapeutics, wide-ranging public health practices, use of a variety of other preventive and therapeutic measures, remarkable discoveries in microbiology and immunity, general improvement in conditions of life, and their attendant effects of decreasing the spread and the consequences of infection all came together, particularly after World War II. Only then could infectious disease became a specialty, in the sense that a subgroup of physicians became particularly knowledgeable about the increasing number of therapeutic and prophylactic means for preventing and treating such disease.

Those physicians who continued their primary interest in infectious disease became the source of a substantial proportion of the research that produced new approaches, or investigated the efficacy of older methods. Such physicians necessarily became the repository of knowledge about diseases that had once been common and understood by all physicians and now had become relatively uncommon. Practitioners faced with syndromes suggestive of typhoid fever, or faced with the intricacies of treating enterococcal endocarditis, or bewildered by the array of infections that might accompany antineoplastic, immunosuppressive therapy, often became uncertain of diagnosis and treatment and sought the advice of specialists. Advances in understanding became a special province of these specialists and were transmitted by them to the rest of the profession. The third phase was therefore the professionalization of the infectious diseases specialist as differentiated from other clinicians.

These three divisions are artificial. Each must be discussed in relation to concurrent changes in medical research and practice. However, in this chapter, particular emphasis will be given to the third and most recent division because it represents a more recent trend and because it demarcates the recognition of infectious diseases as a discrete and identifiable subspecialty of medicine. This recognition was one more sign of the maturing of American medicine, and implicitly recognized the main advances in infectious disease. This phase occurred as the great depression, the political turmoil following it, and World War II weakened European medical investigation. The consequent primacy of American medicine is only now beginning to be challenged by the regeneration of European strength and by the emergence of Asiatic dynamism.

Colonial and Postcolonial Infectious Disease

The colonial and postcolonial periods were hardly the times for major American advances in science or medicine. The United States, distant from European culture, was concerned with its own growth and expansion, dealing with the frontier and the indigenous population, protecting itself from inimical European powers, and absorbing wave after wave of settlers and immigrant workers as well as foreign capital. Such a setting offered little room for specialization or for investigation and training in medicine. Most medical practice, as in Europe, was provided by an assortment of "empirics", comprising those who carried along village wisdom or a minimum of apothecary training, midwives, clergy, and some who had served apprenticeships with established medical practitioners. Few had university training or medical degrees, although all began to be called "doctor" by the populace. When medical societies sprang up, membership tended to be limited, as in England, to those who had received medical degrees. In 1765 John Morgan had argued, at first unsuccessfully, for the separation of medicine from pharmacy; there were also attempts to separate physicians from surgeons from apothecaries, but as in England, the separation was relevant only to the more affluent minority, who could afford and have access to the more specialized practitioners.

Important physicians in the colonial days and for many decades thereafter were locally significant but seldom influenced the growth of medical knowledge. For example, although Benjamin Waterhouse's name frequently arises because of his advocacy of inoculation against smallpox, and Cotton Mather, Zabdiel Boylston, and many others were ardently in agreement, this advocacy has only local significance; the basic ideas had arisen elsewhere. The more educated physicians were in touch with authorities in Britain and the Continent, from where the new advances were coming.

A noteworthy early event was the famous controlled experiment conducted in 1802 by Waterhouse, a group of other physicians, and the Board of Health in Boston. Nineteen "volunteer" boys (including two whose fathers were on the Board) were vaccinated, and then housed on an island (now a part of the city) in the harbor. Twelve of the boys and a physician's son who had previously been vaccinated were inoculated, along with two unvaccinated boys, with fresh smallpox matter. All were housed together in one room. The two control boys became seriously ill; the vaccinated boys remained healthy. Then the thirteen healthy boys who had been vaccinated, plus the remaining seven who had not been part of the experiment, were inoculated again with infectious material, and all were housed in the same room with the two boys who had contracted the disease. No new cases appeared. This heroic experiment added little to what was already known but was helpful in convincing a skeptical public. It would hardly be countenanced today.[1]

Medical schools, journals, and societies in Philadelphia, New York, and Boston were repositories of the medical wisdom of the time. The more affluent physicians and students traveled to Europe either to medical school or to walk the wards of teaching hospitals. As in Britain, most hospitals attempted to exclude patients with fevers; others had "foul wards" for patients with fevers and with venereal disease. These wards were hardly the favorites among students or teachers. Thus there was little progress in separating the fevers, although there was substantial awareness and concern with basic hygiene and sanitation, perhaps representing the early influence of French teaching, in which public hygiene and public health were separated from the rest of medicine. The early American medical journals quoted extensively from British and continental publications.

Secular Decline in Mortality from Infectious Disease— Nineteenth Century

For a century after the Revolution, the earlier patterns changed relatively little. The frequently quoted papers of Holmes on puerperal sepsis stand out. However, although they were masterpieces of incisive and satirical prose and careful reasoning, they drew all their information from sources that had already been published, much of the original work having come from Europe.[2]

The reformist thrusts of the early and middle nineteenth centuries were accompanied by the beginning of systematic recording of rates of disease and causes of death in many communities. Although there is much to suggest that mortality rates in London were already declining, and that rates of certain diseases in the United States may have been somewhat lower than in England, documentation of these trends is limited to small communities. The documentation after 1850 is more complete, especially in England, and demonstrates the most remarkable change in the social history of disease. In the United States similar trends were observed in those communities that kept records. Beginning in the second half of the nineteenth century, are recorded regular declines in mortality and in deaths due to such common diseases as tuberculosis (*Figure 4.1*), diphtheria (*Figure 4.2*), pertussis (*Figure 4.3*), rheumatic fever (*Figure 4.4*), measles, puerperal sepsis, and others. The decline was independent of the introduction of specific preventive and therapeutic measures, although there can be no argument concerning the value of various vaccines, antisera, and antibiotics. Dramatic evidence of the decline, from data collected from 1900 onward, can be seen in Table 4.1, with data that begin after the decline was well under way.[3]

What accounts for these extraordinary changes? The usual explanation, under the general term "improved standard of living" with its accompanying improvements in sanitation, water supply, availability of food, and so on, should not blind us to the absence of adequate biological understanding of the specific means by which these reductions were brought about. Furthermore, it is often overlooked that, despite the sorry state of the poor in many communities, and despite the obvious fact that most severe illnesses were

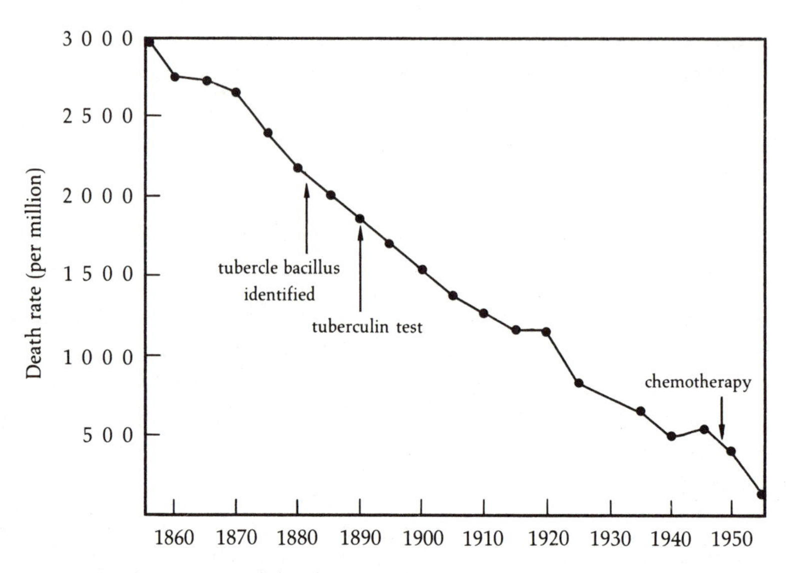

Figure 4.1. Mean annual death rate from respiratory tuberculosis in England and Wales. (Kass 1971.)

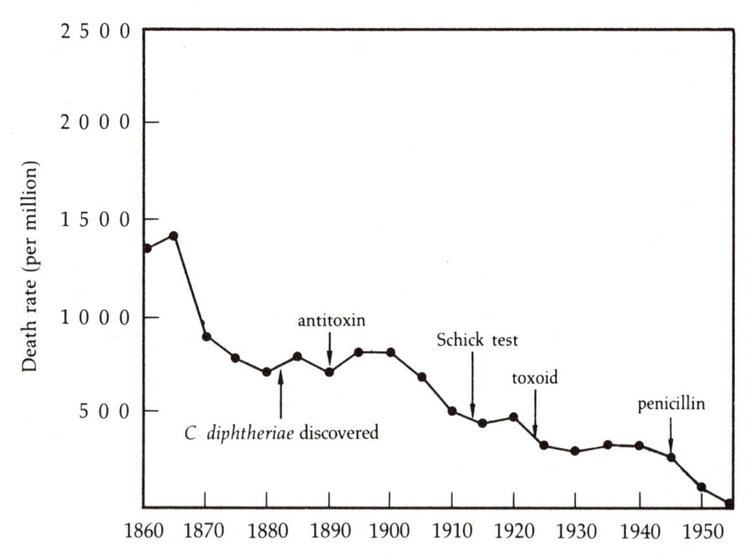

Figure 4.2. Mean annual death rate from diphtheria in children under 15 years of age in England and Wales. (Kass 1971.)

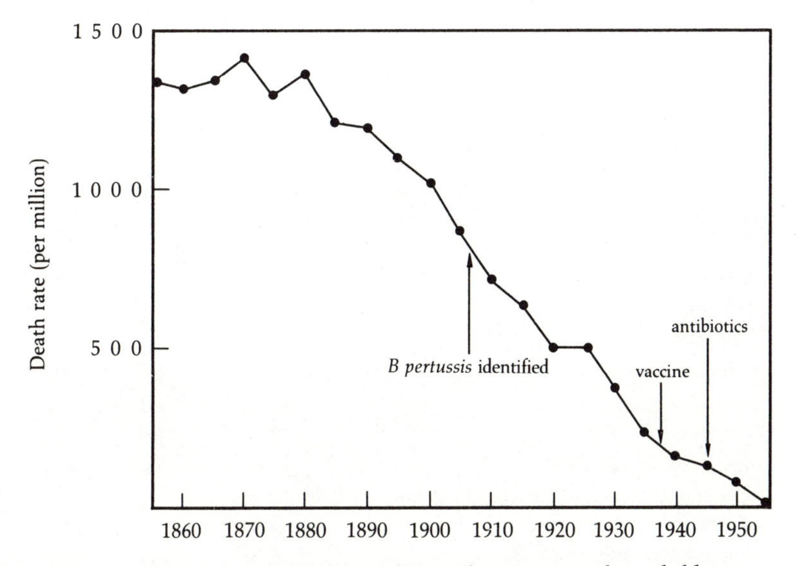

Figure 4.3. Mean annual death rate from whooping cough in children under 15 years of age in England and Wales. (Kass 1971.)

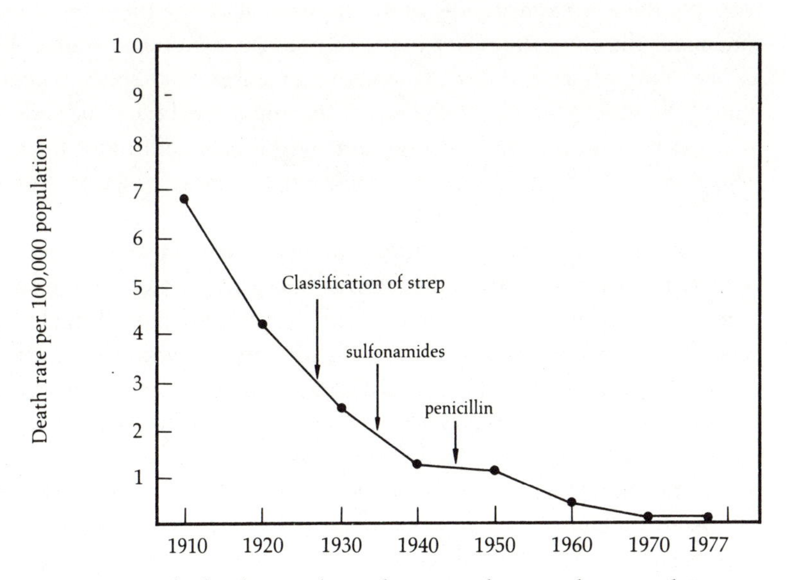

Figure 4.4. Crude death rates from rheumatic fever in the United States, 1910–1977.

TABLE 4.1.
DEATH RATES FOR COMMON INFECTIOUS DISEASES IN THE UNITED STATES IN 1900, 1935, AND 1970

	Mortality Rate per 100,000 Population		
	1900	*1935*	*1970*
Influenza and pneumonia	202.2	103.9	30.9
Tuberculosis	194.4	55.1	2.6
Gastroenteritis	142.7	14.1	1.3
Diphtheria	40.3	3.1	0.0
Typhoid fever	31.3	2.7	0.0
Measles	13.3	3.1	0.0
Dysentery	12.0	1.9	0.0
Whooping cough	12.0	3.7	0.0
Scarlet fever (including streptococcal sore throat)	9.6	2.1	0.0
Meningococcal infections	6.8	2.1	0.3

From: H. F. Dowling, *Fighting Infection* (Cambridge, MA: Harvard University Press, 1977).

more common, and more likely to be fatal, among the poor, the least well off were also the major beneficiaries of the improved statistics: the striking and continuous changes in mortality from, for example, tuberculosis, cannot be ascribed only to the number of families that raised their socioeconomic status from poverty to relative comfort. There must have been some decline in mortality from tuberculosis even among the poor to account for the steady decline in rates at a time when most people were at the lower income levels.

One explanation that has not received much attention, and will be developed in detail elsewhere, is the effect of household service. By the later years of the nineteenth century in England, over 40 percent of all employed persons were in household service. It was this form of employment, even more that in the factories, that sponged up the large numbers of people who had fled the farms after the agricultural depressions. Whatever the inequities of personal service, to most employees such service meant greater regularity of meals, a bed that was not necessarily in a room that was shared with many others, and an insistence by the employers on certain standards of personal hygiene and environmental cleanliness. In the United States, there were not the same legal and sociological imperatives as in Britain, but there were many immigrants and cycles of economic depression. Large numbers of individuals (the numbers less well documented than in Britain) entered household service. In Britain most of the population performed some type of household employment before reaching age twenty-five—similar figures are not available in the United States, but the numbers were undoubtedly substantial. The decrease in opportunities to become infected, by separation of the poorer individuals from their large families and crowded households, is a public health measure that has not received the historical attention that it deserves, although the effect of crowding and numbers of persons per household in increasing the spread of disease has been documented for decades.

Suffice it to say that as the declines in specific infectious diseases occurred, an increasingly prosperous community organized itself to bring the benefits of medical advances forward more expeditiously. By the early decades of the twentieth century, most major cities had clinics for immunization, hospitals were increasing in number and many were specifically designated for infectious diseases or for special groups (such as children) who were especially likely to suffer from such diseases. Courses in hygiene were introduced into schools and universities, while preventive medicine and medical microbiology became installed in the training of medical personnel. This can be illustrated with just a few of the many examples that might be given; intrinsic in these examples is the realization that most of the early discoveries relating microbes to disease were made in Europe.

Early American Studies of Microbiology

Although Austin Flint had written in compelling fashion, in 1874, of the "Logical Proof of the Contagiousness and Non-contagiousness of Disease,"[4] the first demonstration of bacteria in American scientific literature was a review by L. A. Stimson in the *New York Medical Journal* (where Flint's article had appeared a year earlier) with a brief version in *Popular Science Monthly*. The article quoted literature on the European demonstration of bacteria and mentioned especially the discovery of large bacilli in the blood in instances of anthrax. In 1877 two articles in the *Boston Medical and Surgical Journal* summarized Lister's important work on antiseptic surgery.[5]

Firsts are a precarious and uncertain guide to medical or any other history, but a few mentions of pioneering achievements indicate important advances in microbiology in the United States. Thomas J. Burrill was probably the first to introduce bacteriology into the formal university curriculum. In 1880 Burrill published his observations that *Micrococcus amylovorus* caused pear blight, and he demonstrated the effect with a botanical analogue of what was later known as Koch's postulates, reproducing the disease repeatedly in plants with the bacteria that he had isolated.[6] He had already introduced bacterial studies into his course in botany at the University of Illinois during the year or two before his discovery was published. Erwin Smith, a later leader in plant microbial studies, in his obituary of Burrill, stressed the latter's leadership but also his fate as a scientist—extinction by promotion as Burrill assumed administrative duties in his university. In the medical area, William Henry Welch at Bellevue Medical College and T. Mitchell Prudden at Columbia University set up bacteriological laboratories during the later years of the same decade. By 1885, when Welch began his studies at the new Johns Hopkins Hospital, he could report that twenty-six medical graduates were working in his laboratory and that several original investigations, including his own and those of George M. Sternberg, were presenting new discoveries that could rival those of the Europeans. Daniel E. Salmon began work in the Division of Animal Industry in 1879 and five years later was named chief of the renamed Bureau. Promptly he took on Theobald Smith as his associate, and within a few years their discovery of the hog cholera bacillus, now known as *Salmonella cholerae suis,* was announced.[7]

Smith's illustrious career and his unusual perceptivity demand better biographical treatment. He discovered, in addition to the work with Salmon, the differences between bovine and human tubercle bacilli, elucidated the cause of cattle fever and the role of arthropods as vectors, studied flagellar and somatic antigens after recognizing their differences, and discovered anaphylaxis and countless other phenomena of disease.[8] Sternberg, who was an Army officer, was given "courtesy" space by Welch and an appointment at Johns Hopkins. He was probably the most influential microbiologist of the later decades of the nineteenth century given his discoveries of the pneumococcus, his work on the yellow fever commission, his studies on thermal death points of bacteria and on the standardization of disinfectants, and his publication of the first comprehensive Manual of Bacteriology in 1892.[9]

Courses in bacteriology in medical schools began to appear in 1885, usually as part of the course in pathology, and teachers at Johns Hopkins, Harvard, George Washington University in Washington, D.C., Postgraduate Medical School of Chicago, the Universities of Michigan, Wisconsin, and Iowa State College of Agriculture, and the Massachusetts Institute of Technology gave pioneer courses before 1900. The names of Welch, Prudden, William Thompson Sedgwick, Herbert Conn, Frederick Novy, Harold C.

Ernst, H. M. Biggs and, of course, Theobald Smith, are but a few of the noteworthy ones in these pioneering efforts, and the epochal contributions of Walter Reed and his brave associates were reported in 1902.[10]

Meanwhile, Max von Pettenkofer had received funds in 1878 from the Bavarian government to open in Munich the first research institute to investigate microbiological diseases. Andrew Carnegie in 1884 funded Welch's laboratory in the Bellevue Medical College where he and G. H. F. Nuttall discovered, in 1892, the gas bacillus that bears the name *Clostridium welchii.*

Simultaneously these discoveries were being translated into action, although at varying rates. Boards of health began with one established in Boston in 1799 headed by Paul Revere, but the proliferation of these was slow. By 1867, the Association of Boards of Health recorded only a little over one hundred boards. The first hygienic laboratory, specifically funded as such, was at the University of Pennsylvania in 1892, and the first municipal laboratory was established in Providence in 1888. However, by 1914 all states except Wyoming and New Mexico had public health laboratories. Nationally, the Hygienic Laboratory, from which came the National Institutes of Health (NIH), was approved by Congress in 1901.[11]

Specific discoveries in microbiology and immunity were largely the province of Europeans, but American progress was slowly gathering momentum, particularly as young scientists returned from Europe bearing the results of the newest discoveries there. Botanists, pathologists, public health, and sanitary workers as well as physicians and veterinarians laid claim to the field of microbiology. All were correct. Medical microbiology tended slowly to orient itself within pathology. The latter field had been reluctantly recognized in Europe as a separate medical discipline, and the earliest chairs had been created in France and London in the first decades of the nineteenth century. The relatively new specialty of pathology, still trying to establish itself, did not leap at the prospect that the vital and exciting discoveries arising from its offspring should prompt a separation from it.

As the specialized knowledge grew in complexity, however, the separation of microbiology as a separate discipline became inevitable. In 1899 the laboratory section of the American Public Health Association was organized with Theobald Smith as its chairman. In the same year the Society of American Bacteriologists was founded, branching away from its parent American Society of Naturalists, with W. T. Sedgwick and H. J. Conn as the first president and secretary, respectively. Two years later the more medically oriented Association of American Pathologists and Bacteriologists was formed with William T. Councilman and Harold Ernst as president and secretary, respectively. The American Association of Immunologists began meeting in 1914.

Journals, at first broadly medical, became more specialized. The *Journal of the Boston Society of Medical Sciences,* started in 1896, became the *Journal of Medical Research* and in 1901 became the official journal of the Association of American Pathologists and Bacteriologists, later evolving into the *American Journal of Pathology.* The *American Journal of Public Health* began as the *Journal of the Massachusetts Association of Boards of Health,* became in 1906 the *American Journal of Public Hygiene,* in 1911 the *Journal of the American Public Health Association,* and in 1921 assumed its present title. The *Journal of Infectious Diseases* was founded in 1904 by Ludwig Hektoen, at the John McCormick Institute for Infectious Diseases, affiliated with the University of Chicago. The *Journal of Experimental Medicine* began in 1896 and was taken over by the Rockefeller Institute nine years later. The *Journal of Immunology* and the *Journal of Laboratory and Clinical Medicine* began in 1915, and the *Journal of Bacteriology,* published by the Society of American Bacteriologists began in 1916. The latter society was later renamed the Society of American Microbiologists, and now publishes *Infection and Immunity, Journal of Clinical Microbiology, Antimicrobial Agents and Chemotherapy* and *Journal of Applied Bacteriology,* as well as *Microbiological Reviews* and other notable journals.

This brief survey implies some of the changing pressures. Public health soon was perceived to be a broader field than the control of infection, which was its first major concern. Bacteriology became an inadequate title for societies, journals, and laboratories as advances in other aspects of microbiology came forward. New journals and societies in tropical medicine and parasitology bespoke still more specialization. The recent proliferation of immunological and virological journals is adequate testimony to the explosive growth of these fields.

Nobel Prizes are a marker of achievement, although the vagaries of committees have caused many important contributions to be overlooked. The first Nobel Prize in physiology or medicine was awarded in 1901 to Emil von Behring for his development of diphtheria antitoxin, followed by Ronald Ross for his work on malaria. In 1905 Robert Koch received the coveted prize for his work on tuberculosis, and two years later Charles Laveran was recognized for his investigations of protozoal disease. In 1908 Paul Ehrlich and Elie Metchnikov shared the prize for their work on humoral and cellular immunity. Of the first twelve awardees, six worked with pathogens or with immune processes related to microbial diseases. None was an American.

However, the momentum was gathering. The United States, increasing in economic and intellectual strength, was beginning to assert itself, while the economic and political crises in Europe were beginning to undermine the scientific leadership that had been established there. In the United States, the land grant universities, the growing scientific strength of the independent institutions of higher learning, the endowment of special research laboratories such as the Rockefeller and McCormick Institutes, and the creation and increasing recognition by the public of the value of city, state, and national public health departments and their laboratories were all factors in making America a world leader in medicine.

Microbiology was now widely taught as an undergraduate university discipline. Principles of isolation of pathogens and of immunological response became common undergraduate fare for the scientifically minded student and became basic to the education of students in the health professions. Although mortality and morbidity from infectious disease were declining, these diseases were still common enough to be major causes of hospitalization and absenteeism and, in certain occupational, age, and economic groups, they were still major causes of morbidity. The understanding, and later the treatment, of infectious disease required prompt identification of microorganisms with frequent use of serotyping and other specialized tests. The administration of antisera and the treatment of complications of infection and of infectious complications of surgery required skill, the integration of laboratory services, and close clinical supervision. Every clinician, for practical purposes, had to be aware of these treatments. However, with the development of complex tools such as the large number of pneumococcal antisera and the need to isolate and subtype each strain of pneumococcus, and with the wider use of pneumothorax and thoracoplasty for tuberculosis and fever therapy for late syphilis, specialized clinical centers began to veer away from the mainstream of general clinical medicine. Young physicians wishing to acquire specific skills in these fields sought out individual institutions or established proponents of the various methods of treatment.

Additionally, a new awareness was creeping into the field of microbiology that was destined to have far-reaching impact. The study of pathogenic microbes and the immune response was uncovering new principles of biology that had ramifications far beyond infectious diseases alone. The study of mechanisms of pathogenicity stimulated major discoveries in carbohydrate chemistry so that microbial capsules could be investigated. The antibody response was shown to consist of the assembly of specific globulins, and new methods for the study of the structure and activity of these proteins inevitably affected the growing science of protein chemistry even as the study of antibodies drew from protein chemistry some of the discoveries made in the analysis of unrelated proteins. Physiologic responses to infection demanded better understanding of the loss of fluid and electrolytes in fever and infections; this supplemented the growing knowledge enabling treatment of uninfected patients with unrelated diseases. Public health practices aimed at limiting the multiplication and spread of unwanted microbes were improving the quality of food and water with consequences far beyond the narrower objective of limiting the spread of infectious disease. Studies of cellular responses to pathogens and other foreign substances, investigations of the principles of isolation and sanitation, aseptic surgery, animal husbandry, and plant pathology all responded to the newer knowledge.

Perhaps the most important shift during this unprecedented period was an awareness that had been slowly increasing during the entire nineteenth century, which was the idea that disease was not a predestined lot in life or a retribution for a sinful life, but was a finite occurrence, often environmental in origin, that could be prevented or treated successfully. When a disease could not be successfully prevented or treated, research might uncover the means for doing so. New treatments required reliable and available sera or drugs. Pharmaceutical manufacturing, originally a province for individual pharmacists or charlatans, became a respected and essential field of business with a profit to be made, sometimes from illicit sales, but increasingly often from the application of rigorous standards of manufacture. When private enterprise was slow to respond, used shoddy methods, or exacted a price that was considered to be out of the reach of the needy, governmental units were created to supply vaccines, antisera, and other biologic products.

The great depression of the early 1930s and the war that followed produced the next important period in infectious disease. The era of specific chemotherapy had been ushered in by Ehrlich's development of organically bound arsenicals for the treatment of syphilis and of other substances for treatment of protozoal diseases. Because many of the organic compounds that bound heavy metals, and might release them to the detriment of invading microorganisms, were dyes, Ehrlich and his successors continued to investigate empirically the action of dyes against microbes.

In 1935 Gerhard Domagk publicly announced the dye Prontosil, which had been developed by chemists of the I. G. Farbenindustrie.[12] He showed that the administration of the dye to experimental animals cured them of streptococcal infections. This was applied to human infections with similar results. There was a strange delay in the patenting of the discovery, and one can speculate that perhaps the astute chemists of the huge chemical company had already discovered what was later found by the Trefouels and their colleagues at the Pasteur Institute. Prontosil was broken down in the body, releasing into the urine a simple derivative of the well-known sulfanilamide. The next years led to the development of a wide array of derivatives of sulfanilamide which extended its range of effectiveness, decreased its toxicity, and spawned a major sector of the pharmaceutical industry that continues to grow. Today sales of sulfonamides and related compounds are over $50 million annually.

Stimulated by World War II, a group in Oxford led by Howard Florey reexamined a number of potentially useful antimicrobial products, including a product of a Penicillium mold that had been discovered by Alexander Fleming. The latter discovery had not been exploited, in part because Fleming's vision of its value seems to have been limited, and in part because the material itself was labile and difficult to isolate and purify. Ernst B. Chain, Edward Abraham, and their associates undertook a detailed investigation of this material, called penicillin by Fleming. Soon attention was focused on this peculiar product produced by certain strains of the Penicillium mold. As its chemical and therapeutic properties began to be discerned, the development of penicillin passed to the United States where the resources were available for large-scale manufacturing.[13]

Meanwhile, another stream of investigation was being carried on by Selman Waksman, René Dubos, and others, who were all trained in soil microbiology and concerned with factors governing the interaction of the diverse microbial species of soil. Antimicrobial substances, called antibiotics by Waksman, were found, but the first ones isolated by Dubos were too toxic for systemic use. The discovery of streptomycin by Waksman and his associates and the finding that it was active against many bacteria that were relatively resistant to penicillin, such as the tubercle bacillus, made it appear likely that searching into diverse sources of microbes could uncover clinically useful antibiotics.[14] Furthermore, advances in chemical analysis offered possibilities of altering the antibiotic molecules to make them more effective or less toxic, or even just enough different to create a niche in the marketplace. The discoveries of chloramphenicol, the tetracyclines, the erythromycins, the various substituted penicillins, the entire series of cephalosporin derivatives, the rifampins, and many other antibiotics have followed. These discoveries have been broadened to include antineoplastic and antiviral agents, have stimulated work in the protozoal and helminthic fields, and have stimulated also the discovery of nonantibiotic antimicrobial drugs such as trimethoprim and the oxyquinolones. That these have been the most important life-saving drugs in medical history cannot be doubted. They also have had powerful effects on animal husbandry, agriculture, and various technical achievements such as tissue culture. The present market for antibiotics in the United States is approximately $300 million, without taking into account the expense of dispensing and administering these invaluable drugs.

Several trends began to appear in postwar American investigations related to infectious disease. One was the discovery that microbes were an extraordinary tool for the study of cellular phenomena that were not directly related to infectious disease. A major field of exploration emerged from the realization that microbial DNA could be transmitted by appropriate techniques to other cells and carry into the recipient cells genetic information conferring new properties. Apart from proving once and for all that DNA was the repository for genetic information, these experiments provided tools for the investigation of myriad biochemical events and spawned new industries as well as new visions of what might be possible in plant and animal cells. Although currently the number of practical consequences remains limited, the outlook is a stimulating one that has captured the imagination of both the scientific and the industrial communities.

The recognition of the genetic potential of microbial products was accompanied by other major discoveries. New viral agents for disease were being found regularly, and the detailed structure of such viruses was being increasingly understood. Vital to these discoveries was the development of tissue culture methods that made the exploration and identification of viral agents simpler and more efficient than the older methods of isolation. Although John Enders, Thomas Weller, and Frederick Robbins shared the Nobel Prize in 1954 for the discovery that poliomyelitis virus grew in cultures of non-neurologic tissue, making feasible the development of the later vaccines, it could be argued that an even greater contribution was their method of tissue culture that permitted isolation of viruses from crude materials, such as fecal extracts, with relatively little contamination from bacteria.

The appearance of antimicrobial agents, with their remarkable effects, led many prominent medical scientists to the conclusion that problems in infectious disease were essentially solved. The overall theoretical structure was in place, seemingly magical new therapeutic compounds were isolated, and it remained only for the application of these principles to be worked out so that infectious diseases would be conquered. Accordingly, many microbiologists, considering that problems in infectious disease were essentially solved, shifted their attention to the use of bacteria as models for various cellular functions. This shift in attention carried with it the sense, often transmitted to younger individuals, that work in the pathogenesis of infectious disease was essentially derivative, and that the important new discoveries were to be made in other fields. Leaving aside the biological inevitability that new diseases were certain to appear, it was overlooked that the mechanisms whereby illness was produced were understood for no single pathogen. Meanwhile, new techniques were uncovering immunologic principles that were reshaping the understanding of both infectious and noninfectious disease. Furthermore, for many diseases, including malignant and severe degenerative ones, infectious agents were increasingly being considered as etiologic sources.

Another trend was discernible during the early decades following the advent of specific antimicrobial therapy. The development of new drugs and their marketing naturally fell to industry, causing those who remained active in the field of evaluation of antimicrobial therapy to be increasingly constrained to work with industry, often, therefore, to be considered with some disdain by academic colleagues who regarded such involvement with distaste. Some of the distaste has disappeared in recent years, as the development of new genetic techniques has opened important and lucrative opportunities—powerful stimuli to changing the tastes of many of the earlier detractors.

For individuals interested in infectious disease, the years between 1950 and 1970 were sometimes troubling. World War II had brought large armies into contact with bacterial, viral, protozoal, and helminthic diseases in developing countries, and the inadequacy of the highly heralded mechanisms of control and treatment of many infectious diseases had been exposed; however, the full impact of this realization was not always grasped. Some investigators continued to be interested in the problems of protozoal and helminthic diseases, but found that support for research in the so-called tropical diseases was becoming less favorably looked upon, particularly as these diseases became infrequent in industrialized countries. Support by peer groups for research in resistance to antimicrobial drugs, mechanisms of action of these drugs, and their pharmacological actions also diminished. These fields were considered within the purview of commercial or applied interests.

Departments of microbiology in schools of medicine began to change their interests and names away from a connotation of medical involvement. Departments that had once called themselves departments of microbiology, or medical microbiology, or microbiology and immunology, increasingly took on names with molecular connotations, indicative of the changing emphasis. Meanwhile, immunologic research was stimulated by the discoveries of the role of lymphocytes, which had been suggested but not proved decades earlier, and by greater understanding of mast cells, eosinophiles, mononuclear cells, and research into the nature of cell-mediated immunity. Biochemical studies of phagocytes and mediators and detailed study of the structure and different classes of antibodies became commonplace. Immunology as a special field became sufficiently strong that in many institutions separate departments were created, thereby removing some of the homelessness created when immunology was cast from those departments of microbiology that had oriented themselves around microbial physiology and genetics.

A new problem arose in teaching. It was becoming increasingly difficult for students to receive sufficient tutelage in the principles of medical microbiology to prepare them for the clinical events or for the necessities of hospital and public health work that continued to require attention. Yet 15 to 30 percent of patients in hospitals presented some type of infectious disease-related problem, and about a third of all patients received some antimicrobial treatment. Clinicians who had retained an interest in infectious disease were called on to teach medical microbiology to students, but not always with most desirable results, because such clinicians sometimes stressed applied clinical material at the expense of broader principles that might be more valuable to the student in the future.

In schools of public health a parallel series of developments could be discerned. Epidemiology, perhaps the basic science of public health, had begun as a science for studying infectious disease in large populations. However, shifting mortality patterns diverted attention to the cardiovascular and malignant diseases, which had now displaced infectious disease as the chief causes of death and disability.[15] New epidemiologic methods were needed that did not depend, as infection did, on the isolation and identification of specific etiologic agents, since these were unidentified in most chronic diseases. Methods that required statistical manipulations of association and inquired into the interaction of many variables began to be developed, and those who became competent in these newer methods often sought a new identification for themselves by stressing that they were teaching and utilizing methods specifically relevant to noninfectious disease.

The result of these many interacting changes in the social behavior of the academic and scientific world, with its capacity to shape the directions of funding and of academic appointments, led younger aspirants away from infectious disease, and by 1950 to 1960 major departments of microbiology and of medicine had shifted their emphasis away from the study of the pathogenesis of infectious disease. Departments of pediatrics and some departments of preventive medicine continued an interest in infectious disease research. When I was seeking a fellowship for training as a clinical investigator in infectious disease, in 1948–49, I considered seriously only three departments of medicine in the entire country.

Symptomatic of the changing perceptions, the National Institute of Allergy and Infectious Diseases, which represented the discipline that had once been the basis around which the entire National Institutes of Health had been formed, became one of the more poorly funded institutes, and even within it increasing sums were being allocated to immunologic explorations and away from infectious diseases as such. To this day there is no study section in infectious diseases.

For practical purposes, the industrial requirement that new antimicrobial drugs be evaluated was one of the few stimuli left to continuing clinical investigation in infectious disease, although a relatively small number of dedicated and productive investigators were still examining problems in pathogenesis and resistance in infectious disease.

Organizational Structures in Infectious Disease

The strains were aggravated by another development. The major conferences that were devoted to the examination of antimicrobial drugs were tending to disregard problems in pathogenesis, pathologic physiology, epidemiology, or other aspects of infectious disease. Perhaps the most widely attended conference on antimicrobial drugs was the annual meeting held in Washington, D.C., and initiated in 1971 by Henry Welch, who was at that time in the antibiotics division of the Food and Drug Administration and editor of a new journal devoted to work in the antimicrobial drug field.

Since the annual meeting was to have an important but relatively limited scope, a number of investigators in infectious disease, interested in other aspects as well, convinced Maxwell Finland, already recognized as the leading figure in the investigation of antimicrobial drugs, to call an informal dinner meeting during the course of the antibiotics meeting. The after-dinner discussions consisted of informal presentations by many investigators who reported on their current work in nonantibiotic-related aspects of infectious disease. The dinners, attended at first by twenty or thirty people, grew in popularity and were ultimately attended by as many as one hundred medical scientists. It began to be evident that a more formal organization was needed, one that would devote itself to the scientific study of infectious diseases at the broadest level, not excluding antimicrobial drugs but not making them the exclusive focus. Meanwhile, informal groups were discussing similar needs at various other national meetings, and a convergence of these views was bound to occur.

Several courses of action were discussed at these informal meetings, including the formation of a special division of the Society of American Microbiologists. Many felt, however, that although there was an obvious coincidence of interests with the Society, the latter group had a much broader scope and membership, and there was fear of loss of the specific identity of those interested in infectious diseases. Ultimately, at one of the dinner meetings accompanying the antibiotics conferences in Washington, a committee was appointed by Finland. Lowell Rantz chaired it, and I was its secretary. The committee investigated the several organizational possibilities, informally polled those who had been at the dinner meetings, recommended that a new society be formed, and requested the secretary to prepare a list of possible members. The membership was to be drawn from among medical microbiologists, clinical investigators, public health workers, governmental agencies, and industry, without regard to the nature of their specific degrees or training but with emphasis on their scientific productivity and interests in infectious disease as broadly defined.

A list of approximately 250 was drawn up. A postal questionnaire indicated support for the formation of a new organization, and the committee called a meeting at the Airlie House in Warrenton, Virginia, in 1963, just preceding the antibiotic meeting in Washington. Rantz and I suggested a unique format, which was accepted, with only four speakers on each of two days. It was hoped that this format would permit detailed presentations and extended discussions and be sufficiently different from other meetings that the new group would set its own distinctive tone and style.

The first meeting was attended by about 125, or about half of those initially approached. There was some opposition to the new society, and several senior figures in the field either did not respond to the invitations or refused to attend the first meeting. Nevertheless, the group resolved to form the Infectious Diseases Society of America (IDSA), the title so chosen to indicate that membership from all of the Americas was invited.[16] Finland was elected the first president, to serve for one year, Rantz to be president-elect, and

Kass as secretary for five years. Unfortunately, Lowell Rantz died before becoming president. John Enders became the second president, and the Society was launched as a selective organization in which elected membership required notable publication and activity in the field and in which failure to attend meetings would be penalized by discharge from the organization. The IDSA grew by about between thirty-five and fifty members each year, and membership was restricted to those who had made substantial contributions to the field. By 1971, changing pressures brought a revision of the membership structure. Meetings were increasingly popular, and attendance was restricted to members and a limited number of guests, who could come only if the sponsoring member also attended the meeting. Failure to attend three consecutive meetings without an excuse acceptable to the Council led to removal from the Society. Foreign guests, however, were always welcome. These practices tended to keep the Society small and intimate, and made election to membership an important academic recognition, but had certain other disadvantages.

Growing numbers of trainees were seeking entry into the field. Officers of the Society were being called on by Congress and other governmental groups to advise them on various governmental concerns in the field of infectious diseases. Allocations of funds to the National Institute of Allergy and Infectious Diseases was increasingly viewed as a matter of the utmost concern to the Society. A broadening perception of the function of the Society was becoming more popular, and there was pressure to move away from the more restrictive format of membership, to broaden the base of membership, and to become more directly involved in the many political and social issues that were affecting the research and teaching of infectious diseases. In 1979, after a searching inquiry by a committee chaired by Sheldon Wolff, the Society adopted a two-tier membership process by which more senior contributors to the field became Fellows, and those who had published contributions, but were not judged ready to become Fellows, were elected as Members. This new format, of course, added immediately to the membership rolls and the Society now has over 2,000 members, with fifty to one hundred new Members and Fellows added annually. Additionally, the Society added the category of Corresponding Fellow, which made it possible for foreign colleagues to attend the meeting as full participants rather than as guests. Honorary membership continues to be a special category, largely reserved for outstanding foreign contributors to the field.

Rather than single out specific contributions from individuals in infectious disease, I have chosen to list the officers and awardees who have re-

TABLE 4.2.
PRESIDENTS OF THE INFECTIOUS DISEASES SOCIETY OF AMERICA

1964	Maxwell Finland
1965	John Enders
1966	Harry Dowling
1967	Charles Rammelkamp
1968	Walsh McDermott
1969	Albert Sabin
1970	Edward Kass
1971	Robert Austrian
1972	Gordon Meiklejohn
1973	Leighton Cluff
1974	George Jackson
1975	Dorothy Horstmann
1976	Edward Hook
1977	Theodore Woodward
1978	Harry Feldman
1979	Jay Sanford
1980	Floyd Denny
1981	Sheldon Wolff
1982	Sydney Finegold
1983	Abraham Braude
1984	Theodore Eickhoff
1985	Paul Quie
1986	Richard Hornick
1987	Calvin Kunin
1988	Jack Remington

ceived special recognition from the Infectious Diseases Society. These are listed in the accompanying table and give an overview of those who have provided the leadership within the Society (*Table 4.2*).

In 1978 the *Journal of Infectious Diseases*, published by the University of Chicago Press, and edited at that time by James Moulder, decided to review its own status. The journal had enjoyed a distinguished history since its founding in 1904 by Ludwig Hektoen. Hektoen was director of the John McCormick Memorial Institute for Infectious Diseases affiliated with the University of Chicago. For many years, Hektoen and the associate editor, Edwin O. Jordan, edited the journal, which was in the forefront of publications in the field. The Institute from which it sprang was abolished and slowly the fortunes of the *Journal* declined until, at the time that Moulder solicited the inquiry, the subscription list numbered approximately 1,700 subscribers, the great majority of which were institutions. There were doubts about the wisdom of continuing to publish at all. The University of Chicago Press appointed a committee to review the status of the *Journal* and to suggest either discontinuation of publication or an alternative format that would reverse the trend in readership. One of the members of the committee, the late A. F. Rasmussen, Jr., also a member of the IDSA and a close personal friend, discussed with me, while I was secretary of the Society, some of the possibilities, including the suggestion that the Infectious Diseases Society might be ready to publish a journal. I presented this to the Council.

The officers were, of course, concerned lest our fledgling group assume an obligation that it could not fulfill. The then president, Walsh McDermott, along with the secretary, explored the budgetary implications, and discussed several alternatives. By the next meeting, when Charles Rammelkamp had become president, an arrangement had been worked out with Jean Sacks, then Journals manager for the University of Chicago Press, whereby the Press would continue to publish the journal, but as a monthly with an entirely new format. Kass would become editor, with K. F. Austen, John Enders, William McCabe, Morton Swartz, Louis Weinstein, and later Bernard Fields as associate editors. The editorial office would be moved to Boston, and editorial meetings held regularly to ensure full discussion and peer review.

The scientific standards of the journal assured, the Press supported the new venture and an amicable and productive relationship between the Press and the Society has continued. The *Journal of Infectious Diseases* now has over 8,500 subscribers throughout the world, and is, by general opinion, the leading journal in this field. The first editors served for eleven years, after which the editorial office moved to the University of Illinois (Chicago) with George G. Jackson, second secretary and later president of the IDSA, as editor. At present, Martha Yow is editor, and the editorial office is at Baylor University School of Medicine in Houston. Each editor has been strongly supported by outstanding associate editors, and by a national and international editorial board, symbolizing the wide range of interest and the quality of the performance of the *Journal.*

The *Journal* had begun its second life by publishing reviews and symposia as well as research reports. By the time that I had completed the second five-year term as editor, pressure for publication of high quality research reports was making it difficult to find space for review articles. Also, an increased number of special supplements was putting heavy pressure on the editors and the staff. Therefore, I suggested that the Society publish a second journal, *Reviews of Infectious Diseases.* I agreed to start it, with associate editors Neil Blacklow, John David, Sherwood Gorbach, Alice Huang, Dennis Kasper, and Jerome Klein. In 1979 the first issue was published and the subscription list is now about 6,000 subscribers. Both journals of the Society are still growing. New journals in infectious disease have followed in many countries, and a new American journal devoted entirely to pediatric infectious disease is functioning successfully.

Subspecialty Certification in Infectious Diseases

The growth of the infectious diseases community occurred at a time when governmental and other agencies were becoming increasingly concerned about the growing costs of medical care and were beginning to set salary and training standards. Inevitably, specialists and subspecialists received added financial and structural recognition. The demand for consultation from infectious disease specialists increased; many diseases that had once been common and readily treated by all physicians had become so uncommon that diagnosis and treatment was considered the domain of specialists. In addition, the correlation of clinical findings with laboratory reporting was becoming more demanding. More sophisticated microbiological function led to the isolation of organisms that were relatively unfamiliar except to the specialist. Increasing resistance to antimicrobial drugs posed problems of choice. The proliferation of antimicrobial drugs presented an almost bewildering array of possibilities, with life-threatening consequences in many instances if the wrong choice was made. Immunosuppressive disorders, induced or spontaneous, and an aging population brought increasing numbers of patients with complex problems of infection and resistance. The need for specialists in infectious diseases was being perceived as never before.

A subspecialty board in infectious disease was established under the aegis of the American Board of Internal Medicine, chaired initially by Jay P. Sanford. By 1984, 1,534 physicians had passed the subspecialty board examinations. Candidates for the examination must have passed the examination for the American Board of Internal Medicine and have received at least two years of subspecialty training in infectious diseases. Approximately 250 diplomates are added to the subspecialty list annually. There are now 149 training programs in infectious disease in the United States, and programs exist in forty-one of the fifty states. The rate of growth has been so rapid that there is concern among thoughtful observers whether, with such continued growth, all of the infectious disease specialists can be absorbed into the medical system. There is hardly a better example of the dynamic nature of American society: a field that was barely represented only a few decades ago is now in danger of being oversupplied.

The earlier meetings devoted to antimicrobial agents were superseded by the Interscience Conference on Antimicrobial Agents and Chemotherapy (ICAAC) under the sponsorship of the American Society of Microbiology. Leadership in this endeavor was supplied by those interested primarily in antimicrobial agents, with representation from industry, government, and academia. A liaison committee between ICAAC and IDSA has coordinated the two meetings, which have been held in tandem in the same location so that those who were interested and eligible could attend both. Gladys Hobby was particularly instrumental in the setting up of ICAAC. She edited the annual volume that carried the proceedings of the meeting, and, when the volume became large enough, converted the annual volume into the journal *Antimicrobial Agents and Chemotherapy* and was its first editor. The annual meeting of ICAAC now draws 7,000 to 8,000 participants. The meeting, although principally oriented around antimicrobial agents, presents many brief papers on pathogenesis, epidemiology, and other aspects of infectious disease. The program is worked out in collaboration with representatives of the IDSA, which has retained its format of a limited number of lengthier reviews with extended discussion.

The breadth of infectious disease is such that it becomes impossible to list all of the organizations that are relevant to its activities. The American Epidemiological Society regularly provides a forum for presentation and discussion of new advances in epidemiology of infection, as does the larger and somewhat less elitist Society for Epidemiologic Research. The American Public Health Association and the combined meetings of the American Federation for Clinical Research, the American Society for Clinical Investigation, and the Association of American Physicians have major subsections in which relevant presentations are a major part of the meetings and where there is much competition to be on the program; the same is true for major medical organizations such as the American Medical Association and the American Colleges of Physicians, pediatrics and other relevant specialties, and the many special research groups within the various subspecialties.[17]

The role of the national government in stimulating research in infectious disease has been critical throughout the entire history of infectious disease in the United States. The National Institutes of Health (NIH), the Centers for Disease Control (which began as the Communicable Diseases Center), the Food and Drug Administration to a somewhat lesser but important degree, and many other governmental agencies have been essential resources providing intramural funds for major investigations within their own walls and in governmental installations throughout the world; particularly in the case of the NIH, they have provided the major share of funding for all infectious diseases research. The Walter Reed Army Institute of Research and the Naval Medical Center have contained strong and productive units in infectious disease research, and the Department of Defense has provided many contracts to academic centers for investigation. The Armed Forces Epidemiologic Board (AFEB) was a major coordinating group for infectious disease research carried on in and outside the military. Its achievements in the understanding of streptococcal disease, rheumatic fever, meningococcal disease, acute respiratory disease, influenza, and numerous other infectious diseases have been of major importance.

The Epidemic Intelligence Service (EIS) of the Centers for Disease Control (originally the Communicable Disease Center) has become a national and international resource. Founded and brought to maturity by Alexander Langmuir, it has educated hundreds of young physicians in the intricacies of epidemiologic investigation and analysis, solved innumerable outbreaks, defined new diseases as they appeared, and put into perspective outbreak after outbreak. Virtually every health department has at some time sought its assistance, as have increasing numbers of countries. A comparable international service is now being organized in collaboration with the World Health Organization.

Infectious disease and related research has received its share of international and national honors. The list of Nobel Prize winners contains many lessons, particularly for Americans. Only one prize had been won by an American before the fourth decade in which the prizes were awarded. In succeeding decades, this country garnered the major share of the prizes in all fields—undoubtedly a tribute to the academic and financial strength and political will to see science flourish. But the United States benefitted enormously from the losses of others. As of 1984, twenty-one of fifty-four American Nobel laureates were born in other countries, and several more received their awards in other countries but came to the United States to continue their work. Of all of the fields of study that were honored in Physiology and Medicine, eight awards were for work in immunology; four each in microbiology, antimicrobial therapy, and parasitology; two in virology; and several of those in biochemistry and genetics utilized microbial models or materials that were dependent on earlier microbiological investigation. To this list should be added the cautionary one of those who did not receive the award. Who could argue that O. T. Avery and his associates, René Dubos, K. F. Meyer, Michael Heidelberger, Theobald Smith, Walter Reed, and many others, excluding those still working actively and still eligible, did not do work of comparable importance?

Even this cursory survey, leaving out many important groups and organizations, and doing little justice to the vigorous leadership and the personal impact of many able and devoted participants, indicates the growth and the new vitality that the study of infectious disease has enjoyed. Such a survey, by concentrating on the United States, also fails to do justice to the key roles of international organizations such as the World Health Organization, the United Nations, the many international health foundations and organizations in many countries, the international scientific organizations, and the international network of industrial and pharmaceutical firms. They have all, in their respective ways, conducted and sponsored numerous investigations and many field trials of vaccines and new drugs. To tell the story of the relatively recent conquest of mortality from cholera, and the life-saving role of oral rehydration, required a lengthy and fascinating volume by van Heyningen and Seal. To offer in similar detail a description of the individuals, the institutions and the work, even of the past fifty years, would require an encyclopedic effort that would be enlightening and of great historic significance.

Much remains unsaid in this overview, but several conclusions can be drawn. The first is that in a field as vital to human survival and health as infectious disease, the problems will continue to be vast and the vistas virtually unlimited. The second is that in every active field of science new phenomena are uncovered that may change perceptions in other fields, and even create new ones. The study of infectious diseases illustrates this principle abundantly. The third is that in infectious disease the hard mills of the clinic and of the community are the final determinants of progress. The fourth, a corollary to the third, is that academic seers, despite their achievements, have proved to be hardly more perceptive in reading the future than have the crystal ball gazers of lesser background. We can confidently look ahead to further understandings of natural phenomena and of the prevention and treatment of human disease, and we can be confident also that infectious disease will produce its share of that progress.

I am grateful to Paul B. Beeson and Robert Petersdorf for permitting me to use some of the data that they have collected, to Amalie M. Kass for much careful editing and advice, and to Katherine Hayes for her assistance.

NOTES

1. This extraordinary escapade is one of the first controlled clinical experiments in American history. The details can be found in "Report of the Board of Health, December 16, 1802," *Boston Med Surg J* 45 (1901): 445, and it is summarized in *Medicine in Colonial Massachusetts* (Boston: Colonial Society of Massachusetts, 1980), 92–93.

2. Oliver Wendell Holmes, "The Contagiousness of Puerperal Fever." This famous paper was published in the *New England Quarterly Journal of Medicine and Surgery* 1 (1843): 503–30. Only one volume of the journal was ever published. The paper by Holmes has often been reprinted; an especially good reprinting is in *Medical Classics* 1 (1936): 211–43. Holmes summarized the many case reports that had accumulated suggesting the spread of puerperal sepsis from patients who had a variety of septic diseases; only the attending doctor or the instruments seemed to account for the spread. When the paper was initially read to the Boston Society for Medical Improvement, the Society urged Holmes to publish it. Immediately, Charles Delucena Meigs of Philadelphia, a distinguished obstetrician, attacked Holmes, holding that no gentleman would be so unclean as to spread the pestilence, and ascribed the disease to Providence. Holmes wrote his second paper, entitled "Puerperal Sepsis as a Private Pestilence," as a riposte. It can be found in the *Medical Classics,* as above, following the first paper. Holmes attacked the stultifying atmosphere that accepted personal views over carefully collected observations, showing the influence of his studies with Pierre-Charles-Alexandre Louis in France. His devastating attack on Meigs took the form of an explanation to students of why they should not be unduly confused by the claims and counterclaims with respect to puerperal sepsis, pointing out that "We do not deny that the God of battles decides the fate of nations; but we like to have the biggest squadrons on our side, and we are particular that our soldiers should not only say their prayers, but also keep their powder dry."

To the medical students, in a studied attempt to help them from their presumed state of confusion, he indicated that they often confounded belief with evidence, and that they often did not consider a point settled, no matter how strong the evidence, while there was still controversy. "They have not learned that error is got out of the minds that cherish it, as the taenia is removed from the body, one joint, or a few joints at a time. . . . They naturally have faith in their instructors, turning to them for truth, and taking what they may choose to give them; babes in knowledge, not yet able to tell the breast from the bottle, pumping away for the milk of truth at all that offers, were it nothing better than a Professor's shrivelled forefinger."

3. Thomas McKeown, *The Modern Rise of Population* (London: Edward Arnold, 1976); Edward H. Kass, "Infectious Disease and Social Change," *J Infect Dis* 123 (1971): 110–14; Harry F. Dowling, *Fighting Infection* (Cambridge, MA: Harvard University Press, 1977).

4. Austin, Flint, "On the Logical Proof of the Contagiousness and of the Non-contagiousness of Disease," *NY Med J* 19 (1874): 113–33. See also L. A. Stimson, "Bacteria and their Influence upon the Origin and Development of Septic Complications of Wounds, *NY Med J* 22 (1875): 113–15.

5. Joseph Lister, "On a New Method of Treating Compound Fractures, Abscess, etc., with Observations on the Conditions of Suppuration," *Lancet* 1 (1867): 364–73, 418–20. The method consisted of wrapping the wound with fabrics that had been saturated with dilute carbolic acid, the diluent being either water or oil.

The method ran into stormy opposition in London, but was tested by several American surgeons, including Jackson at the Massachusetts General Hospital, with excellent results. See also, Lister's lecture, "On the Antiseptic Principle in Surgery," in the *British Medical Journal,* 21 September, 1867. See also Robert White, "Personal Observations of Lister's Antiseptic Treatment," *Boston Med Surg J* 97 (1877): 235–45 and O. T. Howe and H. L. Morse: "Surgical Cases of Dr. Warren. Cases of Injury to Hand from Explosion: Lister's Dressing and Chondrosarcoma of the Ulva: Lister's Dressing." *Boston Med Surg J* 97 (1877): 371–73.

6. Thomas J. Burrill, at the Illinois Industrial University, later the University of Illinois, described *Micrococcus amylovorus* in 1880 as the cause of blight, especially in pear and sometimes apple trees. From Paul F. Clark, *Pioneer Microbiologists of America* (Madison: University of Wisconsin Press, 1961).

7. D. E. Salmon and T. Smith, "The Bacterium of Swine-plague." *Am Month Microsc J* 7 (1886): 204–5. This was followed, in the same year, with the next discovery, showing the way to a whole series of bacterial vaccines: idem, "On a New Method of Producing Immunity from Contagious Diseases," *Proc Biol Soc Washington* 3 (1886): 29–33.

8. Theobald Smith was one of the most remarkable of all American contributors to understanding infectious disease. In addition to the aforementioned studies with Salmon, he demonstrated that arthropods could carry infectious agents to mammals: "Investigations into the Nature, Causation, and Prevention of Southern Cattle Fever," published in *Bureau of Animal Industry, Eighth and Ninth Annual Reports* (Washington: Government Printing Office, 1891 and 1892; repr. in *Medical Classics* 1 (1937): 379–596. His contributions to tuberculosis, immunity, and many other aspects of infection and immunity are landmarks.

9. George M. Sternberg was an Army physician who was given permission to work at Johns Hopkins Medical School. He was among the earliest to isolate the pneumococcus, studied yellow fever, and made many other important contributions to the early understanding of microbial disease. He also founded the Army Medical School and rejuvenated a rather poorly functioning Army Medical Corps.

10. Clark, *Microbiologists of America* and H. A. Lechevalier and M. Solotorovsky, *Three Centuries of Microbiology* (New York: McGraw Hill, 1965).

11. M. P. Ravenel, ed., *A Half Century of Public Health* (New York: American Public Health Association, 1921).

12. G. Domagk, "A Contribution to the Chemotherapy of Bacterial Infections. Classics in Infectious Diseases," *Rev Infect Dis* 8 (1986): 163–66.

13. Gladys L. Hobby, *Penicillin: Meeting the Challenge* (New Haven: Yale University Press, 1985) and Ronald W. Clark, *The Life of Ernst Chain, Penicillin and Beyond* (London: Weidenfeld and Nicolson, 1985).

14. Selman A. Waksman, *Scientific Contributions of Selman A. Waksman; Selected Articles Published in Honor of his 80th Birthday,* H. Boyd Woodruff, ed. (New Brunswick, NJ: Rutgers University Press, 1968).

15. H. Bostrom and N. Ljundstedt, *Medical Aspects of Mortality Statistics* (Stockholm: Almqvist and Wiksell International, 1981).

16. E. H. Kass and K. M. Hayes, "A History of the Infectious Diseases Society of America, 1962–1987," *Reviews Infect Dis* 1988 (Suppl.) (in press).

17. R. L. Petersdorf, "Whither Infectious Diseases? Memories, Manpower and Money," *J Infect Dis* 153 (1986): 189–95.

5

One Hundred Years of American Gastroenterology

JOSEPH B. KIRSNER

> We are like dwarfs situated on the shoulders of giants. We see more things than the ancients and things more distant. But it is neither due to the sharpness of our sight nor the greatness of our stature. It is simply because they have lent us their own.
>
> *Bernal of Chartres (12th century)*

The 1880s were a watershed in American medicine. Science and medicine began to interact more closely, initially via the emergence of bacteriology, and subsequently as the rise of the university-based medical school and new laboratories awakened public interest in scientific medicine and stimulated early medical philanthropy.[1,2] Considerable knowledge of the digestive system had been accumulated by 1886. The gross anatomy of the gastrointestinal tract had been largely identified. Investigators had begun to reveal the digestive and metabolic capacities of the pancreas, liver, and gastrointestinal tract. After two thousand years of speculation, gastric function had been partially clarified by the 1803 experiments of a group of medical students at the University of Pennsylvania, by William Prout's identification of hydrochloric acid, and through William Beaumont's physiologic studies (1823–1833) on Alexis St. Martin.

TABLE 5.1.
EARLY AMERICAN GASTROENTEROLOGY BOOKS

1714	Weslen, John. *Primitive Physick or An Easy and Natural Method of Curing Most Diseases.* Philadelphia
1807	Ewell, James. *The Medical Companion or Family Physician*
1807	Gunn. *Domestic Medicine or Poor Man's Friend*
1850	Drake, Daniel. *Diseases of Malaria in the Interior Valley of North America.* Urbana, Illinois: University of Illinois Press
1852	Smith, H. H. *A System of Operative Surgery.* Philadelphia: Lippincott, Grambo and Company
[?]	Massie, J. C. *Treatise on Eclectic Southern Practice of Medicine*
1854	Morgan, William. *The Homeopathic Treatment of Indigestion, Constipation and Haemorrhoids.* Philadelphia: Rademacher & Sheek
1875	Drewery, G. O. *Common Sense Management of the Stomach.* New York
1896	Kellogg, J. H. *The Stomach: Its Disorders, and How to Cure Them.* Battle Creek, Michigan: Modern Medicine Publishing Company
1897	Hemmeter, John C. *Diseases of the Stomach Their Special Pathology, Diagnosis, and Treatment, with Sections on Anatomy, Physiology, Analysis of Stomach Contents, Dietetics, Surgery of the Stomach, etc. (In Three Parts).* Philadelphia: P. Blakiston's Sons
1900	Einhorn, Max. *Diseases of the Intestines.* New York: William Wood
1901	Hemmeter, John C. *Diseases of the Stomach*
1904	Benedict, A. L. *Practical Dietetics 1904—Golden Rules of Dietetics*
1906	Tuttle, J. T. *A Treatise on Diseases of the Anus, Rectum and Pelvic Colon.* 2nd edition. New York: Appleton
1907	Boas, I. *Diseases of the Stomach.* Translated by A. Bernheim. Philadelphia: F. A. Davis
1910	Hemmeter, John C. *Diseases of the Intestines: Their Special Pathology, Diagnosis, and Treatment.* 2 volumes. Philadelphia: P. Blakiston's Sons
1910	Opie, Eugene L. *Disease of the Pancreas.* 2 editions. Philadelphia: Lippincott
1911	Cannon, Walter B. *The Mechanical Factors of Digestion.* New York: Longmans
1911	Cannon, Walter B. *Bodily Changes in Pain, Hunger, Fear and Rage.* 2 editions. New York: Longmans
1911	Aaron, C. D. *Diseases of the Stomach with Special Reference to Treatment.* Philadelphia: Lea & Febiger
1912	Musser, J. H., and A. O. J. Kelly. *A Handbook of Practical Treatment.* Philadelphia: W. B. Saunders
1913	Coleman, Robert. *Diseases of the Stomach, Intestines, and Pancreas.* Philadelphia: W. B. Saunders
1913	Lockwood, G. R. *Diseases of the Stomach including Dietetic and Medicinal Treatment.* Philadelphia: Lea & Febiger
1913	Kemp, R. C. *Diseases of the Stomach, Intestines and Pancreas.* Philadelphia: W. B. Saunders
1914	Niles, G. M. *The Diagnosis and Treatment of Digestive Diseases.* Philadelphia: P. Blakiston's Sons

TABLE 5.1.
(CONTINUED)

1914	Lynch, J. M. *Diseases of the Rectum and Colon and Their Surgical Treatment.* Philadelphia: Lea & Febiger
1914	Stockton, Charles G. *Diseases of the Stomach and Their Relation to Other Diseases.* New York: D. Appleton
1915	Aaron, C. D. *Diseases of the Digestive Organs*
1916	Carlson, Anton Julius. *The Control of Hunger in Health and Disease.* Chicago: University of Chicago Press
1917	Kellogg, J. H. *Colon Hygiene.* Michigan: Good Health Publishing Company
1918	Kellogg, J. H. *Autointoxication or Intestinal Toxemia.* Battle Creek, Michigan: Modern Medicine Publishing Company
1920	Carman, Russell D. *The Roentgen Diagnosis of Disease of the Alimentary Canal.* 2 editions. Philadelphia: W. B. Saunders
1921	Aaron, C. D. *Diseases of the Digestive Organs with Special Reference to Their Diagnosis and Treatment.* Philadelphia: Lea & Febiger
1922	Alvarez, Walter C. *The Mechanics of the Digestive Tract.* New York: Paul B. Hoeber
1922	Case, J. T. *The X-ray Examinations of the Alimentary Tract.* Southmoth, Troy, New York
1923	Lyon, B. B. Vincent. *Non-surgical Drainage of the Gallbladder and Biliary Tract.* Philadelphia: Lea & Febiger
1927	Crohn, Burrill B. *Affections of the Stomach.* Philadelphia: W. B. Saunders
1927	Rehfuss, Martin E. *Diagnosis and Treatment of Diseases of the Stomach with an Introduction to Practical Gastro-Enterology.* Philadelphia: W. B. Saunders
1929	Kantor, John L. *The Treatment of the Common Disorders of Digestion.* St. Louis: C. V. Mosby
1930	Alvarez, Walter C. *Nervous Indigestion.* New York: Paul B. Hoeber
1930	Pottenger, Francis Marion. *Symptoms of Visceral Disease. A Study of the Vegetative Nervous System in its Relationship to Clinical Medicine.* 4 editions. St. Louis: C. V. Mosby
1931	Morgan, William Gerry. *Functional Disorders of the Gastrointestinal Tract.* Philadelphia: Lippincott
1932	Rankin, F. W., Fred Wharton, Arnold Bargen, and L. A. Buie. *The Colon, Rectum and Anus.* Philadelphia: W. B. Saunders
1933	Bloomfield, A. L., and W. S. Polland. *Gastric Anucidity.* New York: MacMillan
1935	Bargen, J. A. *Management of Colitis.* National Medical Book Company
1935	Eusterman, George B., and Donald C. Balfour. *The Stomach and Duodenum.* Philadelphia: W. B. Saunders
1935	Cole, L. G. *Radiologic Exploration of the Mucosa of the Gastrointestinal Tract.* St. Paul: Bruce
1936	Jackson, C., and C. L. Jackson. *Disease of the Air and Food Passages of Foreign Body Origin.* Philadelphia: W. B. Saunders

TABLE 5.1.
(CONTINUED)

1938	Jones, C. M. *Digestive Tract Pain (Diagnosis and Treatment, Experimental Observations)*. New York: MacArthur
1937	Schindler, R. *Gastroscopy, The Endoscopic Study of Gastric Pathology*. Chicago: University of Chicago Press
1939	Soper, H. W. *Clinical Gastroenterology*. St. Louis: C. V. Mosby
1940	Buckstein, Jacob. *Clinical Roentgenology of the Alimentary Tract*. Philadelphia: W. B. Saunders
1948	Alvarez, Walter C. *An Introduction to Gastro-Enterology*. New York: Paul B. Hoeber

The story of Beaumont (1785–1853) and his remarkable observations on St. Martin is a classic chapter in the history of American physiology and gastroenterology.[3,4] Walter B. Cannon, in his 1933 Beaumont Foundation lecture,[5] wrote: "Working in a backwoods Army post, under the most unfavorable conditions, without laboratory aid, with no journals or other literature to consult, with no associates to encourage him and to help him create an atmosphere for research, Beaumont for long periods conducted careful studies on his patient." Beaumont's resourceful studies were the most comprehensive observations of gastric function heretofore performed and influenced gastroenterologic thought significantly.[6] Less well appreciated is the fact that Beaumont's gastric fistula studies were neither the first nor the last; more than a dozen instances of physiologic studies in gastric fistula patients have been recorded in the world literature.

By 1886, fifty years had elapsed since Heinrich Geissler of Bonn, Germany, a glassblower, constructed tubes containing various gases which produced a soft glow with the passage of a high tension electrical discharge. These tubes were the forerunner of the Geissler-modified Crookes tube, utilized by W. C. Roentgen in 1895 to discover the X ray and applied by W. B. Cannon to his physiologic studies of the gastrointestinal tract.[7] By 1886, nitrous oxide, ether, and chloroform had been introduced as anesthetics, accelerating the development of surgery. The surgical idea of antisepsis had been introduced by Joseph Lister, facilitating the initial gallbladder operations in America in 1867 of J. Bobbs and M. Sims. Nearly fifty years also had elapsed since Austin Flint had written on dyspepsia (1841) and on the relationship between gastric atrophy and pernicious anemia; soon thereafter Jackson (1854) and Dalton (1857) performed physiologic studies on bile and on the processes of digestion. In 1879 J. C. Woodward surveyed the terrible diarrheal diseases among Union soldiers during the Civil War and described bacillary dysentery before the discovery of the Shiga, Kruse, and Flexner dysentery bacilli. Reviews of peptic ulcer, dilatation of the stomach and gastric cancer by William Welch in Pepper's *System of Medicine* (1885), C. Herter's "Bacterial Infections of the Digestive Tract," and William J. Mayo's "Acquired Diverticulitis of the Large Intestine" reflected a significant awareness of digestive problems.[8] At the first meeting of the Association of American Physicians on 17 June 1886, president Francis Delafield (1841–1915) discussed "chronic catarrhal gastritis." Reginald Fitz presented his classic study of acute appendicitis at the same meeting[9] and three years later described acute pancreatitis,[10] continuing in America the meticulous clinical analysis advocated by Pierre Louis of Paris fifty years earlier. American textbooks on digestive diseases appeared several years later (*Table 5.1*). Gastroenterology journals were not to appear in America for several decades (*Table 5.2*).

TABLE 5.2.
SOME EARLY GASTROENTEROLOGY (AND GI-RELATED) JOURNALS

1895	*Archiv fur Verdauungskrankheiten mit Einschluss der Stoffwechsel Pathologie und der Diatetik* (I. Boas) (*Gastroenterologia* in 1939)
1899	*Transactions American Proctologic Society*
1902	*Japanese Journal of Gastroenterology*
1903–1934	*Transactions of the American Gastroenterological Association*
1907	*Archives Français des Maladies de la Appareil Digestif et du Maladies de la Nutrition* (A. Mathieu)
1911	*American Journal of Gastroenterology* (until 1914)
1914–1916	*Review of Gastroenterology* (A. Bassler)
1916	*American Journal of Gastroenterology* consolidated with the *Proctologist* (until December 1916)
1934	*American Journal of Digestive Diseases and Nutrition* (B. S. Cornell)
1935	*Revista de Gastroenterologia de Mexico*
1936	*Proctology*
1943	*Gastroenterology*
1946	*GEN* (Venezuela)
1954	Resumption of *American Journal of Gastroenterology* (S. Weiss)
1960	*Gut*

Increasing Medical Specialization—Late Nineteenth Century

Advances in American medicine accelerated during the last quarter of the nineteenth century and the early years of the twentieth century. The physical examination had become a "sophisticated method with an array of bedside instruments,"[11] fostering specialism.[12] Those responsible for training new physicians strove to keep pace. Although William Osler is credited with creating the clinical clerkship at Johns Hopkins, E. D. Fenner of New Orleans probably had preceded him.[13] Graduate medical schools in New York, Philadelphia, and Chicago now provided opportunities for advanced study.[14,15] And, as A. M. Harvey notes, "No single event had a more profound effect on medical education and medical practice than the development of full-time positions in clinical departments, beginning at Johns Hopkins University."[16] From the full-time system emerged the clinical scientist, a clinician who could bridge the gap between the practicing physician and the laboratory scientist. Thus by 1927 the clinical departments at the University of Chicago had adopted this full-time principle, and gastroenterology, under the direction of Walter Lincoln Palmer, was a major section within a department of medicine composed entirely of medical specialties, an arrangement later followed by many academic medical centers.

Early German Gastroenterology and Its Impact On American Gastroenterology By the 1880s, clinical medicine and the medical sciences had reached new heights in Germany, where the relationship between the patient's bedside and the laboratory bench were defined more clearly than anywhere else. Carl Ludwig (1816–1895) in Leipzig and Johannes Müller (1801–1858) in Berlin dominated German science. They were followed by Theodor Schwann, Jakob Henle, Ludwig Traube, Rudolf Virchow, and Hermann von Helmholtz, who were important contributors to gastroenterologic knowledge. F. T. von Frerichs (1819–1888), in his monograph *On Diseases of the Liver*, had described acute yellow atrophy of the liver and other liver diseases. Ottmar Rosenbach (1851–1907), a disciple of Julius Cohnheim, had advocated the physiologically oriented quantitative clinical approach previously advanced by Ludwig Traube (1818–1876) and Frerichs. Theodore Billroth (1829–1894) of Vienna and his students were pioneering new operative techniques for digestive diseases requiring surgery. In Berlin Ismar Boas (1858–1938), a student of Carl Ewald, established the first gastroenterology clinic in 1885 (the Ambulatorium for Gastric and Intestinal Disease), an early forerunner of the American specialty clinic. By 1906, when the Ambulatorium closed, he had instructed more than 1,000 physicians including a hundred "gastroenterologists." Boas is credited with demonstrating the presence of occult blood in diseases of the gastrointestinal tract, and the absence of hydrochloric acid and the presence of lactic acid in carcinoma of the stomach. A prolific writer, Boas established the first specialty journal in gastroenterology, the *Archiv fur Verdauungskrankheiten mit Einschluss der Stoffwechsel pathologie und des Diatetik.*[17] The impact of German biomedical sciences and clinical medicine on the United States was substantial and, through the immigration to America of physicians trained during this time, including J. Hemmeter, Max Einhorn, M. Manges, and J. Kaufmann, accelerated the trend to specialization in gastroenterology.[18]

Increasing American Interest in Gastroenterology Despite progress in other fields of medicine,[19] scientific advance in American gastroenterology lagged. "Stomach specialists" were criticized as preoccupied with the stomach tube. Diagnostic technology was crude and access to the digestive tract remained difficult. Curative treatments were lacking. Samuel Gee's 1888 dictum "Medicine is not a science but an empirical art" was especially applicable to the gastroenterology of the 1880s.

Nevertheless, in 1889 A. J. Baxter[20] of Astoria, Illinois, Chairman of a state Committee on Diseases of the Alimentary Tract, had emphasized the relationship of dyspepsia to nervous tension or to indiscretions in diet. William Osler's (1849–1919) papers on gastric and duodenal ulcer, amebic dysentery, jaundice, cirrhosis of the liver, gallstones, cancer of the stomach, abdominal tumors and "angina abdominis" were outstanding clinical treatises.[21] Publications such as *Diseases of the Stomach* by J. C. Hemmeter of Baltimore and *Diseases of the Stomach and Intestines* by Max Einhorn (1862–1953) of New York in 1897 (*Table 5.1*) heightened clinical interest in digestive disorders and attracted an increasing number of physicians to the field. With this rising interest came a sense of dissatisfaction, among the better educated (often German-trained) gastroenterologic physicians, with the quality of clinical gastroenterology in this country, although new diagnostic instruments and improving surgical techniques had expanded the diagnostic and therapeutic capabilities of the "stomach specialist." Professionalization and the increasingly focused knowledge of the gastrointestinal specialist intensified the desire for public recognition and peer approval.

TABLE 5.3.
FOUNDING MEMBERS OF THE AMERICAN GASTROENTEROLOGICAL ASSOCIATION (3 June 1897)

C. D. Aaron (Detroit)	J. Kaufmann (New York)
A. L. Benedict (Buffalo)*	M. Manges (New York)*
L. Brinton (Philadelphia)*	F. H. Murdock (Pittsburgh)
A. P. Buckman (Indiana)*	C. E. Simon (Baltimore)*
M. Einhorn (New York)	D. D. Stewart (Philadelphia)
H. L. Elsner (Syracuse)	C. G. Stockton (Buffalo)
J. Friedenwald (Baltimore)	T. H. Stuckey (Louisville)*
J. C. Hemmeter (Baltimore)	H. E. Tuley (Louisville)*
A. A. Jones (Buffalo)	

*Early resignation

Formation of The American Gastroenterologic Association In 1886 Heinrich Salzer, a German-educated immigrant to Baltimore, organized the *Gastroenterologische Krankheiten Verein* in an attempt to unite physicians interested in disorders of the digestive system. The effort failed. However, the activities of physicians like Hemmeter, Einhorn, Meltzer, and others trained in gastrointestinal diseases in Germany, and the increasing involvement of American-educated physicians, renewed efforts to create a special digestive disease society. Those efforts bore fruit a decade later.

On 3 June 1897, at the annual meeting of the American Medical Association in Philadelphia, eight physicians[22] interested in the study of the digestive tract met in the office of Dr. David D. Stewart. From the meeting evolved the American Gastroenterological Association (AGA) (*Table 5.3*). The draft of a constitution and bylaws included the objective of "promoting the study of the digestive tract in all its phases."

The initial course of the AGA was uncertain. There was little investigation in digestive disorders. Gastrointestinal diagnoses of the time included such vague entities as gastric neurasthenia, visceroptosis, sluggish bile, and intestinal autointoxication ("intestinal sewage poisoning"). Therapeutic measures such as gastric douches, bitters, stomachics, artificial ferments (malt diastase, pancreatin, papain), sarsaparilla and dandelion as biliary stimulants, abdominal corsets, high colonic enemas, and the insufflation of carbonic acid gas for rectal disease reflected the limited state of gastroenterologic knowledge. Despite the increasing specialism of medicine at the turn of the nineteenth century, internists and other specialists were reluctant to further subdivide the field and there was concern with a "narrow point of view."

Samuel J. Meltzer (1851–1920) was a major figure in the early scientific development of gastroenterology in America. Before immigrating to New York in 1883, he had studied in Berlin and in Konigsberg with Hugo von Kronecker, himself a student of Carl Ludwig. Meltzer investigated the process of deglutition with himself as a subject, and developed the Kronecker-Meltzer theory that swallowed substances are propelled down the esophagus by pressure developed in the mouth rather than by peristaltic waves, a concept later challenged successfully by W. B. Cannon. While in general practice in New York, Meltzer was the obstetrician for the infant Burrill Crohn in 1884 (perhaps destining him for gastroenterology at birth!). Working in George Curtis' physiologic laboratory at Columbia University and in Welch's pathology laboratory at Bellevue Hospital, Meltzer plunged into research on the actions of adrenalin upon blood vessels and the pupillary muscles. He developed a method of artificial respiration by pharyngeal and intratracheal insufflation. He also observed that the local application of magnesium sulfate on the mucosa induced a complete local relaxation of the intestinal wall, and he suggested its use via the duodenal tube in patients with biliary colic or jaundice, in whom biliary secretion could be collected for diagnostic purposes. The relaxation of the sphincter of Oddi, he anticipated, might facilitate the elimination of a calculus of "moderate size."[23] These observations, which were among the earliest illustrating the close relationship between so-called basic science and clinical knowledge, subsequently led to extensive studies of gallbladder and bile duct disease via cytologic and chemical examination of aspirated bile secretion.[24]

According to Meltzer, the future of medicine depended on the application of science to clinical problems. He was a key figure in the founding of some of America's most prestigious scientific organizations, including The American Physiological Society, The American Society for Clinical Investigation (1908), and The Society for Experimental Biology and Medicine (1905), dubbed the "Meltzer-Verein." In 1904 Meltzer assumed the presidency of the fledgling American Gastroenterological Association. He strongly advocated specialist medical science. Speaking to the AGA, Meltzer called for specialization as a means of fostering the science of medicine and gastroenterology even more than its practice. Meltzer, the founder of experimental medicine in America, gave up practice in 1904 and joined the recently established (1901) Rockefeller Institute, where he remained until his death in 1920. Although not involved in the clinical study of digestive diseases, he had exerted a lasting influence on the evolving field of gastroenterology.[25]

The AGA's First Decade The first scientific meeting of the AGA was in Washington, D.C. on 2 May 1898. Charles G. Stockton presided at a gathering of eight members and several visitors. The second meeting in 1899, also in Washington, attracted seven members; the third meeting, in 1900, twelve members. At the sixth meeting, President John C. Hemmeter of Baltimore spoke on "The Use and Abuse of the Imagination in Experiments and Observations in Medicine." The seventh meeting was on 6 and 7 June 1904 in Atlantic City, with twenty-nine members in attendance (down from thirty-nine in the preceding year). Twenty-five percent of the members enrolled during the first seven years had resigned, including two former presidents. The eighth meeting of the AGA in New York on 24 and 25 April 1905 included papers by W. B. Cannon on "Motor Activities of the G.I. Tract" and Lafayette B. Mendel on "The Chemical Processes of Digestion" and attracted a larger audience. By the 10th meeting of the AGA in 1907, the AGA membership consisted of fifty active members and two honorary and two corresponding members.[26]

Gastroenterology was thus one of the earliest specialties to emerge. Its presence, predating that of its future parent internal medicine, did not go unnoticed. An item in the *Journal of the American Medical Association* (1899) reflected the prevailing British attitude toward medical specialism in America and particularly toward proctology. On the defensive, the editorialist quoted the *Journal*'s British counterpart:

> We are at a loss to know whether or not to feel offended at this sarcastic reference to one of our young societies by the *British Medical Journal*. In its issue for April 29, 1899, under the caption 'Specialism in the United States,' it says: 'The development of medical specialism in the United States suggests that in that enlightened republic a condition of things may in time be brought about like unto that which prevailed in ancient Egypt, where the human body was, as it were, pegged out in claims, each of which was allotted to a particular class of specialists. Among the most recent indications of this tendency may be noted the formation of an American Association of Proctologists, which is to devote itself to the cultivation of rectal surgery, a field which it appears has been very much neglected by the physician and the general surgeon. . . . A body whose scientific enterprise extends somewhat higher is the American Gastro-Enterologic Association, which will hold its sec-

> ond annual meeting in Washington on May 2, after the meeting of the Association of American Physicians.'[27]

It may be noted parenthetically that the British Society of Gastroenterology was established in 1937.

AGA Presidential Themes A theme emphasized by most AGA presidents throughout the twentieth century has been the need for more science in gastroenterology, and for scholarly clinical work,[28] a need that continues today. In 1923 David Riesman added that specialists were now advancing medicine even while criticized, by laymen and general practitioners alike, as "faddists." George M. Piersol noted in 1927 that gastroenterologists had "laid themselves open to criticism" by getting "carried away by their subject." He emphasized the importance of a broad medical perspective: "It can be truly said that although a good internist may be a poor gastro-enterologist, a good gastro-enterologist must never be a poor internist." In 1928 W. C. Alvarez of the Mayo Clinic stressed the importance of specialists remaining open to laboratory investigation from "all over the civilized world," even that "made by men outside our ranks."

By the 1940s, the emphasis was on a thorough foundation in internal medicine, an important issue in considering certification in gastroenterology. Walter L. Palmer of Chicago in 1946 recalled the discussion in the 1930s as to a separate board on gastroenterology:

> The view finally prevailed that the specialist in digestive disease should be primarily an internist and secondarily a gastroenterologist. A criticism often levelled at all specialists is their alleged failure to see the patient as an individual. The proper correction for this defect, it seems to me, is not to abandon specialization but rather to train every specialist that he must be first of all a physician.

This principle, in fact, has been the basis for the great majority of training programs in gastroenterology into the 1980s.

In the 1950s and 1960s, as NIH funding levels increased dramatically, presidential messages emphasized the need for quality up-to-date research. In 1954 Dwight L. Wilbur commented,

> Research in gastroenterology is lagging far behind that in most other branches of medicine and particularly far behind researches in disease of the cardiovascular system, cancer, poliomyelitis, diabetes, and many other disorders. In fact, there is evidence of lack of interest on the part

> of medical students and instructors in the basic scientific aspects of diseases of the gastrointestinal tract. . . . This situation has arisen in part because clinical gastroenterology developed early and broke away from internal medicine and the basic medical sciences, because of the difficulty of applying modern quantitative methods in research in gastroenterology, and, because, owing to the lack of emotional or public health appeal of diseases of the gastrointestinal tract, there is no public urge or demand for research.

The Gastroenterology Research Group, formed in 1956 by Joseph B. Kirsner and E. C. Texter of Chicago, later an important forum for research in gastroenterology, was a direct response to this speech.

The Early Twentieth Century

An increasing number of physicians and scientists entered the field of gastroenterology during the early years of the twentieth century (*Table 5.4*). Individually, each contributed substantially to the increasing knowledge of the digestive tract. Collectively, these early contributions involved controlled observation and quantitation by means of instruments developed by Hemmeter, Einhorn, Gross, Turck, and others, including (1) the stomach bucket, (2) string test for peptic ulcer, (3) tests for gastrointestinal (GI) motility, (4) the duodenal bucket to collect duodenal secretions, (5) a duodenal feeding apparatus for peptic ulcer, (6) the pyloric dilator, (7) the simultaneous gastroduodenal aspirator, (8) a jointed long intestinal tube, and (9) a primitive endoscope. In 1889 Einhorn developed the gastro-diaphane, an incandescent light on the end of a soft rubber stomach tube connected by wires to a storage battery used for lighting up the stomach and noting its position, size, and outline. While subsequently rendered obsolete, these instruments reflected typical early activity in the field of gastroenterology.[29]

The experimental achievements of Walter Bradford Cannon (1871–1945) of Harvard heralded a new era in American physiology. Complementing the work of I. P. Pavlov (1849–1936) on gastric secretion,[30] Samuel Meltzer's studies on deglutition, and Roentgen's 1895 discovery of the X ray, and following the suggestion of his physiology professor Henry I. Bowditch, Cannon began to study esophageal peristalsis with a crude X ray apparatus in 1896. In his first experiment, he fed a pearl button to a dog. By the fluoroscopic screen he was able to watch it pass down the esophagus into the stomach; the movement was described as "regular", as reported later by Davenport.[31] Cannon then studied the goose and the cat, immobilizing the

TABLE 5.4.
AMERICAN GASTROENTEROLOGY IN THE TWENTIETH CENTURY: PHYSICIANS AND SCIENTISTS

Outstanding Clinicians	
C. G. Aaron	Ludwig Kast
T. Althausen	Jacob Kaufmann
A. F. C. Andresen	J. A. Lichty
J. A. Bargen	B. B. Vincent Lyon
A. Bassler	John Mateer
W. A. Bastedo	C. McVicar
Henry W. Bettman	T. G. Miller
H. L. Bockus	R. W. Mills
R. Boles, Sr.	Walter L. Palmer
T. Brown	M. Paulson
T. R. Brown	G. M. Peirsall
A. F. Chace	Milton Portis
M. Comfort	Sidney Portis
B. B. Crohn	M. E. Rehfuss
Max Einhorn	David Reisman
G. B. Eusterman	C. Simon
Julius Friedenwald	Albert Snell
J. C. Hemmeter	F. B. Turck
I. R. Jankelson	James Weir
C. M. Jones	F. W. White
Sara Jordan	A. Winkelstein
J. L. Kantor	
Endoscopists	
E. G. Benedict	H. Plummer
Chevalier Jackson	Rudolf Schindler
H. Moersch	P. Vinson
Surgeons	
Donald C. Balfour	John H. Garlock
A. A. Berg	W. W. Keen
Joseph Bloodgood	F. Lahey
J. Deaver	William J. Mayo
R. Elman	Willy Meyer
J. T. Finney	Albert J. Ochsner

TABLE 5.4.
(CONTINUED)

Radiologists	
F. J. Baetjer	J. Mills
Russell Carman	S. Morrison
J. T. Case	H. Pancoast
L. G. Cole	D. D. Stewart
B. Kirklin	
Physiologist-Scientists	
W. C. Alvarez	S. A. Komarov
B. P. Babkin	L. B. Mendel
W. B. Cannon	H. Necheles
A. J. Carlson	Harry Shay
Franklin Hollander	J. E. Thomas
A. C. Ivy	H. B. Williams

animals in a box. He found that he could visualize the stomach and the intestines by giving the animal salts of heavy metals, especially bismuth and later barium, to swallow, either suspended in liquid or mixed with the animal's food. In this way he was able to observe the passage of food from the mouth to the rectum. Cannon later studied at last twelve species of vertebrates and in 1898 published the first comprehensive study of the movements of the stomach during digestion.[32] A later paper described early studies of the digestive tract in humans.[33] An impressive number of papers and monographs followed (*Table 5.5*). The noted physiologist H. W. Davenport has reviewed Cannon's contributions to gastroenterology.[34,35] These include pioneering physiologic studies of the motor activity of the esophagus; physiologic (acid) control of the lower esophageal sphincter and of the pylorus; vagus regulation of the motor activity of the esophagus; the movements of the stomach, small intestine, and colon; the nature and control of gastric emptying; the nature of hunger; the neural organization of emotional expression as observed in the gastrointestinal tract; the impact of emotional activity on gastrointestinal function; and the intrinsic and external innervation of the gastrointestinal tract.

Bertram W. Sippy (1866–1924), a contemporary of Hemmeter, Einhorn, and Friedenwald, was a major figure in Chicago and American gastroenterology during the first quarter of the twentieth century.[36] Trained as a neurologist (like Arthur Hurst) and as an internist, Sippy was a superb clinician and teacher; his students included such prominent gastroenterologists as Ralph C. Brown and Walter L. Palmer of Chicago, and Sara M. Jordan and Edward S. Emery of Boston. Sippy's acid neutralization program for peptic ulcer—utilizing diet and bismuth subcarbonate, sodium bicarbonate and calcium carbonate, and periodic gastric aspiration—was for many years the dominant therapy for peptic ulcer.[37] A feature of the 1915 meeting of the American Association of Physicians was the debate on the management of peptic ulcer: with Sippy defending the medical treatment and W. J. Mayo supporting the surgical approach, the outcome predictably was a draw.

Although full-time academic medicine had been established in America, there were few academic gastroenterology units in medical schools; the New York Post-Graduate Medical School (M. Einhorn, 1888), Mount Sinai Hospital, New York (B. Crohn, 1916), Johns Hopkins (1920s), Harvard (Chester M. Jones of the Massachusetts General Hospital), and the University of Chicago (W. L. Palmer, 1927) were perhaps among the earliest. However, prominent gastroenterologically oriented physicians occupied important hospital and clinical teaching positions. Also, aided by physicians who had served in World War I, "cooperative specialism" gradually emerged as an important trend,[38] leading to the establishment of group clinics throughout the United States which were recognized for their high quality patient care and their clinical studies. Gastroenterology was an important division in the medical and surgical departments of these clinics (for example, the

TABLE 5.5.
WALTER B. CANNON: MONOGRAPHS

The Mechanical Factors of Digestion (1911)
Bodily Changes in Pain, Hunger, Fear and Rage (1915)
The Physiologic Nature of Hunger
Neural Organization of Emotional Expression
The Wisdom of the Body (1932)
The Autonomic Neuro-Effector System (1937)
The Supersensitivity of Denervation Structures—A Law of Denervation (1949)
Digestion and Health (1936)
The Way of an Investigator (1945)
"Neural Organization for Emotional Expression," Chapter 22 in *Feelings and Emotions* (1928)

Mayo, Lahey, Cleveland, and Ochsner clinics); they were developing outstanding clinical specialists long before the appearance of NIH-supported gastrointestinal training programs (1950s).

Other Early Twentieth-Century GI Physiologists Cannon was the first to relate the "pangs" of hunger to contractions of the empty stomach, a relationship Beaumont also had surmised. This observation was extended by Anton J. Carlson (1875–1956) of the University of Chicago in his studies with "F. V.", his laboratory diener, who had required a gastrostomy because of a complete stricture of the esophagus following the ingestion of lye as a child. Carlson, born in Sweden, early on was a carpenter, a student of psychology and philosophy, a minister, and a graduate student in physiology. In 1904 he became a member of the Department of Physiology at the University of Chicago, which included A. B. Luckhardt and R. C. Gerard. Carlson's monograph, *The Control of Hunger in Health and Disease*, published in 1916, included such observations as the inhibition of gastric contractions during periods of fear and reddening of the gastric mucosa and strong gastric contractions during periods of anger.[39] He concluded that hunger usually began with weak gastric contractions, becoming more vigorous, appearing at shorter intervals, and culminating in a spasm of smooth muscle. A tireless teacher and fearless researcher, Carlson had great analytic talent in resolving physiologic problems. His immortal "Vot is de evidence?" left an indelible mark on generations of students.

Walter C. Alvarez (1884–1978) was born in San Francisco in 1884 and graduated from what is now Stanford University Medical School in 1910. From 1913 to 1925, he practiced internal medicine in San Francisco and did research at the University of California. Among the first to use an X ray apparatus to examine the gastrointestinal tract, he went on to Cannon's laboratory where he developed the concept of gradients of motility in the bowel. His Harvard studies, culminating in the *Introduction to Gastroenterology* (1922), helped lay the foundation of modern gastroenterology. In 1925 Alvarez joined the Mayo Clinic. For the next twenty-five years he was active in the clinical and research aspects of gastroenterology. Alvarez pioneered in the diagnosis and care of nervous, neurotic, and psychotic patients with somatic gastrointestinal complaints. This work resulted in his *Nervous Indigestion* (1930), initiating the field of psychosomatic gastrointestinal illnesses. Retiring from the Mayo Clinic in 1952, he devoted the next twenty years to a small clinical practice in Chicago and extensive health education activities.[40]

In the mid-twentieth century and beyond, American physiologists continued to strengthen the scientific basis of gastroenterology. Among them were A. C. Ivy, Frank Mann, Lester Dragstedt, S. A. Komarov, Harry Shay, Franklin Hollander, Jesse Bollman,[41] and, more recently, H. W. Davenport, Morton I. Grossman, and Charles F. Code.

Early twentieth century scientific developments included the discovery of secretin[42] and gastrin.[43] Somewhat later A. C. Ivy of Chicago isolated the hormone cholecystokinin (CCK), which causes the gallbladder to contract (1928). These discoveries facilitated later concepts, such as that of the gastrin-mediated Zollinger-Ellison syndrome, and introduced the new and rapidly developing field of digestive endocrinology.[44]

American Gastroenterology in the Second Quarter of the Twentieth Century

Gastroenterology during the depression years in America was viewed chiefly as a clinical activity. Direct access to gastrointestinal structures remained difficult, limiting the acquisition of accurate information. Controlled studies were infrequent and anecdotal observations and empirical therapy predominated. Osler's 1930 *Textbook of Medicine* listed such now obsolete gastrointestinal disorders as "cirrhosis ventriculi, neuroses of the stomach, diphtheroid (croupous) and phlegmonous enteritis, visceroptosis, nervous colitis, intestinal sand and such hepatic disorders as catarrhal jaundice, chronic angiocholitis, chronic cholecystitis, syphilitic cirrhosis and chronic peritonitis." Disorders such as achalasia of the esophagus, coeliac disease, regional enteritis, ulcerative colitis, and viral hepatitis were not mentioned. Only ten years later (1941), the book *Diseases of the Digestive System*, edited by S. A. Portis of Chicago and involving many of America's leaders in digestive diseases, included authoritative discussions of the physiology, pathophysiology, and the etiology of digestive diseases, as well as considerations of the role of allergy and nutrition and the interactions of the gastrointestinal tract with other bodily systems (cardiovascular, renal, endocrine, metabolic).

The gastroenterologist's approach to the patient in the 1930s and 1940s emphasized a meticulous history, complete physical examination, and relatively simple laboratory studies, such as gastric analysis, limited blood chemistry (serum electrolytes, glucose, proteins and serum amylase); stool examinations (for occult blood, bacterial pathogens, parasites); and procto-sigmoidoscopy with the rigid instrument. Laborious fecal fat analyses were possible in patients suspected of steatorrhea. Many gastroenterologists not only practiced clinical medicine but also functioned as radiologists, using rather primitive X ray equipment. Some continued to dispense medication from their office. In radiology, progress was made in identifying the X ray appearance of esophageal disease, demonstration of the ulcer niche in active benign gastric and duodenal ulcer, and single-column barium examination of the upper gastrointestinal tract and the colon. Roentgen studies of the small bowel were not yet routine. Gastrointestinal mucosal relief studies, under development by Swedish radiologists, were applied by a few American radiologists. Endoscopy of the esophagus and stomach with the semirigid Wolf-Schindler instrument was introduced in 1934 at the University of Chicago by Rudolf Schindler of Munich. Chevalier Jackson of Philadelphia had maintained an endoscopy clinic with rigid instruments, as had Edward Benedict at the Massachusetts General Hospital in Boston. Before long, endoscopy clinics proliferated throughout the country. Techniques also evolved for stomach and later small intestine biopsy. Instruments were being developed for biopsies of the rectum, but an additional two decades elapsed before these resources were fully developed.

The gastric secretory capacity of the stomach, in relation to peptic ulcer and gastric carcinoma, was a major research and clinical focus in the 1930s and 1940s. The mechanism of ulcer pain (acid-pepsin versus spasm) was debated vigorously. Other topics of gastroenterologic interest included the nature of achalasia, the differentiation of benign and malignant gastric ulcer, the surgical treatment of peptic ulcer, the nature and clinical significance of gastritis, regional ileitis, the alleged role of the diplostreptococcus in the etiology of ulcerative colitis, the surgery of inflammatory bowel disease, the earlier diagnosis of gastrointestinal and pancreatic cancer, the role of emotions in digestive diseases, tests of hepatic function, and cholecystectomy for asymptomatic cholelithiasis.

In the 1930s and 1940s, the treatment of gastrointestinal disease continued to be highly empirical. Therapy included soluble antacids (sodium bicarbonate and calcium carbonate) for peptic ulcer, often producing the complications of alkalosis and kidney stones, small amounts of gastric irradiation for peptic ulcer to decrease or eliminate the secretion of hydrochloric acid; and medications of various rationale for ulcerative colitis and regional enteritis. The initial sulfonamides (sulfanilamide, neoprontosil, sulfaguanidine) and antibiotics (penicillin, streptomycin) were tested in various digestive disorders. Nutrition was an important consideration in the management of gastrointestinal problems but resources were limited. Psychogenic, especially psychoanalytical, mechanisms dominated concepts of gastrointestinal disease, and psychotherapy was a major part of the approach to the patient.

Research in gastroenterology during this period included gastric secretion and the search for potent gastric antisecretory drugs; endoscopy; early interest in esophageal and gastrointestinal motility; tests of hepatic function; liver disease (cirrhosis and hepatitis); improved diagnosis of gastrointestinal cancer (utilizing esophageal, gastric, pancreatic, and colonic exfoliative cytology); and the nature of inflammatory bowel disease.

The membership of the AGA increased steadily and included physiologists, pathologists, biochemists, and radiologists. But gastroenterology in the 1930s remained in a transitional stage. The clinical subspecialty of the first quarter of the twentieth century blossomed as a modern investigative discipline only after World War II. Although it lacked full recognition in many American medical schools, nevertheless gastroenterology had gained considerable stature in the major clinics and hospitals of the country. Many recent leaders of the postwar period were recruited to the subspecialty during the 1930s and early 1940s, attracted as much, I surmise, by the personal qualities of their teachers as by the appeal of the field itself (*Table 5.6*).

Major American Gastroenterology Publications The early American medical literature contains few references to digestive subjects other than occasional case reports, often involving abdominal trauma. Beaumont's classic studies on Alexis St. Martin were published in 1833. The experimental observations of Gross on the nature of intestinal wounds appeared in 1843. Early American gastrointestinal surgical contributions similarly reflect slow beginnings, increasing with time. American gastroenterology journals did not appear until the early 1900s.[45,46] Anthony Bassler of New York had founded the first American journal in gastroenterology, *The American Journal of Gastroenterology,* in 1914. However, the American Gastroenterological Association had no official journal in its early years. Since 1903 the papers on the annual meeting had been published in the AGA transactions (now located at the New York Academy of Medicine). In March 1934 the *American Journal of Digestive Diseases and Nutrition* was established by Beaumont S. Cornell of Fort Wayne, Indiana, becoming the official journal of the AGA that August (*Tables 5.2* and *5.7*). Also in 1934 the National Gastroenteroloical Association published its journal, the *Review of Gastroenterology,* which later was absorbed into the *American Journal of Gastroenterology.*

TABLE 5.6.
"RECRUITS" TO THE STUDY OF GASTROENTEROLOGY
IN THE 1930s AND 1940s

T. P. Almy (H. Wolff, S. Wolf, C. M. Jones)
J. E. Berk (J. E. Thomas, H. Bockus)
F. P. Brooks (T. G. Miller)
Hugh R. Butt (A. M. Snell, M. Comfort)
C. F. Code (F. Mann, J. Bollman)
R. M. Donaldson (F. J. Ingelfinger)
J. Fordtran (F. J. Ingelfinger)
M. I. Grossman (A. C. Ivy)
T. R. Hendrix (F. J. Ingelfinger)
F. J. Ingelfinger (T. G. Miller)
K. Isselbacher (F. J. Ingelfinger)
H. D. Janowitz (F. Hollander, A. B. Guttman)
Fred Kern, Jr. (T. P. Almy)
J. B. Kirsner (W. L. Palmer)
T. E. Machella (T. G. Miller)
C. G. McHardy (D. C. Browne)
A. I. Mendeloff (F. J. Ingelfinger)
H. M. Pollard (R. Schindler?)
H. Popper (H. Eppinger, A. C. Ivy)
J. M. Ruffin (C. M. Jones)
M. H. Sleisenger (T. P. Almy)
H. M. Spiro (C. M. Jones)
M. P. Tyor (J. M. Ruffin)
W. Volwiler (C. M. Jones)
S. Wolf (H. Wolff)

In 1937 Walter Alvarez of Rochester, Minnesota replaced Frank Smithies as editor of the *American Journal of Digestive Diseases and Nutrition.* In January 1943, in cooperation with the Williams and Wilkins Company of Baltimore, the AGA launched its new journal, *Gastroenterology,* with Alvarez as editor and A. C. Ivy of Chicago as assistant editor. The editorial board and the editorial council of *Gastroenterology* included many of the leading American gastroenterologists (*Table 5.8*). In the subsequent four decades, *Gastroenterology* has become recognized as the premier journal in this field.

New Gastroenterology Organizations The American College of Gastroenterology (ACG) originated in November 1932 as a development of the increasing clinical interest in gastroenterology. The goals set forth in the certificate of incorporation included advancing the clinical study of gastrointestinal disorders, gastrointestinal research, continuing education, and to further their gastroenterology training. Chapters were established throughout the United States and in several foreign countries. Reflecting the orientation of the College, committees subsequently were appointed on Patient Care, Health Care Delivery, Peer Review, Cost Containment, and Medico-Legal Issues. In the following year, the *Review of Gastroenterology* became the official journal of the Society, with Samuel Weiss as the first editor. In 1954 the name of the journal was changed to its current title, *American Journal of Gastroenterology*. Milton J. Matzner, David A. Dreiling, Arthur E. Lindner, and Martin H. Floch served as subsequent editors. The American College of Gastroenterology grew steadily both in stature and educational impact over the next half century; its membership today exceeds 2,100.[47]

Relationships between the AGA and the College were cool for many years. AGA members regarded themselves as better trained and as more substantial contributors to gastroenterologic knowledge. The College was considered not yet free of the empiricism and dogma of the past. In the 1960s, officials of both organizations came to recognize that the AGA and the ACG each had useful roles in modern gastroenterology. Gradually, members of the AGA became more involved in the teaching activities of the ACG and especially in its annual programs. Beginning in the mid-1980s, an

TABLE 5.7.
INITIAL EDITORIAL COUNCIL—
AMERICAN JOURNAL OF DIGESTIVE DISEASES AND NUTRITION (1934)

B. S. Cornell, Frank Smithies, and W. C. Alvarez, editors

Boris Babkin	A. C. Ivy
Frederick Banting	Chevalier Jackson
Arthur Bloomfield	Sara Jordan
Henry Bockus	Frank Lahey
A. J. Carlson	B. B. V. Lyon
Burrill Crohn	Alton Ochsner
Lester Dragstedt	Martin E. Rehfuss
John T. Finney	Leon Schiff
Julius Friedenwald	Franklin White

TABLE 5.8.
GASTROENTEROLOGY: INITIAL EDITORIAL GROUP (1943)

Editor: W. C. Alvarez
Assistant Editor: A. C. Ivy

Associate Editors

A. H. Aaron	P. Klemperer
J. A. Bargen	F. H. Lahey
H. L. Bockus	F. C. Mann
W. C. Boeck	H. J. Moersch
B. B. Crohn	V. C. Myers
R. Elman	W. L. Palmer
F. Hollander	J. M. Ruffin
S. M. Jordan	R. Schindler
J. L. Kantor	D. L. Wilbur
B. R. Kirklin	

Editorial Council

Irvin Abell	L. G. Cole	A. A. Jones	M. M. Portis
A. F. R. Andresen	E. N. Collins	C. M. Jones	J. P. Quigley
L. Arnold	G. R. Cowgill	N. W. Jones	M. Rehfuss
B. P. Babkin	C. W. Dowden	J. W. Larimore	V. C. Rowland
C. J. Barborka	L. R. Dragstedt	J. M. Lynch	A. Sachs
W. A. Bastedo	E. S. Emery, Jr.	B. B. V. Lyon	L. Schiff
E. B. Benedict	G. B. Eusterman	T. J. Mackie	H. F. Shattuck
A. A. Berg	J. H. Fitzgibbon	L. Martin	D. V. Silverman
J. M. Blackford	E. B. Freeman	J. G. Mateer	V. E. Simpson
L. Block	E. H. Gaither	T. G. Miller	A. M. Snell
R. B. Boles	L. C. Gatewood	W. G. Morgan	W. H. Stewart
J. L. Borland	F. D. Gordon	H. Nichols	H. M. Soper
R. C. Brown	R. H. M. Hardisty	M. Paulson	J. E. Thomas
T. R. Brown	S. Harris	G. M. Piersol	F. J. Van Liere
J. T. Case	C. G. Heyd	J. T. Pilcher	M. G. Vorhaus
			F. W. White

official committee representing both organizations has begun to meet regularly to consider issues of mutual interest.

The American Association for the Study of Liver Diseases The motivation for the establishment of an organization focused on the liver developed after World War II among physicians and scientists meeting at the Drake Hotel in Chicago to attend the annual meetings of the Central Society for Clinical Research. In 1948 several physicians decided to convene a small meeting in the library of the Hektoen Institute for Medical Research of the Cook County Hospital. After several such gatherings,[48] the American Association for the Study of Liver Disease (AASLD) was incorporated in the state of Illinois in March 1949. In its early years the format was a clinical pathological conference in the morning, scientific sessions in the afternoon, and a symposium and dinner in the evening.[49] As the association grew, the programs expanded to serve a membership now close to 1,000. Programs reflect the rapid accumulation of knowledge of the liver in health and disease, transmitted by means of the well-attended annual meeting, a comprehensive teaching course, Digestive Disease week, and the association's journal, *Hepatology*. Recently the AASLD has established the American Liver Foundation to raise money in support of research and education. Relationships between the AASLD and the AGA have been cordial and supportive throughout.

AGA Progress The AGA gradually achieved stability and leadership in the United States, improving the qualifications for gastroenterologic specialists and upgrading the caliber of clinical diagnosis and therapy. John C. Hemmeter[50] (1863–1931), in reviewing the programs of the AGA during its first thirty years, classified more than 50 percent of the papers as "publications that were pivotal, of exceptional merit in creating an entirely new view of some aspect of digestive disease." David Riesman[51] (1867–1940) of Philadelphia, surveying the history of gastroenterology for the first thirty years (1897–1927), concluded that gastroenterology had "builded well" and that "it should be taught as a regular part of the medical curriculum." It was not to attain that status until the 1950s.

Julius Friedenwald[52] (1866–1941) had reviewed the progress of the AGA in 1941 and characterized the AGA as having a modest beginning, increasing success, and currently a "most important stimulus to clinical and laboratory research in gastroenterology." After World War II the AGA began to occupy a more central role. Franklin W. White[53] (1869–1950), looking back over fifty years in 1947, noted, "it is a far cry from the early meetings in a small room on a side street in Atlantic City with ten or fifteen members present and eight or ten papers, to the meeting this year, with forty-four papers and an attendance of 400 to 500 members and guests. . . . Gastroenterology has been built up by the work of many men in many fields—chemistry, physiology, pathology, roentgenology, clinical medicine and surgery. . . . There were early difficulties . . . gradually overcome by honest work and high ideals."

The expanding base of gastroenterologic knowledge is reflected in Moses Paulson's 1969 *Gastroenterologic Medicine*, encompassing more than 1,600 pages, 496 illustrations, and eighty-five contributors. Since then the number of books on gastroenterology and related subjects has proliferated enormously. *Gastrointestinal Disease* (1983), edited by M. H. Sleisenger and J. S. Fordtran, incorporated ninety-five authors, 1,850 pages of text and references, and includes topics unheard of before 1950: immunology and diseases of the gastrointestinal tract, gastrointestinal peptide hormones, neurology of the gut, short bowel syndrome, sexually related intestinal disease, carcinoid syndrome, effects of systemic and extraintestinal disease on the gut, dissolution of gallstones, vascular diseases of the bowel, nutritional deficiency in gastrointestinal disease, and a dazzling array of modern diagnostic procedures. The 1985 Bockus *Gastroenterology*, under the chief editorship of J. Edward Berk of Irvine, California, includes 4,730 pages in seven volumes, 3,736 illustrations, and 304 contributors, a spectacular testament to the growth of gastroenterologic knowledge.

My personal memories of the annual AGA meetings begin in 1937. Programs before World War II were devoted largely to clinical observations and case studies. Beginning in the mid-1950s, however, carefully designed investigations and laboratory research presentations became more numerous. A tremendous increase in the number of papers and programs occurred only after 1966, expanding rapidly into the current format of "Digestive Disease Week." This program incorporates multiple organizations (*Table 5.9*) in a one week extravaganza of many day-long meetings, each focused on an interesting aspect of gastrointestinal disease, encompassing basic research, controlled clinical studies, scholarly clinical reports, endoscopy, and abdominal surgery. The meeting is supported by an extensive display of exhibits and scientific posters and quantities of up-to-date information sufficient to satisfy all scientific and clinical interests.

Formal Subspecialty Recognition of Gastroenterology In the 1930s, the pressure for formal specialty certification increased as hospital and medical

TABLE 5.9.
1985 ANNUAL MEETING OF AMERICAN GASTROENTEROLOGICAL ASSOCIATION

Participating Groups
Gastroenterology Research Group
Society for Surgery of Alimentary Tract
American Society for Gastrointestinal Endoscopy
American Association for Study of Liver Diseases
Inflammatory Bowel Disease Forum
AGA Councils: Aging and GI Tract; Clinical Epidemiology; Nerve/Gut Interaction
Medical Student Research

school appointments and membership in the more prestigious medical societies often were determined by such certification. Albert F. R. Andresen of Brooklyn, New York, played a leading role in this effort on behalf of the American Gastroenterological Association.[54] In June 1933, the AGA and the AMA Sections on Gastroenterology and Proctology each appointed a committee to consider the formation of an American Board of Gastroenterology. A constitution and bylaws were adopted and officers were elected: Albert F. R. Andresen, President; Franklin W. White, Vice President; the Secretary-General and Treasurer posts went to Ernest H. Gaither and Frank Smithies, respectively. The Board of Regents included Henry L. Bockus, George B. Eusterman, Adolph Sachs, and Sidney Simon. The Gastroenterology Committee requested the establishment of a certifying Board of Gastroenterology, a recommendation initially rejected by the Advisory Board for Medical Specialties, formed in 1934 in Philadelphia. Walter L. Palmer of Chicago recalls the basis of this initial negative response as the desire to first establish the American Board of Internal Medicine.

An appeal to the American Medical Association resulted in a reversal of the decision, and approval for a gastroenterology certifying board was granted. However, the leadership of the AGA held back because of the conviction that gastroenterologists should first be thoroughly qualified in internal medicine. Further action, therefore, was delayed until the establishment of the American Board of Internal Medicine in 1936. The parent board then granted specialty approval in June 1940, and the Gastroenterology Board set forth requirements for admission to the certifying examination. The authorization by the medical department of the United States War Department in June 1940 to establish positions for certified gastroenterologists in its general hospitals throughout the United States and abroad significantly enhanced the specialty status of gastroenterology. The AMA committee on Medical Education and Hospitals, approving residencies and fellowships in gastroenterology in 1948, further emphasized its specialty status. The American College of Gastroenterology subsequently participated in the certifying examinations. At the initial examinations on 18 April 1941 in Boston, four of eight candidates passed.[55] My own certification in gastroenterology at the 1942 oral examination was dependent, the same day, on passing an oral examination in internal medicine. These were in turn conditional on earlier passing a comprehensive written examination in internal medicine. This relationship to internal medicine has been maintained and most training programs in gastroenterology accept only candidates already trained in internal medicine. By 1985 more than 4,000 candidates successfully negotiated the certifying process.

During and After World War II

During World War II, gastroenterologists, like all other medical and surgical specialists, were preoccupied with military-related health problems. As a board-certified gastroenterologist in one general hospital in the European Theater (January 1944–May 1945), I dealt with functional digestive disorders, peptic ulcer, bacillary and amebic dysentery, other enteric infections, and hepatitis. As the gastroenterologist for another general hospital functioning in Japan (September 1945–June 1946), I found the gastrointestinal problems similar except for more enteric infections and more hepatitis. Clinical studies were not possible in Europe because of military activity or in Japan because of the requirements of an occupying military force. In America, gastroenterologic interest continued in the "usual problems" of peptic ulcer, inflammatory bowel disease, and hepatic disease, with early attention to nutrition.

The post-World War II period (1946—) marked the beginning of an impressive expansion of medicine and its specialties.[56] Major advances in scientific knowledge and in medical, surgical, diagnostic, and therapeutic technology produced substantial improvements in diagnosis and therapy, kindling the philanthropic interests of both the government and the public. The public subsidy of graduate medical education via the G.I. Bill of 1944 accelerated specialism in gastroenterology, as in all other specialties, and in other professions as well. Interest in Board certification in all subspecialties, as an endorsement of excellent qualifications for hospital appointments and membership in various societies, increased greatly,[57] further encouraged by the National Institutes of Health through its support of research and training programs in gastroenterology.

Medical schools throughout the country, now increasingly aware of the importance of gastroenterology, established sections, divisions, and even departments of gastroenterology. New ideas, new methods, and new instruments rapidly expanded the technological resources of the gastroenterologist, catalyzing interest in gastroenterologic research and creating an enhanced sense of professional identity. The more complicated technology being applied to the study of digestive diseases necessitated more sharply focused education and training, and gradually evolved into comprehensive training programs of two and three years' duration.

A new generation of gastroenterologists, maturing during and just before the war, assumed leadership in American gastroenterology in the post-World War II period. Henry L. Bockus (1894–1984), a student of Max Einhorn, carried on his work at the Graduate Hospital of the University of Pennsylvania. His clinical gastroenterology program trained hundreds of America's leading clinical gastroenterologists. Walter L. Palmer (1896—), a student of B. W. Sippy and a superb clinician, teacher, and clinical scientist, established one of the first academic departments of gastroenterology in the United States at the University of Chicago in 1927. I joined him in 1936. Palmer was recognized for his carefully controlled clinical studies in peptic ulcer. His emphasis on the scientific method and on the relationship between research and clinical medicine was one of the major factors in the upgraded academic status of gastroenterology in the United States. Lester Dragstedt, a student of A. J. Carlson at the University of Chicago, began his experimental physiologic studies of gastric secretion in the 1940s, culminating in the operation of vagotomy and pyloroplasty for peptic ulcer.

Outstanding gastroenterologic clinicians of this era included Russell S. Boles, Sara M. Jordan, A. M. Snell, Dwight Wilbur, Julian M. Ruffin, H. M. Pollard, Chester M. Jones, and J. A. Bargen. They were followed by Hans Popper, Gerald Klatskin, T. P. Almy, F. J. Ingelfinger, G. McHardy, J. B. Kirsner, Hugh R. Butt, H. D. Janowitz, K. J. Isselbacher, A. I. Mendeloff, F. Kern, M. H. Sleisenger, F. P. Brooks, among others. NIH-supported training programs in gastroenterology were established in the 1950s, initially at Boston University (F. J. Ingelfinger) and at the University of Chicago (W. L. Palmer and J. B. Kirsner). The number of programs oriented to laboratory research and to scholarly clinical investigation increased over the next decade. In addition, many hospital centers and medical schools established their own quality training programs in clinical gastroenterology.

Gastroenterology and the National Institutes of Health The Division of Research Grants of the NIH was established in 1947 and soon began to facilitate research in many areas of medical science. For gastroenterology, the National Institute of Arthritis, Metabolic and Digestive Diseases became a significant growth factor in the early 1950s, supporting an increasing number of research projects, training programs, and fellowships. With the establishment of the General Medicine Study Section, the impact of the NIH on gastroenterology, as on many other medical areas, was profound.[58,59] The NIH, operating through a system of study sections, committees, and councils, maintained high standards of objectivity, minor criticisms notwithstanding. Judging by my own consultative relationships with the NIH over a period of approximately fifteen years (1955–1970), the freedom and creativity of investigators and the independence of American medical schools were not restricted. Unhampered by limiting traditions, the NIH recognized, in cooperation with medical schools and scientists generally, the need to strengthen lagging, poorly supported medical and basic science areas. Developed at a time of perceived need—the 1950s and 1960s—with their shortages of investigators and teachers and limited medical school budgets, the extramural programs of the NIH and the General Medical Study Section of the National Institute for Arthritis, Metabolic, Digestive and Kidney Diseases proved of incalculable value in the rapid development of the medical sciences, including gastroenterology, and were a major growth factor for the field.

American Gastroenterology in the 1970s and 1980s

Important changes continue to characterize American gastroenterology in the 1980s,[60] modifications reflecting expanding knowledge and improving diagnostic technology. More training time is directed to the application of diagnostic methods, especially endoscopy and imaging procedures. Research activity has increased and has become more complicated, but continues to lag behind other medical specialties in terms of major breakthroughs. The enlarging clinical scope of gastroenterology, dominated by improving endoscopy and imaging techniques and increasingly complicated research, which now involves cells, cell membranes, genes and oncogenes, immunology and neuroendocrinology, has changed the training objectives for new generations of clinical and academic gastroenterologists. Training programs for individuals interested and qualified for investigative careers now extend for three to five years and often necessitate lengthy training in basic research laboratories. Clinical gastroenterology continues to be preoccupied with the familiar problems of acid-peptic disease, gastroesophageal reflux, hepatitis, cirrhosis of the liver, cholelithiasis, pancreatic disease, inflammatory bowel disease, and cancer. The major new clinical problem for the American gastroenterologist probably is the acquired immune deficiency disease (AIDS) and its impact on the digestive tract, especially the virulent and multiple superinfestations so resistent to current therapy.

The American Gastroenterological Association, the American College of Gastroenterology, and the American Association for the Study of Liver Disease have become major forums for gastroenterologists and related clinical and scientific disciplines. By mid-1986 the AGA membership approximated 5,000. In 1948 there were only two residencies, seventeen fellowships, and one postgraduate course. In 1985 the number of gastroenterology training programs in the United States and Canada exceeded 250, including more than 1,000 post-medical residency physicians in active training. Thus, once underway, specialization in gastroenterology in America developed at a rate exceeding trends elsewhere in the world. At its 1985 annual meeting in New York, the AGA attracted approximately 5,200 physicians, surgeons, scientists, and other health professionals who listened to nearly 1,000 scientific papers and viewed innumerable posters and research displays. Similarly, the American College of Gastroenterology, emphasizing clinical gastroenterology, provided the other major forum for gastroenterology in America. Concurrently, the number and the scope of GI organizations increased steadily (*Table 5.10*).

An important corollary development, reflecting the uniquely American philanthropic interest of the public was the formation of lay organizations, affiliated with physicians and societies oriented to a particular aspect of gastroenterology, often for the purpose of fund-raising (*Table 5.11*). The mounting importance of digestive diseases as a national health problem in the United States resulted in two major reviews under the auspices of the American Gastroenterological Association in 1967 and 1974. In 1973, the status of the AGA and its future were comprehensively reviewed by a presidential commission. Yet another review was undertaken by the AGA Governing Board in 1986. Gastroenterology, in less than 75 years, had developed into one of the most successful subspecialties of American internal medicine. The eight 1897 founding members of the AGA could hardly have anticipated this remarkable growth of gastrointestinal medicine in the United States, but probably they would not have been surprised.

Technology and Its Impact: Gastrointestinal Tubes Gastric tubes, originating in ancient times with the vomiting feather (pinna) have progressed

TABLE 5.10.
EARLY AMERICAN GI ORGANIZATIONS

1886	Gastroenterologische Krankheiten Verein, Baltimore (H. Salzer)
1897	American Gastroenterological Association
1899	American Proctologic Society (T. C. Martin)
1914	AMA Section on Gastroenterology and Proctology (American Medical Association established 1847)
1915	New York Gastroenterological Association (A. Bassler)
1920	Southern Gastroenterological Association
1920s	Eastern Gut Club
1932	Society for the Advancement of Gastroenterology
1938	National Gastroenterological Association (American College of Gastroenterology [1954])
1940	American Board of Gastroenterology (A. F. R. Andresen)
1941	American Gastroscopic Club (R. Schindler)
1948	Inter-American Association of Gastroenterology
1949	American Association for Study of Liver Disease (H. Popper)
1954	American College of Gastroenterology (see above)
1956	Gastroenterology Research Group (J. B. Kirsner, E. C. Texter)
1958	Organisation Mondiale de Gastroenterologic (World Organization of Gastroenterology, Washington, D.C.)
1960	Society for Surgery of the Alimentary Tract (W. H. Cole, R. Turell, J. M. Waugh)
1961	American Society for GI Endoscopy (continuation of American Gastroscopic Club)

through an interesting evolution, including the whalebone "stomach cleanser" of the American Indian (1600s) and the stomach aspirating tubes of John Hunter in London and Alexander Munro in Edinburgh. The use of the stomach tube in America probably began with Philip S. Physick of Philadelphia in the early years of the nineteenth century. Physick passed a large flexible catheter into the stomachs of three-month-old twins with whooping cough who had received an overdose of laudanum. With a syringe he injected ipecac and warm water, withdrew the stomach contents, and repeated the process with warm water alone. One patient recovered. American contributions to intubation methodology were renewed with Max Einhorn in 1890, J. C. Hemmeter in 1896, and M. Gross, A. L. Levin, and M. E. Rehfuss, each of whom created devices to examine the stomach and duodenum. B. B. Vincent Lyon of Philadelphia introduced duodenal drainage in the diagnosis and treatment of gallstones. Nasogastric suction for the ileus of peritonitis was initiated in 1911. In 1925 Robertson Ward of San

Francisco advocated continuous gastroduodenal aspiration for the management of intestinal obstruction. In 1931 O. H. Wangensteen and his colleagues at the University of Minnesota began their classic studies on intestinal intubation in the management of obstruction and in postoperative abdominal care. Their work stimulated many useful contributions, including the double-lumen tube of T. G. Miller and Osler Abbott in Philadelphia and the Cantor tube of Meyer Cantor in Detroit. Important contributions were made later by Ian Wood and his colleagues in Australia; by J. Tomenius of Sweden in the development of the gastric biopsy tube with a guillotine cutting device, providing full-thickness gastric mucosal tissue; and by Margot Shiner of London in the evolution of the small intestinal biopsy tube.

TABLE 5.11.
OTHER DIGESTIVE DISEASE ORGANIZATIONS

American Celiac Society
American Digestive Disease Society
American Hepatic Foundation
American Liver Foundation
American Society for Parenteral and Enteral Nutrition
American Society of Colon and Rectal Surgeons
Center for Ulcer Research and Education Foundation
Children's Liver Foundation
Coalition of Digestive Disease Organizations
Cystic Fibrosis Foundation
Dean Thiel Foundation
Federation of Digestive Disease Societies
The Gail I. Zuckerman Foundation
The Gastro-Intestinal Research Foundation of Chicago
Gluten Intolerance Group
International Association for Enterostomal Therapy, Inc.
Lifeline Foundation, Inc.
National Foundation for Ileitis and Colitis
The North American Society for Pediatric Gastroenterology
Pediatric Liver Research Foundation
Society of American Gastrointestinal Endoscopic Surgeons
Society of Gastrointestinal Assistants, Inc.
United Ostomy Association

Gastrointestinal Endoscopy Gastric endoscopy had had an uncertain beginning earlier in the nineteenth century, when P. Bozzini (1806), A. Kussmaul (1867), J. Mikulicz, C. Ewald (1875), and F. Riegel (1881) had utilized rigid tubes to peer down the esophagus and glimpse the interior of the stomach, not infrequently at great risk to the patient. The establishment of gastroscopy at the University of Chicago with the arrival of Rudolf Schindler (1888–1968) from Munich in 1934 marked the close of an introductory era of instrumental development and the beginning of an accelerated growth period in endoscopic development and application. The direct visualization of the interior of the esophagus and stomach had begun in Europe. Early intubation efforts by laryngologists seeking a method to examine the larynx directly also helped set the stage for later developments. The early efforts of German endoscopists failed, despite the collaboration of the opticians Max Nitze and Josef Leiter (creators of the electrically lighted cystoscope in 1881) because of an inadequate optical system and light source. By 1911, optical systems had been improved and miniature electrical bulbs had been constructed, enabling H. D. Elsner in Germany to utilize a rigid instrument carrying a light bulb at the distal end, and by means of mirrors, prisms, and lenses to transport satisfactory images to the eyepiece of the instrument.

Schindler, noting the dominant role of the stomach in the disability of so many soldiers, began in 1920 to develop his own modification of an instrument created by G. Wolf in Berlin, aided by cooperative sword-swallowers. However, the endoscopic procedure was difficult. Accidents occurred, with occasional fatalities. In 1928 Schindler, in cooperation with the optical firm of G. Wolf in Berlin, began the construction of the semi-flexible gastroscope, an accomplishment completed in 1932. The new instrument revolutionized gastroscopy. Schindler immigrated to the United States in 1934 and, with his wife Gabrielle as his assistant, established an active endoscopy training program at the University of Chicago. Its impact was immediate and far-reaching. Here hundreds of physicians and surgeons from all parts of the United States and many foreign countries gathered to observe and learn upper GI endoscopy. Each observation—the normal stomach, gastritis, peptic ulcer, tumors, the postoperative stomach, the relationship between the visual and histological findings—became a research project.[61] Modifications of the Schindler instrument came rapidly, including the rubber finger tip, biopsy forceps, endoscopic photography, and, most significantly, the advent of fiberoptics.

Basil Hirschowitz, now of Birmingham, Alabama, played an important role in the development of the fiberoptic endoscope, including visualization of the duodenum and, most importantly, the use of a more flexible, safer instrument facilitating an easier examination for the patient. As related by Sir Christopher Booth, the fiberoptic story actually began with a British gastroenterologist at St. George's Hospital in London, Hugh Gainsborough, who encouraged Harold Hopkins of the Imperial College of Science and Technology to develop the idea of a coherent glass fiber bundle for transmitting an optical image along a flexible path.[62] With his graduate student N. S. Kapany, he was able after two years to produce a successful image transmitting bundle.[63] Sir Francis Avery Jones, quickly recognizing the importance of this development, then encouraged his student, Basil Hirschowitz, to pursue Hopkins's accomplishment. The initial fiberscope, a "rather thick forbidding rod," was passed in Hirschowitz himself.

Eventually, an instrument for the examination of the esophagus, stomach, and duodenum was produced for clinical application. The initial results were published in the *Lancet* in 1961.[64] Hirschowitz subsequently immigrated to the United States and the University of Michigan. American efforts to further develop fiberoptic instruments included commercial firms such as Optics Technology and educational institutions such as the Illinois Institute of Technology. The firm of American Cystoscope Makers at first declined to participate in this effort. In 1963 the Illinois Institute of Technology Research Institute and Louis Streifeneder at the Eder Instrument Company produced the first prototype fiberoptic sigmoidoscope in this country. The Eder program was halted by their inability to obtain the appropriate glass fibers. In 1968 the AMCI, led by Bergein Overholt of Knoxville, Tennessee, developed an American flexible sigmoidoscope and subsequently a fiberoptic colonoscope. The flexible fiberoptic sigmoidoscope was first used successfully in America in 1963.[65]

In Japan, Professor Tadayoshi Takemoto, in cooperation with the Olympus Company and the Machida Company, developed improved fiberoptic endoscopes, revolutionizing the entire endoscopy field.[66] Subsequently, technological developments, especially by the Japanese, have further revolutionized upper and lower GI endoscopy. Most recently, an intestinal fiberoptic endoscope has been produced and utilized by the Japanese. All these developments culminated in the development of a new field of gastrointestinal endoscopic therapy. The American Society for Gastrointestinal Endoscopy, originating in Chicago in 1941 as the American Gastroscopic Club, has grown steadily, with a current membership approximating 3,500, and today it is a major force in American gastroenterology. Its annual meeting and postgraduate course, part of Digestive Disease Week, attract thousands of endoscopists and gastroenterologists from the entire world.

Scientific Knowledge and Technology in the Growth of Gastroenterology The steady expansion of scientific knowledge in gastroenterology, as Christopher Booth has indicated, has dramatically reduced the world mortality from cholera, clarified the role of gluten in celiac disease, and increased our understanding of the etiology and different types of hepatitis.[67] To these advances might be added awareness of the critical importance of hydration and fluid balance in the management of diarrheal states in the underdeveloped countries, increased knowledge of the chemistry of bile and the dissolution of cholesterol gallstones, the evolving new fields of gastrointestinal immunology and intestinal neuroendocrinology, mechanisms of intestinal transport and absorption, the role of nutrition, the genetics of digestive disease, eating disorders, other psychogenic illnesses, and the expanding knowledge of the liver in health and disease.

In gastroenterology the technical advances have been equally remarkable. In addition to aseptic surgery, anesthesia, the discovery of X rays and new drugs, Booth includes endoscopy, liver biopsy, gastric and intestinal biopsies, fiberoptic endoscopic instruments, peritoneoscopy, splenic angiography, and more sophisticated imaging procedures, including the gamma camera, digital vascular imaging, ultrasonography, computerized axial tomography of the abdomen, and magnetic resonance imaging. In therapy, the list might include therapeutic endoscopy, use of the laser beam, and such drugs as newer antibiotics, H2 blockers, anti-inflammatory agents and parenteral hyperalimentation. Booth notes that "a good deal of modern medicine (and gastroenterology) depends more on technology than on science." He raises important questions, which need to be resolved in the immediate future, regarding safety, efficacy, and cost-effectiveness.[68]

A. Keller[69] has noted that most types of scientific endeavor need someone with a practical hand, seldom the original theorist. "Most technologies are created by individuals with a clear understanding of a wide range of scientific facts and their implications. Science was not the prime originator of technology, not even the catalyst. But modern technology would be impossible without scientific training and comprehension of the nature of things." But surely both science and technology are indispensable and interdependent. Advancing scientific knowledge and ingenious technology each have contributed significantly to the development of gastroenterology as a medical specialty.

Concluding Comments

The growth of gastroenterology in America during the past century may be summarized in the terms of J. M. Eisenberg[70] and Rosemary Stevens,[71] whose perceptive observations have clarified the process of medical specialization in America. The development of gastroenterology as a distinctive medical field has paralleled the course of other medical subspecialties in this country, albeit at a slower rate (*Tables 5.12, 5.13*). Gastroenterology sought progress, professional identity, and recognition by seeking to become

TABLE 5.12.
EARLY AMERICAN DEVELOPMENTS TOWARD SPECIALIZATION IN GASTROENTEROLOGY IN THE UNITED STATES

1. Early American Research
   - W. Beaumont, gastric function (A. St. Martin)
   - R. Dunglison, GI physiology
   - J. Jackson, digestion of fats
   - J. Dalton, physiology of bile, gastric secretion
2. Early American Clinical Studies
   - A. Flint, gastric atrophy and pernicious anemia (1860), "dyspepsia" (1866)
   - J. Woodward, diarrhea and dysentery (1879)
   - R. Fitz, acute appendicitis (1884), acute pancreatitis (1889)
   - W. J. Mayo, diverticulitis colon (1887)
3. Early American Surgery
   - Ether anesthesia (Morton, Warren)
   - Surgical Advances (Physick, Gross, Halsted, Fenger, Murphy, Mayos, Others)
4. Further development, clinical application of stomach tubes, endoscopes, and other instruments
5. Application of X rays to study of GI tract (Cannon, Hemmeter)
6. Cholecystography (Graham, Cole, 1924)
7. Early Specialty Hospitals
   - 1800+ Mental Hospitals
   - 1824 Massachusetts Eye and Ear Infirmary
   - 1832 Boston Lying In Hospital
   - 1836 New York Hospital for Skin Diseases
   - 1858 Illinois Eye and Ear Infirmary (Chicago)
   - 1886 Gastroenterologische krankheiten Verein (H. Salzer, Baltimore)
8. American immigration of German-trained gastroenterologists, including Max Einhorn, J. C. Hemmeter, J. Kaufmann, and M. Manges

TABLE 5.13.
ADMINISTRATIVE EVOLUTION OF MEDICAL SPECIALISM IN THE UNITED STATES

1850	Emergence of "the inexorable law of specialization" (David J. Davis)
1865	AMA Convention in Boston, Committee on Ethics Report on Specialism
1866	Medical specialism generally acknowledged
1869	AMA specialties: "legitimate fields of practice"
1870s	Specialism in Europe Postgraduate education in specialties (Harvard)
1897	Concerns about skill and knowledge of specialists (G. B. Johnston)
1907	Need for proper education of specialists (G. Shambaugh) (Minnesota program: eye, ear, nose, throat)
1915	American College of Physicians
1916	American Board of Ophthalmology
1921	Council on Medical Education and Hospitals: Certification of specialists
1933	Formation of Medical Specialty Boards American Board Internal Medicine
1940	American Board of Gastroenterology
1940	U.S. War Department recognition (gastroenterology in all general hospitals)

From: R. Fitz, "The Rise of the Practice of Internal Medicine as a Specialty," *N Engl J Med* 242(1950): 569; D. J. Davis, "The Rise of Medical Specialism," in *The History of Medical Practice in Illinois*, vol. I: 1850–1900 (Chicago: Illinois State Medical Society, 1955), 91–98.

more "scientific." Key factors in this evolution included the development of instruments (e.g., the stomach tube, gastroscope, colonoscope); the discovery of the roentgen rays and later many innovative imaging techniques; the emergence of bacteriology and the germ theory of disease enabling the more precise diagnosis of gastrointestinal infections; the introduction of anesthesia and asepsis, facilitating the development of abdominal surgery; the increasing scientific knowledge of gastrointestinal function in health and disease, providing an indispensable knowledge base; and the contributions of hard-working and highly motivated scientists and physicians.

Knowledge of the digestive tract during the past one hundred years thus represents a continuum of information accumulated at an ever-quickening rate, over centuries, and involving many outstanding individuals, obviously motivated by those remarkable "serving men" of Rudyard Kipling: "Who, what, how, why, when and where."[72] These circumstances, concurrent with advancing biological and natural sciences and increasing specialization in medicine and surgery, including the establishment of specialty organizations, encouraged well-trained physicians and scientists with particular interest in the digestive tract and with specialized technological skills, to unite for the purposes of increased communication and exchange of ideas, improved quality of gastroenterologic diagnosis and therapy, and both public and peer recognition.

As to the future, gastroenterology faces several important problems: (1) the hazard of losing the "human touch" and evolving into a guild of specialized technologists with an excessively narrow medical focus, (2) the possibility of diminishing numbers of investigators, limited budgets, and decreased gastroenterologic research, and (3) the general danger of stifling bureaucratic over-regulation. Regardless of the substantial progress in medicine as a whole and of gastroenterology in particular, not all of the difficulties of sick people can be resolved by technology. Human illness is a product of multiple causes and multiple mechanisms, including life stresses. The blending of religion, philosophy, and healing in ancient history probably was no accident. Medicine and gastroenterology today hopefully will not overlook this important link, for as Howard Spiro has declared, "man is still more than his body."[73]

A second hazard is the recurrent tendency of gastroenterologists, especially technologically oriented gastroenterologists, to dissociate from the parent discipline of internal medicine. Superior gastroenterologic clinical practice is simply not possible without a solid foundation in the broad field of internal medicine, especially in view of the intricate interrelationships of the gastrointestinal tract with virtually all bodily systems.

The third peril relates to the changing nature and increasing demands of modern research. As Herman and Singer have indicated, advancing knowledge and changing technologies have lengthened and intensified research training. Increasing professionalization in research already has increased competition for funds, so that the part-time clinical investigator is now at a serious disadvantage in competition with the full-time reseacher. These trends, the more limited budgets of academic departments of medicine, and the decreasing interest in research careers among current gastroenterology fellows pose a significant problem for the future of gastroenterologic research.[74]

A hazard, for all of medicine, is the current continuing proliferation of administrative limitations on the care of the sick in the United States, measures instituted primarily on the expectation of "cost containment," a worthy though illusory objective, but spawning increasing numbers of equally costly administrative health care programs of unproven benefit to sick people. Medicine in America, after one hundred years, once again is changing. Whereas in the past the trend was toward lofty objectives, increased knowledge through scholarly clinical study, perceptive laboratory investigation, and quality patient care, the trend today appears to be in the opposite direction: cost containment above all other considerations, even to the point of rationing essential health services[75] and endangering the quality of patient care.

Finally, in G. Vico's terms, gastroenterology these past one hundred years can be characterized as having made "intelligible advances" rather than "progress towards perfection."[76] It is sobering to realize that, despite the impressive developments of the past century, we still do not know the cause and the pathogenesis of most disorders of the gastrointestinal tract. We have indeed traveled long and far, but not far enough. Marvelous opportunities yet await the gastroenterologists of tomorrow.

This study was supported in part by the Gastro-Intestinal Research Foundation of Chicago.

NOTES

1. B. J. Stern, *American Medical Practice in the Perspective of a Century* (New York: The Commonwealth Fund, 1945).
2. Russell C. Maulitz, "Physician versus Bacteriologist: The Ideology of Science in Clinical Medicine," in *The Therapeutic Revolution*, M. J. Vogel and C. R. Rosenberg, eds. (Philadelphia: University of Pennsylvania Press, 1979).
3. W. S. Miller, "William Beaumont, M.D. (1785–1853)," *Ann Med His* 5 (1933): 28–51.
4. J. J. Bylebyl, "William Beaumont, Robley Dunglison and the Philadelphia Physiologists," *J Hist Med* 25 (1970): 3–21.
5. W. B. Cannon, "Some Modern Extensions of Beaumont's Studies in Alexis St. Martin," *J Mich State Med Soc* 32 (March–May 1933): 155–64, 215–224, 307–16.
6. J. S. Meyer, *Life and Letters of Dr. William Beaumont* (St. Louis: C. V. Mosby, 1939).
7. W. B. Cannon, "Early Use of the Roentgen Ray in the Study of the Alimentary Canal," *JAMA* 62 (1914): 1–3.
8. J. Bordley III and A. M. Harvey, *Two Centuries of American Medicine* (Philadelphia: W. B. Saunders, 1976).
9. R. H. Fitz, "Perforating Inflammation of the Vermiform Appendix With Special Reference to its Early Diagnosis and Treatment," *Trans Assoc Am Physicians* (1896): 107.
10. R. H. Fitz, "Acute Pancreatitis," *Boston Med Surg J* 120 (1889): 215, 219.
11. E. C. Atwater, "Internal Medicine in the Education of American Physicians," in *The Education of American Physicians*, R. L. Numbers, ed. (Berkeley and Los Angeles: University of California Press, 1980), 143–74.

12. G. Rosen, "Changing Attitudes of the Medical Profession to Specialization," *Bull Hist Med* 12 (1942): 343–54.

13. E. D. Fenner, "Introductory Lecture," *New Orleans Medical News and Hospital Gazette* 3 (1856): 577–600.

14. Bordley and Harvey, *Two Centuries of American Medicine.*

15. C. D. Haagensen and W. E. B. Lloyd, "The Doctor's Dilemma," in *A Hundred Years of Medicine* (New York: Sheridan House, 1943), 375–412.

16. Bordley and Harvey, *Two Centuries of American Medicine.*

17. J. D. Boyle, *I. Boas—First Gastroenterologic Specialist* (in preparation).

18. J. C. Hemmeter, "German-American Influence on Medicine and Surgery," *Medical Library and Historical Journal* 4 (Sept. 1906).

19. Charles Rosenberg, "The Practice of Medicine in New York a Century Ago," *Bull Hist Med* 41 (1967): 223–53.

20. George H. Coleman, "Internal Medicine," in *History of Medical Practice in Illinois* (Chicago: Biographical Publishing, 1922), Chapter 8.

21. F. Cunha, *Osler as a Gastroenterologist* (San Francisco: 1948).

22. The physicians attending were Max Einhorn (New York), John C. Hemmeter (Baltimore), David D. Stewart (Philadelphia), Allan A. Jones (Buffalo), Frank H. Murdoch (Pittsburgh), A. P. Buchman (Indiana), Lewis Brinton (Philadelphia), and Charles D. Aaron (Detroit).

23. S. J. Meltzer, "The Disturbance of the Law of Contrary Innervation as a Pathogenic Factor in Diseases of the Bile Ducts and the Gallbladder," *Am J Med Sci* 153 (1917): 469–77.

24. B. B. V. Lyon, "Diagnosis and Treatment of Diseases of the Gallbladder and Biliary Ducts—Preliminary Report of a New Method," *JAMA* 73 (1919): 980–82.

25. A. McGeehee Harvey, "Samuel J. Meltzer, 'Pioneer Catalyst in the Evolution of Clinical Science in America,'" *Perspect Biol Med* (spring 1978): 431–40.

26. J. D. Boyle, "The American Gastroenterological Association: History of its First Seventy-Five Years," *Gastroenterology* 65 (1973): 1023–1106.

27. "Minor Comments," *JAMA* 32 (1899): 1066.

28. F. P. Brooks and American Gastroenterological Association, *AGA Presidential Addresses,* 1983.

29. J. Friedenwald, "On the Development of Gastroenterology in America," *Medical Record* (1909): 1–27. *AGA Presidential Address,* 1909. Important events in the development of gastroenterology.

30. I. P. Pavlov, *The Work of the Digestive Glands,* W. H. Thompson, trans. (London: C. Griffin, 1910).

31. H. W. Davenport, "The First Walter Bradford Cannon Lecture Before the Society of Gastrointestinal Radiologists," *Am J Roentg Rad Ther Nucl Med* 119 (1973): 235–40.

32. W. B. Cannon and A. Moser, "The Movements of the Food in the Oesophagus," *Am J Physiol* 1 (1898): 435–44.

33. W. B. Cannon, "Early use of the Roentgen Ray in the Study of the Alimentary Canal," *JAMA* 62 (1914): 1–3.

34. H. W. Davenport, "Walter B. Cannon's Contribution to Gastroenterology," *Gastroenterology* 63 (1972): 878–89.

35. H. W. Davenport, "The First Walter B. Cannon Lecture," *Am J Roentg Rad Ther Nucl Med* 119 (1973): 235–40.

36. W. L. Palmer, "Dr. Bertram W. Sippy's Contributions to Medicine," *Proc Inst Med Chicago* 27 (1968): 75–84.

37. B. W. Sippy, "Gastric and Duodenal Ulcer: Medical Cure by an Efficient Removal of Gastric Juice Corrosion," *JAMA* 64 (1915): 1625–30.

38. S. J. Reiser, *Medicine and the Reign of Technology* (Cambridge, England: Cambridge University Press, 1978).

39. A. J. Carlson, *The Control of Hunger in Health and Disease* (Chicago: University of Chicago Press, 1916).

40. S. Hyman, Chicago, personal communication, 1986. On dyspepsia see G. H. Brieger, "Dyspepsia: The American disease? Needs and opportunities for research," in *Healing and History,* Charles Rosenberg, ed. (New York: Science History, 1979), 179–90.

41. W. J. Meek, "The Beginnings of American Physiology," *Ann Med Hist* 10 (1928) : 111–25.

42. W. M. Bayliss and E. H. Starling, "Preliminary Communication on the Causation of the So-Called 'Peripheral Reflex Secretion' of the Pancreas," *Lancet* 1 (1902) : 813.

43. J. S. Edkins, "On the Chemical Mechanism of Gastric Secretion," *Lancet* 2 (1905) : 156.

44. M. I. Grossman, "A Short History of Digestive Endocrinology" in *The Gastrointestinal Hormones and Pathology of the Digestive System,* M. Grossman, V. Speranza, N. Basso, et al., eds. (New York: Plenum Press, 1978), 5–10.

45. J. M. Armstrong, "The First American Medical Journals" in *Lectures on the History of Medicine* (Philadelphia: W. B. Saunders, 1926–1932), 357–69.

46. H. B. Shafer, "Early Medical Magazines in America," *Ann Med Hist* 7 (1935) : 480–91.

47. M. H. Kaplan and Officers of the American College of Gastroenterology. Based on information provided by Daniel Weiss, retired Executive Director of the College (November 1985), with the assistance of M. H. Kaplan, David A. Dreiling, and R. J. Priest, and in cooperation with Walter H. Jacobs, President, and John P. Papp, President Elect.

48. The initial discussants, in addition to Hans Popper, included the following: J. L. Bollman and H. R. Butt (Rochester, MN), P. Gyorgy (Philadelphia), F. W. Hoffbauer (Minneapolis), L. Schiff (Cincinnati), and R. B. Capps, A. C. Ivy, R. M. Kark, F. Schaffner, and J. B. Kirsner (all of Chicago).

49. H. Popper, "History of the American Association for the Study of Liver Disease," *Hepatology* 2 (1980) : 874–78. Excerpted in part by permission of the author and the AASLD.

50. J. C. Hemmeter, *History of Thirty Years Activity of the American Gastroenterological Association, Transactions of the AGA* (Baltimore: Waverly Press, 1928), 5–7.

51. David Riesman, "The History of Gastroenterology 1897–1927," in *High Blood Pressure and Longevity and Other Assays* (Chicago and Philadelphia: John C. Winston Company, 1937), 649–56.

52. Julius Friedenwald, "The Early History of the American Gastroenterological Association: Its Aims, Adversities, Aspirations and Success," *Gastroenterology* 42 (1962) : 722–31.

53. F. W. White, "The Fiftieth Anniversary of the American Gastroenterological Association," *Gastroenterology* 9 (1947) : 499.

54. White, "Fiftieth Anniversary of the AGA."

55. A. F. R. Andresen, "History of Board Certification in Gastroenterology," *Gastroenterology* 27 (1954) : 244–255.

56. L. S. King, *Medical Thinking—A Historical Preface* (Princeton: Princeton University Press, 1982).

57. R. Stevens, *American Medicine and the Public Interest* (New Haven: Yale University Press, 1971).

58. J. B. Kirsner, "The Impact of the National Institutes of Health Upon Gastroenterology in the United States," *Gastroenterology* 46 (1964) : 53–61.

59. J. B. Kirsner, "Reflections on Education in Gastroenterology in the United States," *Scand J Gastroenterol Suppl* 9 (1970) : 17–22.

60. N. J. Greenberger, "Changes in Gastroenterology 1960–1985: Lessons from the Past and Implications for the Future," *Gastroenterology* 89 (1985) : 933–38.

61. R. Schindler, *Gastroscopy* (Chicago: The University of Chicago Press, 1937).

62. C. C. Booth, "What has Technology Done to Gastroenterology?" *Gut* 26 (1985) : 1088–94.

63. Harold Hopkins and N. S. Kapany, "A flexible fibrescope, using static scanning," *Nature* (Jan. 1954), 39–41.

64. B. I. Hirschowitz, "Endoscopic Examinations of the Stomach and Duodenal Cap with a Fiberscope," *Lancet* 1 (1961) : 1074–78.

65. B. F. Overholt, "The History of Colonoscopy," in *Colonoscopy*, R. H. Hunt and J. D. Waye, eds. (Chicago: Yearbook Medical Publishers, 1981), 1–7. (Reproduced by permission from the author and the editors.)

66. C. C. Booth, "Technology and Medicine," *Proc Soc London* 224 (1985) : 267–85.

67. Booth, "Technology and Medicine."

68. Booth, "What Has Technology Done to Gastroenterology?"

69. A. Keller, "Has Science Created Technology," *Minerva* 22 (1985) : 160–82.

70. J. M. Eisenberg, "Sculpture of a New Academic Discipline—Four Faces of Academic General Internal Medicine," *Am J Med* 78 (1985) : 283–92.

71. Rosemary Stevens, *American Medicine and the Public Interest* (New Haven: Yale University Press, 1971).

72. R. Kipling, "The Elephant's Child—1909," cited by R. Asher, "Six honest serving men for medical writers," *JAMA* 208 (1969) : 83–87.

73. H. M. Spiro, *Clinical Gastroenterology* (New York: MacMillan, 1983).

74. S. S. Herman and A. M. Singer, "Basic Scientists in Clinical Departments of Medical Schools," *Clin Res* 34 (1986) : 149–58.

75. J. B. Kirsner, "The Changing Medical Scene (1929–1985)," *Perspect Biol Med* 29 (1986) : 227–42.

76. G. Vico (1668–1744), *The New Science*. Trans. from ed. 3, 1744, by Thomas Goddard Bergin and Max Harold Fisch (Ithaca, NY: Cornell University Press, 1948).

6

A Century of American Rheumatology

THOMAS G. BENEDEK

This chapter presents a survey of the evolution of rheumatology into a clinical and scientific subspecialty. The ways in which relevant scientific knowledge accrued and the kinds of new information which encouraged specialization are emphasized. The development of its organizational structure is treated in less detail.

In the 1880s pediatrics was beginning to be separated from adult medicine, but no compartmentalization was taking place within nonsurgical adult medicine. Frederick C. Shattuck, professor of medicine at the Harvard Medical School, commented in 1897:

> Specialism is a natural and necessary result of the growth of accurate knowledge, inseparably connected with the multiplication and perfection of instruments of precision. It has its drawbacks, absurdities even. . . . A few years ago a recent graduate and ex-hospital interne asked me, apparently seriously, to give him the name of a specialist in rheumatism. We can afford to laugh at these things.[1]

Shattuck might as well have chosen another category of diseases whereby to illustrate the impracticality of specialization at that time, but he considered a specialist in rheumatism the most unrealistic.

Rheumatic Diseases in 1885

Although no reliable prevalence of data from the nineteenth century exist, "rheumatic" patients undoubtedly were sufficiently plentiful and their diseases were sufficiently chronic that a practitioner could have limited himself to their care. Rheumatic fever in both children and adults would have occupied a large share of his practice. Directly infectious forms of arthritis also would have been prominent, particularly Pott's disease and "white swelling" (tuberculosis of the vertebral column and of peripheral joints). He would be seeing cases of neuropathic arthropathy due to syphilis, but none resulting from the principal modern cause, diabetes mellitus, because no diabetic lived long enough to suffer this complication. Owing to the poorer nutrition and shorter life span, he would see rickets and its consequent deformities but little osteoporosis.

When our nineteenth-century "rheumatologist" encountered cases of osteoarthritis, rheumatoid arthritis, ankylosing spondylitis, and gout, he had great difficulties in differential diagnosis, in part because he was unaware of the clinical distinctions and in part because of the lack of technological assistance. The diagnosis of gout was confused by the inclusion of a miscellany of complaints as "irregular" or "retrocedent Gout." According to Longstreth (1882), "acute rheumatoid arthritis is, in my experience, the most difficult condition to distinguish from acute rheumatism."[2] Juvenile polyarthritis had not yet been described and undoubtedly was diagnosed as rheumatic fever. Ankylosing spondylitis was considered to be either Pott's disease or osteoarthritis of the spine. There also was terminological confusion. For example, in the 1880s rheumatoid arthritis often was called osteoarthritis,[3] or even rheumatoid osteoarthritis.[4] We may assume that the disease we recognize as osteoarthritis occurred less frequently because of the shorter life expectancy.

The rarer connective tissue diseases were probably not recognized. The one that had been known the longest was scleroderma; polyarteritis had recently been described in Europe, whereas polymyositis had not been recognized at all; systemic lupus erythematosus had not been differentiated from discoid lupus erythematosus. Hypertrophic pulmonary osteoarthropathy also was unknown, and when it was described a few years later the disease differed from the one with which we are familiar: it was not associated with lung cancer, which then was a rarity, but with chronic pulmonary infections (*Table 6.1*).

TABLE 6.1.
FIRST AMERICAN REPORTS OF VARIOUS MUSCULOSKELETAL DISEASES

Disease	*Author*	*Location*	*Year*	*Ref.*
Ankylosing spondylitis	H. P. Wilson	Baltimore	1856	5
	E. H. Bradford	Boston	1883	6
Scleroderma	A. B. Arnold	Baltimore	1869	7
	W. F. Day	New York	1870	8
Reiter's disease	E. H. Bradford	Boston	1883(?)	6
	F. E. Simpson	Chicago	1912	9
Gonorrheal arthritis	E. A. Chancellor	St. Louis	1883	10
Polymyositis	G. W. Jacoby	New York	1888	11
Pulmonary osteoarthropathy				
(infectious)	F. A. Packard	Philadelphia	1892	12
(neoplastic)	E. M. Hasbrouck	Salisbury, MD	1898	13
Systemic lupus erythematosus	W. Osler	Baltimore	1895	14
Juvenile polyarthritis	H. Koplik	New York	1896	15
Polyarteritis nodosa	F. R. Sabin	Baltimore	1901(?)	16
	A. R. Lamb	New York	1914	17

Diagnoses depended almost entirely on the history and physical examination. The best established laboratory technics were bacteriological and even these were confined to a few research laboratories. Whatever rheumatologic diagnosis was made, what treatment could have been offered in 1885? Dietary manipulation, opiates, and quinine had been prescribed nonspecifically for a long time, but colchicum was the only drug that was acknowledged to have a specific beneficial effect, albeit limited to acute gout. The pharmaceutical revolution had just begun. Salicin, extracted from willow bark and from meadowsweet, had been introduced in the previous decade, followed by salicylic acid and sodium salicylate.[18,19] Although these drugs caused considerable gastric irritation, they were quickly recognized as superior, particularly for the treatment of rheumatic fever.[20] The practitioner might also find a surgeon who would drain and irrigate a chronically distended joint.[21]

A substantial literature was available for purchase or, if the physician lived in one of the few large cities, in a medical library. Little of the writing was by American authors. Indeed, there was only one American rheumatologic treatise: *Rheumatism, Gout, and Some Allied Disorders,* by Morris Longstreth of Philadelphia (1882).[22] Aside from English books and

TABLE 6.2.
MEDICAL RHEUMATIC DISEASE ADMISSIONS TO MASSACHUSETTS GENERAL HOSPITAL, 1877–1899[26]

"Rheumatism"	900
Gonorrheal arthritis	16
Gout	24
Rheumatic gout	3
Tabes with Charcot joint	1
Mean per year	41

journals, many French and German texts were available in translation. A leading physician would probably have obtained some training in Europe and be able to read the publications in the original. They offered countless therapeutic impressions but no controlled evaluations.

The predominant area of medical research in the 1880s was bacteriology, and the most important demonstrably infectious form of arthritis was due to the tubercle bacillus. It was several years after Koch's discovery in 1882 until this microbe became generally accepted as the cause of extrapulmonary tuberculosis.[23] "Tuberculosis of bones and joints is such a common affection that a large percentage of the clinical material of the surgeon and the general practitioner is made up of such cases." Thus did Nicholas Senn begin his monograph of 1892, *Tuberculosis of Bones and Joints,* the first major American work on the subject.[24] While it may have been up to the general practitioner to diagnose osteoarticular tuberculosis, treatment, such as it was, was in the realm of the orthopedic surgeon. For example, of 1,662 cases of joint diseases admitted to the Hospital for the Ruptured and Crippled, a primarily orthopedic hospital in New York, between 1871 and 1876 51.7 percent were diagnosed to have "vertebral caries," that is, spinal tuberculosis.[25] On the other hand, of 944 cases of joint diseases admitted to the medical services of the Massachusetts General Hospital between 1877 and 1899, no case was identified as tuberculous (*Table 6.2*).[26]

The first accurate rheumatologic microbiology was the culture of gonococci from knee effusions in two cases of gonorrhea by Luigi Petrone (Bologna, 1883).[27] The many successes of the new science led to the belief that a microbial cause might be found for most diseases. This resulted in the persistence of a paradigm regarding the etiology of rheumatic fever and rheumatoid arthritis, begun in 1887 by Alfred Mantle, an English physician. He was not alone in the belief that rheumatic fever and rheumatoid arthritis were merely different expressions of "rheumatism," but also believed that he had discovered the causative germs in blood and joint fluid cultures.[28] The normal bacterial flora of the throat was not understood, nor was the difference between acute rheumatic carditis and bacterial endocarditis. Hence, various organisms that were cultured from the throat and/or blood were implicated in the etiology of rheumatic fever. In regard to rheumatoid arthritis, aside from Mantle's hypothesis, the advocacy of a bacterial cause was reenforced by the 1893 report by Max Schüller, a German surgeon, of a distinctive bacillus in cultures from blood and joints.[29]

The Status of Rheumatic Diseases in 1910

In 1910 a diagnostician was equipped with descriptions of major rheumatic diseases that had been unknown in 1885, access to more publications, and most importantly, roentgenology. Although there were some important American reports, such as Osler's studies (1895–1904), which began to define systemic lupus erythematosus,[30,31] the European literature remained the most influential. The most comprehensive American text was *Diseases of the Bones and Joints* by Goldthwait, Painter, and Osgood, three Boston orthopedic surgeons, first published in 1909.[32] Its surgical orientation influenced the space allotted to the various topics: 253 pages (37%) to tuberculosis, ninety-six pages to rheumatoid and osteoarthritis and nontuberculous spondylitis, twenty-four pages to rickets, and eleven to gout. Osler and McCrae's seven-volume *Modern Medicine* was published in the same year. This general work, written from the standpoint of the internist, included an excellent fifty-seven-page chapter on "arthritis deformans," thirty-six pages on gout, and only two pages on tuberculous arthritis.[33]

Numerous attempts to classify diseases have been undertaken with varying degrees of complexity since the pioneering work of Boissier de Sauvages in the mid-eighteenth century. In regard to "chronic rheumatism" he designated fifteen varieties.[34,35] Many classifications were proposed in Europe during the nineteenth century, but the first significant American effort was made by Joel E. Goldthwait in 1904.[36] It had some scientific basis in that it was based in part of the appearance of the synovium. However, the ill-defined category of "infectious arthritis" included all diseases that did not fit into the other four designations. It reflected the confidence then held in the predominantly microbial cause of diseases (*Table 6.3*). The absence of a category of neuropathic arthropathy may be indicative of the swing away from excessive reliance on neurologic causal explanations. Two years later P. W. Nathan (New York) created a more elaborate scheme, which, however,

TABLE 6.3.
CLASSIFICATION OF ARTHRITIDES—J. E. GOLDTHWAIT, 1904[37]

Goldthwait's Designation	*Modern Equivalents*
Chronic villous arthritis	Traumatic or mechanical degenerative arthritis
Atrophic arthritis	Rheumatoid arthritis
Hypertrophic arthritis	Osteoarthritis, ankylosing spondylitis
Infectious arthritis (most common)	Septic arthritis, miscellaneous cases, probably mainly rheumatoid
Chronic gout	Tophaceous gout

primarily differentiated "inflammatory or infectious" from "trophic" joint diseases based on the acuteness or indolence of the clinical course.[37] The most scientific early classificatory work, by Nichols and Richardson (Boston, 1909), was based on a study of twenty-seven autopsies and thirty-eight surgical specimens from cases of "arthritis deformans." They concluded that, pathologically, there are two forms of nontuberculous arthritis. As "proliferative arthritis" they designated a disease which begins with inflammation of the synovium and affects the articular cartilage secondarily, and called the disease in which the primary lesion is in the cartilage "degenerative arthritis."[38] They did not use "proliferative" and "degenerative" as synonyms for rheumatoid and osteoarthritis, respectively, but rather concluded that these are the two ways articular tissues respond to nontuberculous injury. This pioneering investigation employed more rigid criteria than Goldthwait had used, but its importance was not appreciated for many years.

Most difficult to explain is the virtual disappearance of the diagnosis of gout. For example, between 1889 and 1903 only forty-two cases were admitted to the Johns Hopkins Hospital with this diagnosis. All were men and, of the thirty-nine who had experienced more than one attack, nineteen had tophi. Evidence of gout was found in 0.33 percent of autopsies.[39] This diagnosis was even rarer at the Massachusetts General Hospital: only nine cases of gout were found among 1,033 medical admissions for rheumatic diseases from 1893 to 1903.[40] Herrick (Chicago) was unusual for a physician in 1906 when he stated that he had seen seven cases in the previous five months and felt that "gout is commoner in the United States than is generally believed."[41] In keeping with this observation, about nineteen cases were diagnosed annually at the Cook County Hospital (Chicago) between 1914 and 1919.[42]

During the first decade of the twentieth century clinical laboratories were established in some of the larger hospitals, and diagnostic bacteriology, rudimentary biochemistry, and hematology became available at least to the physicians who were affiliated with these institutions.[43] Analyses for uric acid were the first chemical determinations that were relevant to rheumatology. Salkowski (Königsberg) in 1871 devised a gravimetric assay.[44] However, this and its numerous modifications all were too insensitive to detect uric acid in blood. Their application was limited to urine and the results were difficult to interpret. As of 1910 no better technique had been discovered.

The principal additions to rheumatologic knowledge in this period resulted from the introduction in 1896 of diagnostic radiology. No discovery in the history of medicine has been employed so widely so rapidly. The first American roentgenogram was published eleven weeks after Roentgen's initial report of his discovery,[45] and the first American book about radiology appeared nine months after the latter event.[46] How widespread the taking of X ray pictures was in the first few years is uncertain, particularly because the practice was not limited to physicians. Physicists and tube manufacturers, among others, also provided this service. Most of the descriptive discoveries were being made in Europe and only two skeletal diseases first reported in the United States were diagnosed with the assistance of radiology. Robert Osgood (Boston, 1903) described aseptic necrosis of the tibial tuberosity.[47] Aseptic necrosis of the capital femoral epiphysis (hip) was reported by Albert Freiberg (Cincinnati, 1905)[48] and Arthur Legg (Boston, 1910).[49] X ray therapy of arthritides also lagged behind European trials. The first reported cases were two men with rheumatoid arthritis who underwent irradiation of several joints in 1905 and 1906 in Philadelphia with temporary improvement.[50]

Medical therapy now included a wider range of analgesics. Aspirin was introduced in 1899 and partially replaced sodium salicylate.[51] Of several p-amino phenol derivatives that had been introduced in the 1880s, phenacetin had become the most popular.[52,53] However, many clinicians favored physiotherapy over any medicinal treatment for chronic arthritis. The literature may not give a representative impression because so large a proportion of the publications on the treatment of arthritis was by surgeons.

The Status of Rheumatology in 1935

The most fundamental advance between 1911 and 1935 was the elucidation of the cause of rheumatic fever. Furthermore, synovial fluid began to be examined, and the erythrocyte sedimentation rate was introduced and applied to identify inflammatory types of arthritis. A method to assay the uric acid content of blood was devised and gradually improved. The one therapeutic advance, although still controversial at the end of this period, was the use of gold compounds to treat rheumatoid arthritis. This also was the time in which rheumatologic organizations were founded.

The unusual concentrations of observable military personnel that are characteristic of wartime often have supplied new medical insights. Thus, although rheumatic fever principally is a disease of childhood, it was diagnosed in 24,770 U.S. soldiers between April 1917 and December 1919, comprising 27 percent of all rheumatologic cases.[54] While there was agreement that rheumatic fever was an infectious disease and that streptococci probably played some role in its pathogenesis, the inconsistency of the bacteriological findings remained baffling. Three hypotheses were formulated: (1) a bacteremia of a rheumatogenic micro-organism selectively localized in the symptomatic sites; (2) the disease was produced by a rheumatogenic toxin made by certain bacteria; (3) the affected tissues responded allergically to a component of some bacteria.[55] The solution of the problem emanated mainly from New York, particularly from Homer Swift and his colleagues at the Rockefeller Institute and Alvin Coburn and his associates at Columbia University.

Swift began his studies in 1916 and by 1928 concluded that the most likely cause of rheumatic fever is an allergic response to repeated streptococcal infections. He believed that nonhemolytic strains probably were the most virulent.[56,57] Coburn's investigations were begun a decade later. He succeeded in identifying the hemolytic streptococcus as the critical microbe, at first from epidemiologic inferences.[58] These were then supported by the application of recent research in streptococcal physiology: the classification of streptococci into serologic types by Rebecca Lancefield (New York, 1928)[59] and the antistreptolysin test for the immunologic response to a streptococcal enzyme by E. W. Todd (London, 1932).[60,61] Coburn concluded that rheumatic fever is caused by an immunologic response to type-A hemolytic streptococci and that a particularly strong antistreptolysin titer is evidence of this.[62] The latter supposition was erroneous, but Coburn, nevertheless, had provided a firm foundation for further pathogenetic and therapeutic research.[63]

The early serologic studies of rheumatoid arthritis are of historical interest not only because they led to the discovery of the rheumatoid factor, but also because they formed the theoretical bridge from the early hypotheses of rheumatoid arthritis as an infectious disease to the contemporary autoimmune hypotheses. As was the case with rheumatic fever, it was debated whether the cause was a primary, presumably hematogenous, infection or a reaction to a remote localized infection. The idea that a "focus of infection" of various sorts may cause rheumatoid arthritis was popularized by Frank Billings (Chicago, 1912), although it did not originate with him.[64,65] It was Billings who introduced the confusing term "chronic infectious arthritis" for rheumatoid arthritis. Although bacteria were believed to have been recovered from joints, blood, or "foci" fairly often, no type was found consistently. The closeness of the association of the two bacterial hypotheses was shown by Russell Cecil (New York, 1929) in the introduction of the first of many papers on the "bacteriology of the blood and joints in chronic infectious arthritis" by stating that "the most important contribution to the etiology of chronic arthritis was made by Billings and his co-workers nearly twenty years ago." Cecil's group therefore began in 1927 to make cultures from the teeth and tonsils and later also from blood and joints of arthritis patients. A "typical strain of attenuated hemolytic streptococcus" was obtained in about two thirds of the cultures from either blood or joints of cases of rheumatoid arthritis.[66] Rabbits were immunized with the "typical strains" and an agglutinin test was developed with the resulting antiserum. About one half of rheumatoid arthritis patients exhibited an agglutination reaction.[67]

The validity of these intriguing results was first challenged by Dawson and Boots, Cecil's colleagues at Columbia University. Their attempts to duplicate the bacteriologic studies yielded consistently sterile cultures.[68] Nevertheless, they did confirm that serum from rheumatoid patients frequently agglutinates hemolytic streptococci, even in high dilution. This laboratory actually obtained agglutination reactions more frequently than Cecil had reported, and demonstrated that whether or not the cultures had been obtained from cases of rheumatoid arthritis was immaterial.[69] Another line of evidence that countered Cecil's hypothesis was the demonstration by Myers and Keefer (Boston, 1934) that rheumatoid arthritis is not associated with the elevated antistreptolysin titers previously shown in hemolytic streptococcus infections.[70] Hence, by 1935 the streptococcal etiology of rheumatoid arthritis had been convincingly disproved, but the meaning of conflicting findings remained to be interpreted.

One useful laboratory test that was introduced during this period was the erythrocyte sedimentation rate. The phenomenon was discovered in Sweden in 1917, but its application to differentiate between inflammatory and noninflammatory musculoskeletal complaints was not reported in the United States until 1928.[71] The results were confirmed by Dawson and Boots in 1930. They found accelerated rates of sedimentation in 62 percent of cases of rheumatoid arthritis, 10 percent of osteoarthritis, and none of "fibrositis."[72] Although this simple test came into routine use, some investigators cautioned against great reliance on the results because it is not sufficiently disease-specific.

After several decades of disappointing experience with urinary uric acid determinations, the clinical value of a serum assay was slow to be accepted. In 1912 Otto Folin at Harvard devised the first practical analytical method sufficiently sensitive to detect uric acid in blood.[73] In a comparison of blood from gouty and nongouty individuals, mean values of 4.3 ± 0.9 mg% and 2.2 ± 0.4 mg%, respectively, were obtained.[74] These are 40 to 50 percent of "true" values. Despite its deficiencies the method was adequate to demonstrate the uricosuric effect of cinchophen.[75] Thus, the beginning of quantitative clinical pharmacology may be considered to date from a rheumatologic investigation in 1913. Folin and other biochemists during twenty years made various improvements of this colorimetric technique. For example, Berglund in 1925 obtained mean values of 8.7 ± 1.8 mg% from seventeen cases of gout and 3.7 ± 1.0 mg% from nineteen cases of rheumatoid arthritis. This author summarized the uncertain status of a uric acid determination as follows:

> Now there are clinicians in England, in Germany, and in other places who see a great many cases of gout, rheumatoid arthritis, muscular rheumatism, migraine, and other headaches, and who are rather liberal with the diagnosis of irregular gout. For many of these very experienced physicians the blood uric acid is a symptoms [*sic*] without great significance.[76]

The most obvious material for study identified with rheumatology is synovial fluid. Certain of its characteristics had been described by Paracelsus in the sixteenth century.[77] But, aside from the bacteriologic cultures which began to be made in the 1880s, it received little scientific attention before the 1920s, largely because it is virtually unobtainable from healthy human joints during life and not consistently available from diseased joints. The early investigations, in part because of small numbers of determinations, gave confusing results. One small study worthy of mention by Allison (Boston, 1926) showed that the glucose content of fluids from cases of tuberculous and gonococcal arthritis is low.[78] The first comprehensive study of synovial fluid was undertaken by David H. Kling (New York) beginning in 1929. His major conclusions, which he reported in a monograph in 1938, were that the viscosity of synovial fluid varies widely and that this is related to the severity rather than the cause of the inflammation.[79] Of greater diagnostic value was the "Ropes test" described in 1947, in which the quality of the coagulum that forms when synovial fluid is added to acetic acid is estimated.[80]

Therapeutics

One may speculate that rheumatology was not yet becoming a subspecialty in the 1930s because the therapy of "rheumatism" had become increasingly chaotic. Diagnostic accuracy had improved very little and, due to the combined effects of improved pharmaceutical manufacturing and inadequate drug control regulations, many more remedies had become available. When there is little agreement among "experts" and any practitioner is likely to obtain as good a result as another, there is no incentive to recognize certain physicians as specialists. With the profusion of medications, drug therapy was held in particularly low esteem. One expert's evaluation of the therapy of rheumatoid arthritis in 1933 does not even mention drugs;[81] another in 1934 only commented in passing that "analgesics such as those of the salicylate group are necessary for the comfort of the patient."[82] Cecil in 1934 questioned sixteen physicians who were interested in rheumatic diseases, most of whom were "professors in leading medical schools," about their therapy for rheumatoid arthritis. "Drugs did not receive honorable mention in a single questionnaire," although all agreed that salicylates are valuable analgesics. Preference was given to rest, physiotherapy, diet, correction of constipation, removal of actual and potential foci of infection, various vaccines, mainly made from streptococci, and blood transfusions.[83] Furthermore, circulatory "stimulants" such as digitalis and nitrites were recommended, along with "specific agents" such as autogenous vaccines, nonspecific stimulants such as foreign protein injections and iodides, "tonics" such as arsenic and strychnine, nutritional supplements, and, with particular emphasis, laxatives.[84] In the words of a future president of the American Rheumatism Association (ARA): "The ideal treatment of this disease [rheumatoid arthritis] will require of the physician an enormous expenditure of nervous energy and the patience of Job, for there must be careful and methodical consideration of each individual problem."[85]

The first rheumatologic drug of the twentieth century considered particularly valuable in the treatment of rheumatic fever and of gout was cinchophen. It was introduced in Germany in 1908, in the United States in about 1912, and remained in extensive use for thirty years. Aside from its specific uses, cinchophen, like the salicylates and phenacetin, became an ingredient of numerous nonprescription analgesic remedies. It was erroneously believed that not only the clinical effects of cinchophen but also its safety were virtually indistinguishable from those of the salicylates.[86,87]

The ambivalence about pharmaceutical therapy may partially explain the reluctance with which gold treatment was accepted. Because of the specificity of the gold compounds, similar only to colchicine in the rheumatologic formulary, they eventually became a factor in the definition of rheumatology as a subspecialty. The reluctance to try gold was not due to the irrational hypothesis which led to its introduction in Europe. At the very same time that gold compounds began to be used in France, Germany, and Austria to treat rheumatoid arthritis, an analogously empirical therapeutic approach was being tried in the United States. An orthopedic surgeon who attended patients at the leprosarium in Louisiana noted that he had seen no cases of coincidental rheumatoid arthritis in patients whose leprosy was being treated with chaulmoogra oil. Based on no more than this, he began in 1930 to treat cases of rheumatoid arthritis with this venerable Asiatic remedy.[88] Despite his optimistic report, this form of therapy did not become popular, and no one knows whether a useful remedy has been ignored.

Jacques Forestier, a physician at the spa in Aix-les-Bains, France, first tried a gold compound (aurothiopropanol sulfonate) to treat rheumatoid arthritis in 1928.[89] The following quotation from his first English language publication about this treatment (1932) demonstrates the analogy with chaulmoogra oil:

> Chemotherapy has always appeared to me likely to be of great help in treating rheumatoid arthritis, since it is efficient in infective diseases, such as syphilis or tuberculosis. A certain amount of similarity between the latter disease and rheumatoid arthritis—i.e., impairment of the general condition, anaemia, leukocytosis, and temperature—led me to believe that some forms of treatment which had proved valuable for tuberculosis could help in the treatment of rheumatoid arthritis. This is why in 1928 I began to treat such patients with gold salts, the method introduced in treating pulmonary tuberculosis by Mollgaard in 1914.[90]

This hypothesis was reinforced by several European investigators who claimed to have cultured variant tubercle bacilli from the blood or joints of rheumatoid arthritis patients.[91] Consequently, Forestier by 1935 had modified his opinion of why gold therapy had resulted in favorable responses in 70 to 80 percent of 550 patients: "Our belief has grown that such a [tuberculous] factor has to be seriously considered in a certain proportion of cases." But "in true tuberculous arthritis . . . it is interesting to point out that gold salts treatment is not quite so successful, and higher dosage is required."[92]

The first American physicians to develop a sustained interest in gold therapy were L. M. Lockie in Buffalo, who began to employ it in 1932,[93] and R. L. Cecil, whose experience began in 1933 following a visit from Forestier.[94] However, after a year of experience Cecil wrote that "patients whom I have treated by this method have never shown very striking results,"[95] and another future president of the ARA stated in 1936 that he found the effect of gold salts "disappointing."[96] By 1937 a series of 900 cases of gold therapy was reported from Leeds, England.[97] The first series of one hundred cases from a single American clinic in New York was not described until 1939.[98] In 1942 Cecil reported on the treatment of 245 cases and had come to endorse it cautiously.[99] There was some difference of opinion about the value of gold therapy for "rheumatoid spondylitis." Forestier believed it to be effective,[100] Cecil the opposite.[101] Both opinions were based on scant data. The initial perception persisted that gold therapy is most likely to be useful in rheumatoid arthritis. The delay in greater acceptance resulted from lingering doubts about gold's benefits versus risks of toxicity.

Institutionalization of Rheumatology

The first American internist to limit his practice to rheumatologic patients was probably Ralph Pemberton in Philadelphia in the 1920s.[102] Before 1927, when Philip S. Hench began a program at the Mayo Clinic, no formal training in the research or treatment of rheumatic diseases existed in the United States. Hench joined the staff of the Mayo Clinic in 1923 after completing his internal medicine residency there. In 1926 he was designated head of a new section devoted to rheumatic diseases and remained its only staff physician until 1935. He spent eight months during 1928 and 1929 in Germany studying laboratory medicine in Freiburg and Munich.[103] However, Hench remained particularly interested in clinical investigation and oriented many subsequently influential rheumatologists in this direction.

Another four new units undertook specialized training in rheumatologic research and treatment in the next decade. The common denominator of three of them was philanthropy. The R. W. Lovett Memorial in 1929 made its first undertaking the funding of a rheumatic diseases unit at the Massachusetts General Hospital (Harvard Medical School). Walter Bauer, an internist who had been interested in metabolic problems, proved to be an excellent choice as its first director. The second rheumatic diseases unit under medical school administration was the Faulkner Arthritis Clinic at the Presbyterian Hospital of New York, owned by Columbia University, founded in 1930 and led initially by Ralph H. Boots and Martin H. Dawson. Both were trained as microbiologists at the Rockefeller Institute. The next unit was established in 1932 at the Bellevue Hospital within the Department of Medicine of New York University. It differed in that the dean of the medical school, John H. Wykoff, determined that rheumatology should be fostered and he organized a program with a unique interdepartmental breadth.[104] Its first and long-time director was Currier McEwen who, like Boots, had a background in rheumatic fever research at the Rockefeller Institute under Homer Swift.

The fifth and last of the pioneer teaching units, the Rackham Arthritis Research Unit at the University of Michigan, was initiated in 1937 in circumstances similar to those at Columbia University and was also being funded in memory of a rheumatoid arthritis patient. Its first chief was Richard H. Freyberg who, like Bauer, had been interested in metabolism and did not have specifically rheumatologic training. The last four units could boast at least two physicians within a year of their establishment. But in a period of severe economic depression the concept of a subspecialty of rheumatology grew slowly. No further specialized units were created until after the Second World War.[105]

Organizations of medical specialists had existed in the United States for nearly ninety years before the founding of an association of rheumatologists.[106] Like other formative aspects of rheumatology, the impetus to organize began in Europe. In 1925 a British Committee on Rheumatism was established, chaired by Fortescue Fox.[107] The recognized international leader of rheumatology soon came to be Jan van Breemen, the director of the Institute for Physical Therapy in Amsterdam. An International Committee on Rheumatism was founded at a meeting held on 26 April 1926 at the rheumatism spa in Piestany, Slovakia, attended by representatives from nine European countries.[108] This was followed six months later by the formation of a national organization in the Netherlands, similar organizations in Germany and Belgium in 1927, and many more in the next two years.[109]

The organizational development of rheumatology in the United States has been complex and has been well described by Smyth, Freyberg, and McEwen in a recent monograph.[110] Briefly, this development may be considered in four divisions: (1) the founding of a professional organization, the American Rheumatism Association; (2) a resultant public fund-raising and

TABLE 6.4.
AMERICAN COMMITTEE FOR THE CONTROL OF RHEUMATISM

Present at First Meeting, 17 March 1928			
Ralph Pemberton	1877–1949	Philadelphia	internist (chairman)
Charles C. Bass	1875–?	New Orleans	internist
Russell L. Cecil	1881–1965	New York	internist
Russell L. Haden	1888–1952	Kansas City, KS	internist
Melvin S. Henderson	1883–1954	Rochester, MN	orthopedist
Joseph L. Miller	1867–1937	Chicago	internist
J. Archer O'Reilly	1879–1951	St. Louis	orthopedist
Robert B. Osgood	1873–1956	Boston	orthopedist
Members Added in 1928/29			
A. Almon Fletcher	1889–?	Toronto	internist
Philip S. Hench	1896–1965	Rochester, MN	internist
George R. Minot	1885–1950	Boston	internist
Cyrus C. Sturgis	1891–1966	Ann Arbor, MI	internist
Hans Zinsser	1878–1940	Boston	M.D. microbiologist

educational organization, the Arthritis Foundation; (3) the establishment of a federally funded research and granting agency, the National Institute for Arthritis and Metabolic Diseases; and (4) a quasi-official certifying body, the subspecialty Board of Rheumatology of the American Board of Internal Medicine.

The immediate stimulus for the establishment of the first American rheumatologic organization, the American Committee for the Control of Rheumatism, came from Louis B. Wilson, the director of the Mayo Foundation. On a trip to Europe in 1926 he learned of interest in organizing efforts to improve the understanding and therapy of the rheumatic diseases. He was asked by van Breemen, Fox, and perhaps others to assist in establishing a committee of physicians in the United States with a similar interest. As a result, a group of five internists and three orthopedic surgeons held its first meeting on 17 March 1928 in Philadelphia, chaired by Ralph Pemberton (*Table 6.4*). In preparation for this meeting Pemberton had visited European organizers in the summer of 1927.[111,112]

The *Journal of the American Medical Association* took notice of the formation of the American Committee by publishing an editorial, written by Pemberton, in July 1928. It concluded as follows:

> there are few other diseases which so readily invite careless and inefficient treatment. . . . The danger of uncritical enthusiasm for new measures is now as great as ever.
>
> Considerable importance therefore attaches to the inauguration of a movement in this country toward solution of the devastating problem of arthritis. In this refractory field early accomplishments of signal value are hardly to be expected. Coordinated and sustained effort must inevitably establish a foundation from which, sooner or later, will spring an awakened sense of responsibility toward arthritic patients, a better understanding of the problem as a whole, decreasing suffering, and a reduction of the large economic loss now born by society.[113]

The primary initial goal of the Committee was to educate physicians in the common rheumatic diseases. In October 1929 it was decided to address this purpose with exhibits to be shown at the national convention of the American Medical Association (AMA). Indeed, at the next five conventions of the AMA there was an arthritis exhibit.[114–118] Except for the exhibit in 1931, these were simple poster presentations defining rheumatoid and osteoarthritis and related gross clinical problems. At the Philadelphia convention (1931) the osteologic collection of the Muetter Museum of the College of Physicians enabled the organizers to make a more elaborate presentation.

The first public meeting, called "A Conference on Rheumatic Diseases," was held in New Orleans on 9 May 1932, immediately preceding the convention of the AMA. The same procedure was followed in Milwaukee in 1933 and in Cleveland in 1934. A survey of the twenty-seven papers presented at the three meetings gives a rough impression of the scientific state of the still unnamed subspecialty. There were thirty-seven authors, of whom three contributed twice (Pemberton, Hench, and Holbrook). Except for solitary papers on gout and on radiologic manifestations, clinical topics were limited to rheumatoid and osteoarthritis. Only one paper in 1934 presented basic research: J. G. Kuhns and H. L. Wetherford of Boston on "the role of the reticuloendothelial system in the deposition of colloidal and particulate matter in articular cavities."[119–121]

At meetings in 1933 the American Committee against Rheumatism formulated the creation of a larger "American Association for the Control of Rheumatism." This was conceived of as an exclusive group of about one hundred influential physicians and laymen to which the Committee was to be advisory.[122] In fact, the charter membership of the "American Association for the Study and Control of Rheumatic Diseases" was 104. Ernest E. Irons was its first president and its first meeting was held in Cleveland in June

1934. The "first annual meeting" simultaneously was the "Third Conference on Rheumatic Diseases." In 1937 the rather cumbersome name was changed to American Rheumatism Association. The idea of exclusiveness was never adhered to, as is shown by the growth of the membership to 226 by 1940. Its leadership showed aggressive initiative and the Association was named host of the seventh International Congress, to be held in 1940. However, because of the outbreak of the war in Europe this Congress was postponed until 1949.

The Status of Rheumatology in 1960

The third quarter century, 1936–1960, saw rheumatology firmly established as a discrete subspecialty of internal medicine. The first use of the term "rheumatologist" I have found appeared in Comroe's *Arthritis and Allied Conditions* in 1940.[123] Both "rheumatology" and "rheumatologist" were first listed in the 1941 edition of Dorland's *American Illustrated Medical Dictionary.*[124] While specialization had multiple determinants, the leading factors undoubtedly were the advent of far more effective therapeutic and diagnostic methods.

The first important events of the period were the discovery of the sulfonamide drugs, particularly their effects in the treatment of gonococcal arthritis and rheumatic fever, followed by the medical circumstances of World War II. Gonorrhea was a very common disease. In the five years from 1923 to 1927, 610 cases of gonococcal arthritis were admitted to Bellevue Hospital, New York. Contrary to the contemporary experience, only seven of the patients were women. Of those who were discharged from Bellevue, 22 percent were hospitalized for longer than one month and another 21 percent were transferred to other hospitals. Many kinds of treatment were employed. Gonococcal vaccines and hyperthermia were the most common forms of therapy, but intravenous Mercurochrome (a mercury and bromine substituted fluorescein), introduced in 1919, also remained popular.[125,126] Forty years later effective treatment had reduced the incidence of arthritis from about 3 percent to about 0.5 percent of cases of gonorrhea and the sex incidence had changed from over 90 percent male to over 70 percent female.

The first reports on the effect of sulfanilamide on gonococcal infections appeared in 1937. C. S. Keefer and W. W. Spink of Boston described the treatment of 140 cases including three with arthritis,[127] and Colston and associates (Baltimore) reported results in eighty cases, including ten of gonococcal arthritis.[128] The results in the arthritis cases appeared to be favorable, with defervescence and symptomatic relief often occurring within two days. But already two years later Keefer sounded some warnings: recurrences of both the febrile arthritis and of gonorrhea may follow withdrawal of the drug; longer treatment than was used at first may be necessary; side effects occur sufficiently often that patients who are receiving sulfanilamide must be followed carefully.[129] Consequently, a therapeutic assessment in 1940 was that oral sulfanilamide and intravenous Mercurochrome were of equal value, and both were safer, although not more beneficial, than fever therapy.[130] The cure rate of gonococcal arthritis with sulfonamide therapy was later estimated to be 70 percent.[131] Its ability to prevent this complication of gonorrhea was demonstrated by military statistics: during World War I gonorrheal arthritis constituted 9 percent of the rheumatic disease diagnoses in the U.S. Army,[132] while only 0.8 percent of the first 5,000 rheumatologic cases admitted to the Army Rheumatism Center in Hot Springs, Arkansas during 1943 to 1945 carried this diagnosis.[133]

Military Rheumatology

During World War I "rheumatic diseases" affected nearly 93,000 American soldiers, or 2.24 percent of Army personnel. Of these, 36 percent received a diagnosis of either rheumatoid or osteoarthritis (not differentiated in the statistics) and 27 percent rheumatic fever.[134] Knowledge of this major category of morbidity prompted the Surgeon General of the Army in 1942 to begin to plan for the care of rheumatically diseased military personnel. As a consequence, World War II spurred the development of American rheumatology in two ways. In the autumn of 1942 the Surgeon General consulted with leaders of the American Rheumatism Association (P. S. Hench, W. P. Holbrook, and W. Bauer) for the planning of "Rheumatism Centers."[135] The government thereby recognized this organization as the representative of a medical specialty. Of greater eventual importance was that many of the physicians who staffed the five centers that were finally established became leading rheumatologists and developed training programs for the next generation.

The first center was activated at the Army and Navy General Hospital, Hot Springs, Arkansas, in 1943. Hench was chief of the medical services and E. W. Boland was chief of the rheumatic diseases section. This section reached a maximum staff of eighteen physicians and a maximum census in excess of 700 patients. During the one and a half years beginning in January

1944, 5,315 patients with musculoskeletal complaints were admitted. Because of the great demand a second even larger general rheumatology center was opened in 1944 near Dallas (Ashburn Army Hospital). Simultaneously, three centers for the treatment of rheumatic fever were activated, two in California and one in Mississippi. Early in 1945 the Ashburn Hospital had 1,661 beds designated for rheumatic disease patients and during the year a total of 3,534 patients occupied these beds. The peak of new cases of rheumatic fever in the Armed Forces occurred in 1944, when 13,400 cases were diagnosed. The average for the four years 1942 to 1945 was 9,821 cases annually.[136,137]

The magnitude of the problem stimulated valuable rheumatologic research in the U.S. military services during and shortly after World War II. It was focused in part on the epidemiology of hemolytic streptococcal infections and their relationship to the occurrence of acute rheumatic fever, and in part on means to prevent this disease. It had already been found in 1938 that sulfanilamide does not alter the course of rheumatic fever[138] and in 1939 that the drug may prevent recurrences.[139] However, it had become evident by 1945 that streptococci develop strains that are resistant to sulfonamides and that these drugs then lose their prophylactic effect. Fortunately, penicillin became available in 1945 in amounts that nearly met the demand. Its greater effectiveness in rheumatic fever prophylaxis when given in adequate dosage was soon demonstrated.[140] A comparison of the prevalence of rheumatic fever in military personnel in the two world wars shows that, as serious as the problem was during World War II, this diagnosis was made in only 10 percent as many Army and 37 percent as many Navy personnel.[141] The extent to which this difference was due to attempts at prevention is uncertain.

The Cardiovascular Diseases Subcommittee of the National Research Council (NRC) in 1943 became concerned with the increased frequency with which the diagnosis of rheumatic fever was being made, particularly in military training camps. The NRC observed that there were no generally agreed upon diagnostic criteria. Recognizing that misdiagnosis could stigmatize individual patients as well as diminish the effectiveness of public health planning, Thomas Duckett Jones, a Boston cardiologist, in 1944 devised a set of five major and seven minor diagnostic criteria. He enunciated the premise that "any single major manifestation with at least two of the minor manifestations would seem to place the diagnosis on reasonably safe grounds."[142] This approach to diagnostic validation was well received and became a model for the diagnosis of other rheumatic diseases. The Jones criteria were revised twice. The first modification, in 1955, mainly altered the importance given to some of the clinical signs, whereas the 1965 revision stressed laboratory evidence of recent streptococcal infection.[143,144]

A lesser accomplishment of military rheumatology was the cautious acknowledgment of Reiter's disease. Peculiarly, the first specific American description of cases was not published until 1942,[145] although several cases of keratodermia blennorrhagica, its cutaneous manifestation, had been described since 1912[146] and some cases of "gonorrheal rheumatism" undoubtedly had been instances of Reiter's disease. The largest of several military reports was a description of twenty-five men who were examined by Hollander at the Ashburn Army Hospital.[147] The reluctance to accept Reiter's disease as a discrete entity was indicated by the hypothesis, advanced by Hench and Boland among others, that gonorrhea may cause or activate rheumatoid arthritis.[148,149] This concept of "post-gonorrheal rheumatoid arthritis" faded out in the 1950s for lack of evidence and as the diagnosis of Reiter's disease became generally accepted. Serologic findings strengthened the evidence for its distinctness, suggesting a genetic predisposition, but an etiologic agent remains to be demonstrated.

Collagen Diseases, Rheumatoid Factor, and Lupus Erythematosus Cell

The foremost conceptual advance of this period was the formulation of the theory of "collagen diseases" by Paul Klemperer, an Austrian-born pathologist at Mount Sinai Hospital in New York. He coined the term in 1942.[150] The existence of connective tissue had been recognized since the 1830s. However, pathologists held that collagen, elastin, and chondrin, collectively called interstitial matter, were physiologically inert proteins.[151] H. Schade, a German biochemist, in 1912 questioned this point of view. Based on studies of the elasticity of various tissues he concluded that ground substance ("interstitial matter") does have unique functions, that cellular components of connective tissue have common characteristics independent of the organ in which they are situated, and that the tissue must be physiologically active.[152] The idea that this disseminated tissue may become specifically diseased originated from later German research, particularly that on the pathogenesis of rheumatic fever by Fritz Klinge. He was impressed by similarities in the histologic changes in the myocardium and synovium, two unrelated tissues in this disease.[153] Klinge's conclusions reflected progressive theory pathologically, but proved to be regressive clinically because he proposed, based on his pathological and experimental findings, that rheumatic fever and rheumatoid arthritis are merely different expressions of "one unified rheumatic event."[154] Because of its multisystem involvement Klemperer first added systemic lupus erythematosus (SLE) to his "disorder[s] of the connective tissue system," and soon included scleroderma as well.[155]

Contrary to some other notable investigators, such as Arnold Rich (Baltimore), Klemperer did not postulate a common etiology for the pathologic similarities of the several diseases which soon became grouped as "collagen diseases." Rich postulated that anaphylactic hypersensitivity may be the common denominator among all of these diseases.[156] Klemperer remained more diffident about pathogenesis and in 1950 also commented perceptively that "a peculiar worship of diagnostic terms has led to an exaggerated popularity of the diagnosis collagen disease. There is danger that it may become a catch-all term for maladies with puzzling clinical and anatomical features."[157] Because the primary abnormalities in these diseases obviously are not limited to the collagenous component of connective tissue, W. E. Ehrich (Philadelphia) suggested in 1952 that they be called instead "systemic diseases of the connective tissue."[158] Indeed, the designation "connective tissue diseases" has gradually replaced "collagen diseases" while uncertainty about which diseases belong in this category has persisted.

The new laboratory techniques of the 1950s and 1960s elucidated the chemistry and structure of connective tissue in great detail. Ironically, this has achieved more to further the understanding of the rare heritable disorders, such as the Ehlers-Danlos and Marfan's syndromes than for the diseases usually encountered by the rheumatologist.

Two simultaneous diagnostic discoveries in 1948 publicized rheumatology among physicians and stimulated basic research: the rheumatoid factor and the lupus erythematosus (LE) cell. The forerunners of the research leading to rheumatoid factor were described in the previous section. The specificity of streptococcal agglutination reactions in rheumatoid arthritis was questioned in the mid-1930s. Allan Wallis (Philadelphia, 1946) provided the final disproof of the pathogenetic role of a strain of streptococci in this disease. He demonstrated that sera from cases of rheumatoid arthritis appear to contain a factor that nonspecifically enhances agglutination reactions and demonstrated this not only with several species of bacteria, but also with collodion particles.[159]

A second line of research began with two fortuitous, independent observations during work with the complement fixation reaction using sheep red blood cells. In the usual reaction between the test serum and sensitized cells hemolysis occurs. Erik Waaler in Oslo performed such a test in 1937 and found that the cells clumped instead of rupturing. The serum came from a patient with rheumatoid arthritis, and this prompted Waaler to carry out a study in which he demonstrated this unexpected reaction in 30 percent of rheumatoid sera and in only 1 percent of controls.[160]

In 1948 Harry M. Rose and colleagues at Columbia University rediscovered this phenomenon. Again, the complement fixation test was being used in a nonrheumatologic investigation. The laboratory technician, who had rheumatoid arthritis, used her own serum as a control and observed agglutination instead of the expected nonreaction. This observation was then pursued by the rheumatologist Charles Ragan and a test that was more sensitive than that of Waaler was developed. According to the original publication, 65 percent of subjects with rheumatoid arthritis and 4 percent of controls exhibited the serologic reaction.[161,162] It became known as the "Waaler-Rose" or "differential sheep cell agglutination test" and was the first test for "rheumatoid factor," a term that was introduced by Ziff in 1957.[163] Numerous modifications were attempted, but as sensitivity was enhanced specificity was lost. Furthermore, the use of biological material such as sheep erythrocytes was both tedious and a source of inconsistency.

Thus, in 1956 J. M. Singer and C. M. Plotz in New York, seemingly independently of Wallis' observation of the agglutination of collodion particles, devised a technique in which inert polystyrene latex particles coated with gamma globulin were agglutinated by serum which contained the rheumatoid factor.[164] This was a substantial improvement later adapted to other serologic tests. However, none of the detection techniques that were devised has fulfilled the hope for achieving a definitive diagnosis. The rheumatoid factor has remained neither sufficiently sensitive nor sufficiently specific. The tests have, nevertheless, been important in several ways. Because the discovery of rheumatoid factor seemed to fulfill the need for a diagnostic test for rheumatoid arthritis it increased the perception that rheumatology has unique attributes. Study of the reaction has furthered the understanding of autoantibodies and, therefore, the scientific basis of much of modern rheumatology. Clinically, the presence of rheumatoid factor, especially in high titer, proved a useful indicator of poor prognosis.[165]

The clinical importance of the discovery of a test for SLE was greater than the discovery of rheumatoid factor, because of both the greater specificity of the LE cell phenomenon and the greater need for a diagnostic tool for SLE. The new test greatly increased case finding and confirmation in a disease that had been considered rare. The reaction which the test demonstrates also was soon shown to be an intimate part of the pathogenesis of the disease.

The designation "LE cell" was coined in 1948 by Malcolm M. Hargraves, a hematologist at the Mayo Clinic, in the first report about this peculiar cell. He stated that "[it] has been called an LE cell in our laboratory because of its frequent appearance in the bone marrow in cases of acute disseminated LE."[166] Actually, Hargraves had observed LE cells in bone marrow aspirates several times between 1943 and 1946, when he made the association between the cells and this disease.[167] Four months after Hargraves' initial report, John R. Haserick, a dermatologist at the Cleveland Clinic, submitted a paper in which he confirmed the spontaneous occurrence of these phagocytic cells in the bone marrow of patients who had acute SLE.[168] In 1949 Haserick found that the LE cells may be demonstrated more easily by incubating normal marrow with plasma from a patient suspected of having SLE, thereby also proving that the inducing factor is in the plasma and not in the marrow.[169] In the same year, in autopsy specimens, Klemperer demonstrated "hematoxylin bodies" that appeared identical with the phagocytosed substance within the LE cells, strengthening the notion that the reaction of the test was related to the pathogenesis of the disease.[170] Numerous techniques to improve the ease and yield of the LE cell reaction were attempted, including the demonstration in 1950 that the active factor is a gamma globulin and that peripheral blood can be used instead of marrow.[171] However, test serum continued to be mixed with cells from another source until 1952, when Hargraves described a more convenient and sensitive technique requiring only incubation of the patient's blood serum and cells, albeit at some loss of specificity.[172]

In 1954 investigators in Switzerland found that isolated cell nuclei can absorb the factor which induces LE cell formation from the serum. They therefore postulated that the factor is an antibody against some nuclear material.[173] This was confirmed and in 1959 the antigenic material was identified as a DNA-histone nucleoprotein.[174] In 1957 G. J. Friou at Yale devised a technique to demonstrate the antibody by indirect immunofluorescence.[175] This permitted quantitation of the reaction. In 1961 J. S. Beck in London showed the presence of at least three distinctive immunofluorescent staining patterns.[176] Subsequently, further refinements led to the discovery of many antibodies relevant to SLE and other diseases and the development of the new discipline of clinical immunopathology.[177]

The third event of the late 1940s did more than any other discovery to interest physicians in rheumatology and to introduce the general public to this subspecialty—namely, the introduction of cortisone and corticotropin. Even though these hormones rapidly came to be used also to treat nonrheumatic conditions, the fact that these "miracle drugs" were first used for rheumatoid arthritis by specialists in the treatment of arthritis continued to focus the cortisone publicity on rheumatology.

Attempts to separate and purify hormones from the anterior pituitary began in the early 1930s and advanced more rapidly than work on the adrenal secretions. The first animal experiments with a corticotropic extract were performed by J. B. Collip in Montreal in 1933[178] and the first clinical trials by K. J. Anselmino in Düsseldorf in 1934.[179] Much purer preparations were isolated by American investigators in 1943.[180,181] More was known about the properties of corticotropin (ACTH) than about cortisone in 1949, although few therapeutic trials had been recorded.

The discovery of cortisone is a unique example of the perseverance of a clinician with unusual clinical insights and brilliant, equally tenacious biochemists. Both lines of investigation began at about the same time, but independently. That the eventual clinical orientation of this work initially was rheumatologic resulted from the happenstance that the clinician, P. S. Hench at the Mayo Clinic, was a rheumatologist. He made two clinical observations which convinced him that rheumatoid arthritis potentially is reversible and that, therefore, the physiologic factor which produces the reversal must be discernible.

In 1929 Hench had observed that a man with rheumatoid arthritis who coincidentally developed hepatitis obtained a remission of his articular symptoms.[182] With additional experience he found that the antirheumatic effect correlated with the severity of jaundice but not with its cause.[183] After twenty years, two weeks before the announcement of the first clinical trial of cortisone, Hench summarized his experience with the rheumatoid arthritis–liver disease interaction and stated that he had observed remissions in twenty-five of thirty cases.[184] Treatment with bilirubin and bile salts had been attempted and found ineffective. Therefore some investigators sought to induce therapeutic jaundice with hepatotoxins that were less dangerous and more consistent than cinchophen, obtaining transient improvement in some cases.[185]

The second observation pertained to the effect of pregnancy. Observations of the amelioration of inflammatory joint diseases during pregnancy are scattered through the medical literature, beginning as early as 1864.[186] However, Hench was the first to study the possibility that there is a causal relationship. Between 1931 and 1938 he observed thirty-eight pregnancies in twenty-two women with joint diseases, of whom seventeen probably had rheumatoid arthritis and two psoriatic arthropathy. Of the twenty-two patients, twenty obtained remissions during thirty-three pregnancies. (The two who did not were cases of rheumatoid arthritis.)[187] This relationship was confirmed by Holbrook, who collected data on ninety-six pregnancies of women who had rheumatoid arthritis. Remissions occurred in eighty-three percent. Consequently, just as jaundice was induced therapeutically, pregnancy was recommended to women who had severe rheumatoid arthritis.[188] Of greater scientific importance than these clinical observations were Hench's conclusions, which pointed the way to research on the adrenal cortex. He wrote in 1938:

> It does not seem illogical to suppose that the agents responsible for both these phenomena are closely related, perhaps identical, and if the agent is a chemical substance, it would appear that it is neither bilirubin nor a strictly female sex hormone. It is interesting to note the close chemical relationship between such diverse substances as cholesterol, ergosterol (the precursor of vitamin D), some of the sex hormones, cortin and bile acids. Further studies are in progress to discover, if possible, the responsible agents for therapeutic purposes. If the potent common denominator of these two phenomena—the ameliorating effects of pregnancy and of jaundice—can be discovered, progress in treatment may be expected.[189]

Within about a decade after 1929, twenty-eight different steroidal compounds were identified in adrenal extracts in laboratories in the United States and Switzerland. Edward C. Kendall at the Mayo Clinic concentrated his work on compounds he designated A, B, E, and F, according to the chronological order of their isolation.[190] It was presumed that these very similar compounds have similar physiologic effects and that their most plausible therapeutic use would be in Addison's disease (adrenocortical failure). The first substance of which a sufficient quantity became available was compound A. When it was used to treat a patient with Addison's disease in 1946, it proved ineffective. On the basis of an observation in 1940 that compound E transiently counteracts the reaction to typhoid vaccine in experimental animals, Hench wanted to try it in patients with rheumatoid arthritis.[191] However, a sufficient quantity did not become available until September 1948, when Merck chemists had devised a partial synthesis of this steroid, so that it no longer needed to be extracted from animal adrenals.[192] The first patient with rheumatoid arthritis began to be treated in September. By April 1949, when the first clinical report was published, sixteen patients had been treated with consistent symptomatic benefit.[193] In 1949 Hench coined the term "cortisone" for compound E, this being a contraction of "corticosterone."[194] The tremendous impact of the early reports about cortisone and the similarly effective ACTH is proved by the conferral of the Nobel Prize for medicine on Philip S. Hench, Edward C. Kendall, and Thaddeus Reichstein only one year following the first clinical report.

In the six years after the short-term efficacy of intramuscularly administered cortisone had been demonstrated in cases of rheumatoid arthritis and SLE, all of the principal pharmaceutical modifications of the hormone were produced. In 1950 it was shown that cortisone is equally effective when taken orally,[195] but ineffective when injected into an inflamed joint.[196] Sufficient quantities of twelve corticosteroids other than cortisone had been produced by 1950 for comparative trials to proceed. Only hydrocortisone (compound F) had an antirheumatic effect.[197] In 1951 Hollander demonstrated that the injection of hydrocortisone acetate into inflamed joints and bursae resulted in rapid decrease of the local inflammation.[198] The first corticosteroid esters, which are absorbed more slowly and exert a more prolonged local effect, became available in 1955.[199] In that year prednisone and prednisolone also were introduced. These were the first synthetic corticosteroid modifications. Because of greater potency and a lesser fluid-retaining effect than results from the natural hormones, these and subsequent synthetic steroids gradually replaced them in rheumatologic therapy.[200]

Gout

Even though effective treatment for acute gout had long been available, this disease continued to be underdiagnosed. In 1928 Hench estimated that at least 40 percent of cases of gout remain misdiagnosed for at least fifteen years.[201] Among one hundred cases of gout collected in Boston in 1946, forty-four patients had symptoms of the disease for from ten to more than thirty years before the proper diagnosis was made.[202] Gout was receiving more attention in the humorous than in the medical literature. This helped to sustain a caricature of the disease and thus, if the patient did not have involvement of the great toe, obvious tophi, or alcoholism, the diagnosis was rarely considered. A "gout poison" was still believed by many to be the cause of disease of various organs, among which only renal impairment is valid.[203] According to an editorial in an American medical journal in 1932, gouty poison also causes neuritis, psoriasis, furunculosis, pharyngitis, laryngitis, bronchitis, asthma, and dyspepsia. Furthermore, "it may select the brain and induce irritability, sleepiness and disinclination to work."

In 1936 Hench commented as follows on the poor sensitivity of most physicians to the recognition of gout:

> If more than 50–70% of his patients have tophi he is too exclusive and is probably omitting cases of bona fide (even if pretophaceous) gout. If less than 35–40% have tophi or if more than 2–5% are females he is too inclusive, diagnosing gout where it does not exist.[204]

By 1938 B. M. Jacobson (Harvard) was able to show that the serum urate concentration of normal men is higher than in women: 4.4 ± 0.9 mg% and 4.0 ± 0.11 mg%, respectively.[205] However, uncertainty about the relationship of hyperuricemia to gout persisted. While, according to Jacobson, only 3 percent of normal adults have a serum urate concentration above 6.0 mg%, this was also true, according to Hench, of only 25 percent of cases of gout.[206] Kinell in 1940 reported serum urate values in nontophaceous cases of gout as low as 1.7 mg% and 2.8 mg% with tophi present.[207] Furthermore, there was disagreement about whether the serum urate concentration changes before, during, or following a gouty attack.

There was less therapeutic experimentation in gout than in other rheumatic diseases, perhaps because of greater reliance on dietary adjustments. During the 1920s cinchophen superceded colchicine as the most commonly prescribed medication for the acute attack. But in the late 1930s, as fear of the hepatotoxicity of cinchophen increased, colchicine resumed its primary position.[208,209] In addition, a low purine diet was frequently recommended. Because of the lack of specific prophylactic therapy, physicians made lifestyle recommendations reminiscent of sixteenth-century prescriptions.[210] According to Comroe (1940), excessive amounts of alcohol should be avoided, as should excessive work, trauma, mental and physical fatigue, while a moderate amount of exercise is desirable.[211]

Diagnostic, biochemical, and therapeutic advances occurred almost simultaneously in about 1950. Attempts to improve the specificity of the uric acid determination by using the enzyme uricase had begun in 1938, but because the result was still obtained from a color reaction, little advantage was gained.[212] The modern technique, which employs the same enzyme but replaces the colorimeter with a spectrophotometer, was devised by Danish biochemists between 1947 and 1953.[213]

Evidence to support the inferences that gout is a metabolic disease had to await the development of isotopic tracer techniques. The earliest such studies in 1943, using heavy nitrogen, revealed that the uric acid that is excreted had not been ingested as such, but was formed from smaller molecules.[214] Between 1947 and 1954 the biosynthesis of uric acid was worked out in detail by biochemists at several American universities.[215] Techniques to determine the uric acid content of the whole body were developed at the same time.[216]

Three principal pharmaceutical advances must be cited: the introduction of both probenecid and phenylbutazone in 1951, which also increased the focus on rheumatologic therapeutics that cortisone and ACTH had just opened, and the introduction of allopurinol in 1963. The usefulness of all of these in the treatment of gout were fortuitous findings. In 1948, in the search for a drug that would retard the excretion of penicillin, carinamide was discovered. It incidentally was found to enhance the excretion of uric acid, although impractically large doses were required.[217] Soon thereafter a derivative, probenecid, was produced, which required only one-twelfth the dose of carinamide and was better tolerated. Probenecid was the first practical uricosuric drug that not only lowers the urate content of the blood, but can also shrink and prevent tophi.[218]

Shortly after probenecid was marketed phenylbutazone became available. Initially this drug was mixed with aminopyrine to improve the solubility of this old febrifuge. But when it was noted that the combination had therapeutic properties in addition to those of aminopyrine, phenylbutazone was evaluated by itself. It rapidly was found to be an excellent alternative to colchicine in acute gout, to be uricosuric, and also to be an effective anti-inflammatory analgesic in other rheumatic and nonrheumatic conditions.[219] Phenylbutazone was the first of the modern "nonsteroidal anti-inflammatory drugs." The latter term was introduced when competitive drugs, which have been designed by pharmaceutical chemists rather than being chanced upon, came into use, particularly in the 1970s.

Allopurinol, an analogue of the uric acid precursor, hypoxanthine, was synthesized in the search for an agent that would facilitate the effect of thiopurine antimetabolites in the treatment of leukemia. Allopurinol was found to inhibit the last two steps in the biosynthesis of uric acid but not other metabolic pathways.[220] Therefore, it has proved to be a safe and effective alternative to the uricosuric drugs to deplete the body's uric acid stores, prevent tophus formation, and diminish the frequency of gouty attacks. According to data collected between 1920 and 1946, tophi were present in 45 percent of cases of gout.[221] Probably because of better diagnosis of nontophaceous cases, tophi were found in 13.7 percent of the cases of gout seen at the Mayo Clinic in 1949. By 1972 the efficacy of the urate-depleting drugs had reduced this to 2.7 percent.[222]

Classification of Diseases

As diseases were increasingly subdivided and the medical vocabulary grew, interest developed in grouping diseases, both for the sake of professional communication and in hope of perceiving meaningful relationships. However, with the eventual exception of diseases having a demonstrably bacterial cause, there was no scientific methodology by which to define many individual diseases. With the advent of specialization, nosology gained importance of another kind, helping to define the scope of the specialty. In 1941 a committee of the New York Rheumatism Association privately published a fairly elaborate "Classification of Diseases of Joints and Related Structures." It was reprinted in 1948 with the mournful introduction, "if the etiology of the various rheumatic diseases were known their classification would be simplified."[223] The 1942 edition of the *Primer on Arthritis* contained another classification, produced by a committee of the American Rheumatism Association, which included the connective tissue diseases that were lacking in the 1941 effort.[224] The most recent classification, published in 1983 in the 8th edition of the *Primer,* shows the progress of four decades, both in its inclusion of newly recognized diseases and in the diagnostic refinement of those known previously.[225] While many diseases still cannot be defined etiologically, descriptive diagnoses have in successive classifications been guided increasingly by scientific criteria.

The innovation which T. D. Jones introduced in 1944 was the specification of various possible attributes of rheumatic fever and a minimum number of these that must be found before the diagnosis may be made with reasonable confidence.[226] A decade later the ARA adopted this technique and by the efforts of expert committees has improved it. Since 1956 criteria studies pertaining to five diseases have been completed: two each on the diagnosis of rheumatoid arthritis, systemic lupus erythematosus, and juvenile polyarthritis, one each for acute gout and progressive systemic sclerosis, and one to define a remission of rheumatoid arthritis.[227–235] In the first study the records of 332 patients who were considered to have typical rheumatoid arthritis by the specialists who contributed them were reviewed and the most consistent findings were categorized, but without the use of a control population.[236] The later investigations have employed the same approach, but with the addition of comparisons with one or more control groups. The follow-up evaluations have resulted in modifications of the preliminary criteria to improve their specificity.[237–239]

Technologic Innovations

While many medical disciplines have matured about the focus of technologic advances that are employed by its practitioners, this has generally not been true of rheumatology. The diagnostic advances that are closely managed by the rheumatologist largely are laboratory procedures—morphologic, biochemical, and immunologic. However, the advent of several technical procedures and their role in rheumatologic practice must be cited briefly.

Polley and Bickel (Mayo Clinic) introduced in 1951 an instrument for the blind punch biopsy of synovium.[240] Its caliber has limited its use to the adult knee. In 1963 Parker and Pearson (Los Angeles) devised a synovial biopsy needle which, because of its smaller size, is more versatile.[241] These instruments are used by rheumatologists, but their principal value has been restricted to the diagnosis of monoarticular arthritis that happens to affect an accessible joint. Use of the blind procedure has been declining since the introduction of arthroscopy.

The first arthroscope was invented in 1931 by M. S. Burman in New York, and in 1934 he and his associates described the internal examination of knees of thirty patients.[242] Probably because of the relatively primitive optics and illumination this instrument did not come to be used by others. The modern arthroscope, with its optics and illumination greatly improved over those of Burman's instrument, was invented in Japan in the late 1960s. It began to be used in the United States in 1971 and rapidly became a mainstay of the orthopedic surgeon, both for diagnosis and some surgery.[243] Orthopedic surgeons could not resist the performance of blind synovial biopsies by rheumatologists, since this procedure does not require an operating room. However, because arthroscopy was developed by orthopedists and these specialists control both training in the technique and usually access to the operating room, few rheumatologists have so far practiced even diagnostic arthroscopy.

The assessment of joint inflammation by radioisotopic scanning was initiated in 1965 by investigators at the Ochsner Clinic (New Orleans) using iodine-131-labeled serum albumin.[244] Other isotopes have been tried since then, and technetium-99, introduced by K. Whaley in Glasgow in 1968, has proved the most generally practical.[245] Although scanning procedures are able to detect inflammation, they do not differentiate its causes.[246] This methodology has remained in the hands of radiologists and specialists in nuclear medicine.

Electromyography first was used in rheumatologic diagnosis in 1950 by

E. H. Lambert (Mayo Clinic) to evaluate patients with dermatomyositis.[247] This technique, which has been greatly increased in its sensitivity with modern electronics, is of unquestioned value in the differentiation of myopathies from neuropathies and in the assessment of residual functional muscle. For reasons that are unclear few rheumatologists have been trained in electromyography, and it is practiced mainly by physiatrists and neurologists.

In the 1950s, with the introduction of methods to assay the serum content of enzymes that are concentrated in muscle cells, the biochemical assessment of muscular diseases also became clinically feasible. Glutamic oxalacetic transaminase (1953), aldolase (1953), and creatine phosphokinase (1959) have received the most use.[248–250] Although these tests at first were applied to muscular dystrophies and other nonrheumatologic myopathies, they soon were found useful in two ways: to assess the response to therapy of inflammatory diseases of muscle such as polymyositis and to help to differentiate inflammatory myopathies from noninflammatory ailments such as polymyalgia rheumatica and fibromyositis.

Further Institutionalization of Rheumatology

Having described the highlights of the scientific development of rheumatology up to about 1960, we must return to the organizational history of the subspecialty, which also matured during this period. In 1946, when the developmental hiatus created by the war had ended and the ARA had a membership of 285, its leadership sought to refocus the organization. For this purpose a Research and Education Committee was established, chaired by outgoing president Paul Holbrook. A subcommittee of New York members recommended that a professional fund-raising firm be consulted about techniques to finance any contemplated activities. The consultant made two principal recommendations: (1) a national voluntary agency should be formed, separate from the ARA, to raise funds in support of research and education; and (2) a national survey should be conducted to assess the status of research, education, and clinical practice in the rheumatic diseases. These recommendations were accepted by the committee and approved by the ARA at its meeting in June 1947. To enhance the credibility of a survey, the cooperation of the National Research Council was solicited and the survey conducted under its auspices.

While the survey was being organized, the other recommendation was also implemented, and in April 1948 the "Arthritis and Rheumatism Foundation" was incorporated in New York. The board of directors consisted of six physicians, including five past presidents of the ARA, and six businessmen. The chairman during the first twenty-two years was Floyd B. Odlum, a California businessman who had rheumatoid arthritis. The first acts of the founding board included enlargement of the board of directors and establishment of a "Medical and Scientific Committee." This group of twelve included four rheumatologists among the several medical specialties that were represented. Except for Morris Fishbein, editor of the *Journal of the American Medical Association* (*JAMA*), all had major academic affiliations.[251]

The objectives of the Foundation, as announced in *JAMA*, included development of a research program, establishment of research and clinical fellowships, development of arthritis centers affiliated with key medical schools throughout the country, promotion of continuing medical education, and creation of clinical facilities for rheumatism patients in connection with general hospitals. Thirty-eight chapters of the Foundation would appear nationally which would integrate programs of investigation and raise funds for local programs.[252]

In the founding year eleven of the planned thirty-eight chapters were established, covering seventeen states and the District of Columbia. By 1958 the Foundation had expanded to fifty-three chapters in forty-three states, and now the entire country is covered by seventy-one semi-independent chapters.[253] A fellowship program to support young physicians and basic scientists for up to three years while they obtained relevant training was begun in 1951 with seven appointments. Support for "senior investigators" for up to five years was initiated two years later. Although the number of fellowships (371 in the first twenty-five years) has remained small in comparison with those funded by the National Institutes of Health, an impressive proportion of the Arthritis Foundation fellows have attained distinguished academic and scientific careers.[254,255]

Both the ARA and the Arthritis Foundation have emphasized the production of educational publications. The principal professional publications have been the *Primer on the Rheumatic Diseases* (since 1934), *Rheumatism Reviews* (since 1935), the *Bulletin on Rheumatic Diseases* (since 1950), and the journal *Arthritis and Rheumatism* (since 1958). The Foundation has also underwritten numerous patient education pamphlets about rheumatic diseases and their treatment.

In 1932, 3,000 copies of a pamphlet entitled *Rheumatism Primer, Chronic Arthritis* were privately printed. Its editor was Russell L. Haden of the Cleveland Clinic.[256] The next edition, *Primer on Rheumatism, Chronic Arthritis*, American Committee for the Control of Rheumatism cooperating with the Committee on Scientific Exhibits 1934, was the first "numbered" primer. It was edited by Edward P. Jordan and printed by the American Medical Association, but published privately.[257] The second to seventh editions (1942–1973) were published in *JAMA*. Each edition has been larger than its predecessor, so that the sixteen pages of 1942 had become 238 pages in the eighth edition (1983), which was published by the Arthritis Foundation.[258] The growth, particularly of the two most recent editions, reflect not only the growth of knowledge, but also the ambitious aims of the editor, Gerald P. Rodnan, as supported by the Arthritis Foundation.

The first of the comprehensive reviews of the English language rheumatic diseases literature was "prepared at the request of the American Committee for the Control of Rheumatism" by a six member committee chaired by P. S. Hench. Hench edited the first nine reviews. The first critical compilation included 465 articles which had been published during 1932 and 1933.[259] In the third review, published in 1937, Hench commented optimistically that although the increasing number of presentations by physicians to county and state medical societies make virtually no pretensions to original research, they are significant in that a broadened view of the problem of rheumatism is reflected. "The general practitioner is no longer willing to ignore rheumatism, content with the sorry gesture of salicylates for his new, and spas for his old, arthritis patients."[260] Indeed, the reviews are useful historical documents which trace in considerable detail the development both of the basic science arm of rheumatology and the growth of rigorous clinical research. The thirteenth was the most comprehensive edition, based on 3,430 articles from 1954 to 1955[261] and the twenty-fifth (last) edition, covering 1979 to 1980, followed in size with 3,312 articles.[262] The reviews, being necessarily always published several years "out of phase" with the summarized material, gradually lost reference value and were discontinued.

The *Bulletin on Rheumatic Diseases* was inaugurated in September 1950 under the editorship of Joseph J. Bunim to foster greater interest in and access to rheumatologic information for practitioners.[263] During each of its first four years the nine issues were limited to two pages. Thereafter more detailed presentations became increasingly frequent, with some issues reaching ten pages. The *Bulletin* has always been provided free of charge with a goal of reaching a much broader medical readership than was anticipated for the *Reviews*.

Until 1958 most rheumatology articles in the American journal literature were scattered through general internal medicine and orthopedic journals. The rheumatology specialty journal most likely to be read was the

Annals of the Rheumatic Diseases, which has been published by the British Medical Association since 1939. The first rheumatology journals to survive for more than a few years have been the French *Revue du Rheumatisme,* begun in 1934, and the German *Zeitschrift für Rheumaforschung,* begun in 1938.[264] Interest in beginning an American rheumatologic specialty journal began in about 1948, but it took a decade for the plan to come to fruition. The major point of dispute during this time was whether American support of the British journal (*Annals of the Rheumatic Diseases*), or perhaps the publication of alternating British and American issues of the *Annals,* might not be sufficient and more economical. However, the ARA decided in 1957 to establish its own journal, and the first bimonthly issue of *Arthritis and Rheumatism* was published in February 1958, edited by William S. Clark. It rapidly became the largest journal in its field. Volume 8 (1965) already exceeded 1,000 pages, and since volume 22 (1979) it has appeared monthly.

In 1949 a bill was introduced in Congress to authorize the creation of a National Arthritis and Rheumatism Institute within the Public Health Service. It was opposed by the Federal Security Agency, which then had authority over the Public Health Service, because the new institute would duplicate some of the functions of the Experimental Biology and Medicine Institute (EBMI), which had been in operation for only a few months. Eventually several bills that pertained to medicine were amalgamated into the Omnibus Medical Research Act of 1950. It incorporated the EBMI into a new National Institute of Arthritis and Metabolic Diseases (NIAMD). This institute was officially established on 22 November 1950 under the directorship of the former director of the EBMI, William H. Sebrell, a nutritionist. Because the Clinical Center (i.e., hospital) of the National Institutes of Health did not open until July 1953, the early work at the NIAMD was limited to the continuation of laboratory investigations and the awarding, beginning in 1952, of a small number of fellowships.[265]

The organization of the NIAMD rapidly increased in complexity, in keeping with the multiple functions it assumed. The extramural grants program, established in 1951, became one of the most influential. Grant disbursement reached one million dollars per year in 1955. By 1961 five million dollars was awarded, and this had reached ten million in 1972. The number of fellowships being awarded was increased substantially beginning in 1962.[266]

In 1953 DeWitt Stetten, Jr., a biochemist, became director of intramural (mainly basic) research and retained this position until 1974. In 1954 J. J. Bunim left the Rheumatic Diseases Study Group of New York University to become chief of the Arthritis and Rheumatism Division of the NIAMD as well as director of the Clinical Center. He retained these responsibilities until his death in 1964.[267]

The Contemporary State of Rheumatology

The most recent period in rheumatology, as in other branches of internal medicine, is characterized by research into what is hoped are fundamental mechanisms of disease at the cellular and subcellular level. We are temporally too close to this work in most cases to judge which of it will have the most lasting importance. However, a few examples may be hazarded.

As recently as 1960, Howard C. Coggeshall could justifiably write that "the aspiration and examination of synovial fluid from arthritic joints has remained the most neglected of all laboratory procedures helpful in the differential diagnosis of arthritis."[268] One retrospective explanation for this neglect is that, aside from bacteriologic culturing, the customary examinations had very limited diagnostic value due to the great overlapping of findings in various diseases. Many thousands of synovial fluids had been examined microscopically for bacteria and cell counts without extra- or intracellular crystals being recognized. This discovery could have been made with an ordinary microscope, although the greater sensitivity of polarizing and phase contrast microscopy was recognized soon after the initial discovery. The observation which initiated the reorientation in the diagnostic importance of synovial fluid was made in 1959 by J. L. Hollander, who found "needle-like crystals of sodium bi-urate in the centrifuged fluid from eight of seventeen joints which were the seat of acute gouty arthritis."[269] This discovery soon was confirmed[270] and in the following six years synovial fluid, examined more with a new focus than with new instruments, yielded further important discoveries.

In 1962 J. E. Seegmiller (NIAMD) found that the injection of microcrystalline uric acid into a joint causes inflammation identical to that of acute gout, whether or not the subject has a history of gout, and that the crystals are phagocytosed by leukocytes.[271] This finally demonstrated the causal relationship between uric acid and gout, and also the effects of physical as well as chemical properties of substances on biologic responses. In the same year McCarty (Philadelphia) demonstrated that crystals of calcium pyrophosphate dihydrate may also occur in synovial effusions, elicit inflammation, and can be distinguished from urate crystals by their different polarization. This was the discovery of "pseudo-gout."[272] In 1966 McCarty and Gatter described a third crystal-induced arthropathy: hydroxyapatite deposition disease.[273] To be detected these nonpolar crystals require the resolution of the scanning electron microscope. So this is a recent example of the requirement for advanced technology for a "new" disease to be identified.

On the biochemical and genetic level, Lesch and Nyhan in Baltimore in 1964 described a pair of mentally defective brothers with a peculiar neurologic syndrome and marked hyperuricemia.[274] A hugely accelerated uric acid metabolism was demonstrated. These observations, made at a time when the relevant basic sciences (enzymology, tissue culture, isotopic tracer techniques) were sufficiently advanced, soon led to a great increase of knowledge of uric acid metabolism, as well as the identification of other heritable anomalies of uric acid metabolism associated with discrete enzymatic defects.[275]

Finally, the discovery of the human lymphocyte antigen (HLA) system must be cited, both because its first successful clinical applications were in rheumatology and because its study involves all levels of research, from epidemiology and nosology to molecular genetics. Leukocyte agglutinins were first detected in 1958 in recipients of multiple blood transfusions.[276] The basic techniques whereby these antigens are now detected were devised in 1964 by immunologists in Los Angeles[277] and New York.[278] The initial clinical hypothesis was that if a greater than chance association is found in a group of individuals who have a certain disease and any of the inherited HL antigens, this may identify an inherited susceptibility to that disease. The first fairly large clinical test of this hypothesis, by F. C. Grumet at Stanford University in 1971, pertained to SLE. A statistically significant association with two antigens was found.[279] However, the greatest impetus to the study of clinical HLA correlations occurred two years later. In a comparison of HLA frequencies in cases of gout, rheumatoid arthritis, and ankylosing spondylitis, an extremely high correlation between one antigen (W-27, now B-27) and ankylosing spondylitis was found, but none with the other two diseases.[280] Concurrently this genetic association was confirmed in England where, in addition, the same association was found only a little less strongly in asymptomatic relatives of the spondylitis patients and in Reiter's disease, which often has a spondylitic component.[281,282] Suddenly there was a new and persuasive line of evidence that ankylosing spondylitis is not a variant of rheumatoid arthritis and that it is genetically predisposed. At first only antigens in the A and B loci of the chromosome were being detected. Then in 1977 Peter Stastny showed an association of rheumatoid arthritis with antigen DRw4, which was absent in cases of juvenile "rheumatoid arthritis."[283]

The difference supported the view of English over American rheumatologists that the juvenile polyarthritis is a disease distinct from rheumatoid arthritis.

The membership of the ARA has continued to enlarge, reaching 1,000 in 1955, 2,000 in 1970, 3,000 in 1978, and 4,000 in 1984. In 1975, with a membership of 2,503, there were eighteen states in which there were less than five members.[284] By 1985, with a membership of 4,259, there were only four such states. The eighteen states in which a total of thirty-nine members lived in 1975 now contain 270.[285]

Two organizational developments occurred in 1965: the ARA and the Foundation were amalgamated and the name of the latter was shortened to "Arthritis Foundation" (AF). The ARA became the scientific section of the AF. Shortly thereafter, the "Paramedical Section of the Medical Council of the Arthritis Foundation" was established. This was both a response to and a stimulus for the growing interest among physical and occupational therapists, nurses, and others in the treatment of rheumatic disease patients. The clumsy name of the organization was changed in 1968 to the "Allied Health Professions Section" and in 1978 to the "Arthritis Health Professions Association." Its membership is approaching 2,000 and its meetings are held concurrently with those of the ARA.[286] As of 1986 the ARA and the AF are again becoming legally separate organizations, primarily for fiscal reasons.

The organization and name of the NIAMD have changed twice and a third reorganization is about to take place. In 1972 it became the Institute for Arthritis, Metabolic and Digestive Diseases (NIAMDD) and in 1981 the Institute for Arthritis, Diabetes, Digestive and Kidney Diseases (NIADDK). The proportion of the funds of the Institute that has been allocated to research and education in arthritic and musculoskeletal diseases has remained approximately constant: 13.6 percent in 1974, 16.0 percent in 1979, and 16.1 percent in 1984, whereas the dollars have increased from 20.1 to 75.3 million.[287] In 1977 "Center Grants" for the support of rheumatic disease departments in medical schools were added. As of 1983, twenty centers were funded in sixteen states. The total federal support for individuals and Arthritis Centers reached $15 million in 1978, $20 million in 1980, and $30 million in 1983.[288] As a result of Congressional action in 1985, the NIADDK will be reorganized as required by the creation of a National Institute of Arthritis, Musculoskeletal, and Skin Diseases.

There were thirty-six rheumatologic training programs in 1956,[289] and these had proliferated to 107 as of 1985.[290] As training also became more formal, the desirability of a certifying subspecialty board began to be debated in the ARA in the early 1960s. By 1941, only five years after the American Board of Internal Medicine was founded, four subspecialty boards were formed for the further qualification of diplomates of the Board of Internal Medicine: in allergy, cardiovascular, gastrointestinal, and pulmonary diseases. Although the practice of certification in a broad area of medicine was well accepted in the 1950s, the apprehension persisted that the recognition of subspecialists by virtue of examination based certification would result in counterproductive isolation. Hence only in 1970 did the ARA leadership request that a subspecialty board of rheumatology, to be administered by the Board of Internal Medicine, be established.[291] Other medical subspecialties had experienced similar conflicts, as is indicated by the fact that in October 1972 the first subspecialty examination was given not only in rheumatology, but also in endocrinology, hematology, infectious diseases, and nephrology. At the first examination 154 of 201 candidates became diplomates in rheumatology. With the examination of 1984 the total has reached 1,863.[292]

Conclusion

In this century, as morbidity and mortality due to infectious agents have increasingly been controlled and the age distribution of the population has shifted upward, the relative prevalence of major rheumatic diseases has changed. Consequently, a large proportion of the clinical problems which confront the modern rheumatologist differ from those which frustrated his predecessor of the 1880s. Due in part to new methodology, such as radiologic examination, but particularly because of the increasing medicinal choices and advances in physical therapy and orthopedic surgery, rheumatic diseases have come to be examined more scientifically and patients have gradually received closer attention. Nevertheless, the development of rheumatology as a subspecialty was restrained to a greater extent than other medical subspecialties. Reasons for this include the difficulty in discovering measurable attributes whereby to define its diseases, a lack of unique technology, and of clearly efficacious treatments.

Rheumatology became transformed from a potential into a recognized subspecialty between 1948 and 1952, the only four-year period during which membership in the ARA doubled (388 to 755). This is attributed to the coincidence during this brief period of the discovery of potent diagnostic and therapeutic methods, as well as the initiation of major support by both governmental and private agencies (*Table 6.5*). In the last quarter century

TABLE 6.5.
SALIENT EVENTS FOR THE RECOGNITION OF RHEUMATOLOGY

Year	Event
1948	Discovery of a test for the "rheumatoid factor"[293] Discovery of the "LE cell"[294] Introduction of streptomycin to treat osteoarticular tuberculosis[295] Establishment of the Arthritis and Rheumatism Foundation[296]
1949	Introduction of cortisone and corticotropin to treat rheumatoid arthritis and systemic lupus erythematosus[297]
1950	Establishment of the National Institute of Arthritis and Metabolic Diseases[298]
1951	Introduction of probenecid to treat chronic gout[299] Introduction of phenylbutazone (nonsteroidal anti-inflammatory)[300] Introduction of intra-articular injection of hydrocortisone[301] First percutaneous synovial biopsy instrument[302] First Arthritis and Rheumatism Foundation fellowships[303]
1952	First NIAMD rheumatology fellowships[304]

rheumatology, like other medical subspecialties, has been oriented toward ever more basic research. Diseases have been discovered, some disease mechanisms elucidated, and the prognosis of many diseases improved. But there still is little etiologically based therapy, and consequently a long scientific road remains ahead.

NOTES

1. F. C. Shattuck, "Specialism, the Laboratory, and Practical Medicine," *Boston Med Surg J* 136 (1897) : 613–17.
2. M. Longstreth, *Rheumatism, Gout, and Some Allied Disorders* (New York: W. Wood & Co., 1882), 178.
3. J. K. Spender, "The Early Treatment of Rheumatoid Arthritis," *Lancet* 1 (1886) : 439–41.
4. A. Hadden, "Rheumatoid Osteoarthritis," *Trans Med Soc State NY* (1886) : 180–87.
5. H. P. C. Wilson, "A Rigid, Anchylosed, Human Skeleton, the Result of Rheumatism," *Med Examiner (Philadelphia)* 12 (1856) : 326–28.
6. E. H. Bradford, "Anchylosis of the Spine: Three Cases Following Rheumatism, Two Being of Gonorrheal Origin," *Ann Anat & Surg (Brooklyn)* 7 (1883) : 279–84.
7. A. B. Arnold, "Three Cases of Scleroderma; with Remarks," *Am J Med Sci* 58 (1869) : 89–91.
8. W. D. Day "Case of Scleroderma or Sclerema, with the Autopsy and Remarks," *Am J Med Sci* 59 (1870) : 350–59.
9. F. E. Simpson, "Keratodermie Blennorrhagique," *JAMA* 59 (1912) : 607–12.
10. E. A. Chancellor, "Gonorrheal Articular Rheumatism," *St Louis Med Surg J* 44 (1883) : 358–65.

11. G. W. Jacoby, "Subacute Progressive Polymyositis," *J Nerv Ment Dis* 13 (1888) : 697–726.

12. F. A. Packard, "A case of Acromegaly, and Illustrations of Two Allied Conditions," *Am J Med Sci* 103 (1892) : 657–69.

13. E. M. Hasbrouck, "A Case of Hypertrophic Pulmonary Osteo-Arthropathy," *NY Med J* 67 (1892) : 665–69.

14. W. Osler, "On the Visceral Complications of Erythema Exudativum Multiforme," *Am J Med Sci* 110 (1895) : 629–46.

15. H. Koplik, "Arthritis Deformans in a Child Seven Years Old," *Arch Ped* 13 (1896) : 161–66.

16. F. R. Sabin, "A Case of Arterial Disease, Possibly Periarteritis Nodosa," *Bull J Hopkins Hosp* 12 (1901) : 195–98.

17. A. R. Lamb, "Periarteritis Nodosa—A Clinical and Pathological Review of the Disease with a Report of Two Cases," *Arch Intern Med* 14 (1914) : 481–516.

18. G. P. Rodnan and T. G. Benedek, "The Early History of Antirheumatic Drugs," *Arthritis Rheum* 13 (1970) : 145–65.

19. W. A. Caldwell, Rational Selection of the Salts of Salicylic Acid for Therapeusis. *Therap Gaz* 12 (1888) : 734–42.

20. C. H. May, "Statistics of Four Hundred Cases of Rheumatism, with Especial Reference to Treatment," *Med Record* 25 (1884) : 57ff.

21. R. F. Weir, "On Antiseptic Irrigation of the Knee Joint for Chronic Serous Synovitis," *Trans Med Soc State NY* (1886) : 376–85; also *NY Med J* 43 (1886) : 204–6.

22. Longstreth, *Rheumatism.*

23. M. Stamm, "Tuberculosis of Bones and Joints," *JAMA* 8 (1887) : 256–62, 285–88.

24. N. Senn, *Tuberculosis of Bones and Joints* (Philadelphia: Davis, 1893), 504.

25. V. P. Gibney, "An Analysis of 1,662 Cases of Joint Disease Examined with Reference to their Causes," *Louisville Med News* 3 (1877) : 185–89.

26. H. F. Vickery, "Chronic Joint Disease at the Massachusetts General Hospital," *Boston Med Surg J* 151 (1904) : 536–37.

27. L. M. Petrone, "Sulla Natura Parasitaria dell'Artrite Blennorragica," *Rev Clin Bologna* 3 (1883) : 94–113.

28. A. Mantle, "The Etiology of Rheumatism Considered from a Bacterial point of View," *Br Med J* 1 (1887) : 381–84.

29. M. Schüller, "Untersuchungen über die Ätiologie der sogennanten chronisch rheumatischen Gelenkentzündungen," *Berl Klin Wchnschr* 36 (1893) : 865–68.

30. Osler, "Erythema exudativum multiforme."

31. W. Osler, "On the Visceral Manifestations of the Erythema Group of Skin Diseases," *Am J Med Sci* 127 (1904) : 1–23, 751–54.

32. J. E. Goldthwait, C. F. Painter, and R. B. Osgood, *Diseases of the Bones and Joints* (Boston: Heath, 1909), 673.

33. W. Osler and T. McCrae, *Modern Medicine: Its Theory and Practice* (Philadelphia: Lea & Febiger, 1909), vol. 6, 501–88.

34. L. S. King, "Boissier de Sauvages and 18th Century Nosology," *Bull Hist Med* 40 (1966) : 43–51.

35. A. Pribram, "Chronischer Gelenkrheumatismus und Osteoarthritis Deformans," in *Specielle Pathologie und Therapie,* H. Nothnagel, ed. (Vienna: A. Holder, 1902), vol. 7, 6.

36. J. E. Goldthwait, "The Differential Diagnosis and Treatment of the So-Called Rheumatoid Diseases," *Boston Med Surg J* 151 (1904) : 529–34.

37. P. W. Nathan, "The Differential Diagnosis of the Diseases Hitherto Grouped Together as Rheumatoid Arthritis, Chronic Rheumatism, Arthritis Deformans, etc.," *Am J Med Sci* 132 (1906) : 857–73.

38. E. H. Nichols and F. L. Richardson, "Arthritis Deformans," *J Med Res* 21 (1909) : 149–205.

39. T. B. Futcher, "The Occurrence of Gout in the United States," *Practitioner* 71 (1903) : 6–16.

40. Vickery, "Chronic Joint Disease."

41. J. B. Herrick, "Differential Diagnosis of Rheumatoid Joint Affections," *JAMA* 48 (1907) : 381–83.

42. C. S. Williamson, "Gout: A Clinical Study of One Hundred and Sixteen Cases," *JAMA* 74 (1920) : 1625–29.

43. C. N. B. Camac, "Hospital and Ward Clinical Laboratories," *JAMA* 35 (1900) : 219–27.

44. E. Salkowski, "Weitere Beiträge zur Kenntnis der Leukämie," *Virchow's Arch Path Anat* 52 (1871) : 58–65.

45. W. J. Morton, "A Röntgen Picture From a Medical Point of View," *NY Med J* 63 (1896) : 333.

46. W. J. Morton and E. W. Hammer, *The X-ray, or Photography of the Invisible, and its Value in Surgery* (New York: 1896), 196.

47. R. B. Osgood, "Lesions of the Tibial Tubercle Occurring During Adolescence," *Boston Med Surg J* 148 (1903) : 114–17.

48. A. H. Freiberg, "Coxa Vara Adolescentium and Osteoarthritis Deformans Coxae," *Am J Orthop Surg* 3 (1905) : 6–14.

49. A. T. Legg, "An Obscure Affection of the Hip-Joint," *Boston Med Surg J* 162 (1910) : 202–4.

50. J. M. Anders, J. Daland, and G. F. Pfahler, "The Treatment of Arthritis Deformans with the Roentgen Rays," *JAMA* 46 (1906) : 1512–14.

51. Rodnan and Benedek, "Early Antirheumatic Drugs."

52. Rodnan and Benedek, "Early Antirheumatic Drugs."

53. Anonymous, "A Substitute for Antipyrin," *Med Record* 35 (1889) : 323.

54. P. S. Hench and E. W. Boland, "The Management of Chronic Arthritis and Other Rheumatic Diseases Among Soldiers of the United States Army," *Ann Intern Med* 24 (1946) : 808–25.

55. H. F. Swift, "Rheumatic Fever," *JAMA* 92 (1929) : 2071–83.

56. H. F. Swift and R. A. Kinsella, "Bacteriologic Studies in Acute Rheumatic Fever," *Arch Intern Med* 19 (1917) : 381–96.

57. H. F. Swift, C. L. Derick, and C. H. Hitchcock, "Rheumatic Fever as a Manifestation of Hypersensitiveness (Allergy or Hyperergy) to Streptococci," *Trans Assoc Am Physicians* 43 (1928) : 192–202.

58. A. F. Coburn and R. H. Pauli, "Studies on the Relationship of Streptococcus Hemolyticus to the Rheumatic Process," *J Exp Med* 56 (1932) : 609–32, 633–50, 651–76.

59. R. C. Lancefield, "The Antigenic Complex of Streptococcus Haemolyticus," *J Exp Med* 47 (1928) : 91–103, 469–80, 481–91, 843–55, 857–75.

60. E. W. Todd, "Antigenic Streptococcal Haemolysin," *J Exp Med* 55 (1932) : 267–80.

61. E. W. Todd, "A Comparative Serological Study of Streptolysins Derived

from Human and from Animal Infections, with Notes on Pneumococcal Haemolysin, Tetanolysin and Staphylococcus Toxin," *J Path Bact* 39 (1934) : 299–321.

62. A. F. Coburn, "Observations on the Mechanism of Rheumatic Fever," *Lancet* 2 (1936) : 1025–30.

63. J. J. Bunim and C. McEwen, "The Antistreptolysin Titer in Rheumatic Fever, Arthritis and Other Diseases," *J Clin Invest* 19 (1940) : 75–82.

64. F. Billings, "Chronic Focal Infections and Their Etiologic Relations to Arthritis and Nephritis," *Arch Intern Med* 9 (1912) : 484–98.

65. E. A. Locke and R. B. Osgood, "Treatment of Non-Tuberculous Chronic Arthritis," *JAMA* 48 (1907) : 388–91.

66. R. L. Cecil, E. E. Nicholls, and W. J. Stainsby, "The Bacteriology of the Blood and Joints in Chronic Infectious Arthritis," *Arch Intern Med* 43 (1929) : 571–605.

67. E. E. Nicholls and W. J. Stainsby, "Further Studies on the Agglutinin Reaction in Chronic Arthritis," *J Clin Invest* 12 (1933) : 505–18.

68. M. H. Dawson, M. Olmstead, and R. H. Boots, "Bacteriologic Investigations on the Blood, Synovial Fluid and Subcutaneous Nodules in Rheumatoid (Chronic Infectious) Arthritis," *Arch Intern Med* 49 (1932) : 173–80.

69. M. H. Dawson, M. Olmstead, and R. H. Boots, "Agglutination Reactions in Rheumatoid Arthritis: I. Agglutination Reactions with Streptococcus Hemolyticus," *J Immunol* 23 (1932) : 187–204.

70. W. K. Myers and C. S. Keefer, "Antistreptolysin Content of the Blood Serum in Rheumatic Fever and Rheumatoid Arthritis," *J Clin Invest* 13 (1934) : 155–67.

71. G. Kahlmeter, "The sedimentation Rate of Erythrócytes in Various Rheumatic Conditions," *Med J Rec* 128 (1928) : 467–69.

72. M. H. Dawson and R. H. Boots, "The Differential Diagnosis of Rheumatoid and Osteoarthritis: The Sedimentation Reaction and its Value," *J Lab Clin Med* 15 (1930) : 1065–71.

73. O. Folin and W. Denis, "A New (Colorimetric) Method for the Determination of Uric Acid in Blood," *J Biol Chem* 13 (1912) : 469–75.

74. O. Folin and W. Denis, "The Diagnostic Value of Uric Acid Determinations in Blood," *Arch Intern Med* 16 (1915) : 33–37.

75. J. S. McLester, "Studies on Uric Acid of Blood and Urine, with Special Reference to the Influence of Atophan," *Arch Intern Med* 12 (1913) : 739–45.

76. H. Berglund, "How Much do We Know About the Relationship Between Uric acid and Gout?" *Med Clin North Am* 8 (1925) : 1635–50.

77. G. P. Rodnan, T. G. Benedek, and W. C. Panetta, "The Early History of Synovia (Joint Fluid)," *Ann Intern Med* 65 (1966) : 821–42.

78. N. Allison, F. Fremont-Smith, M. E. Dailey, et al., "Comparative Studies Between Synovial Fluid and Plasma," *J Bone Joint Surg* 8 (1926) : 758–65.

79. D. H. Kling, *The Synovial Membrane and the Synovial Fluid* (Los Angeles: Med Press, 1938), 299.

80. M. W. Ropes, W. B. Robertson, E. C. Rossmeisl, et al., "Synovial Fluid Mucin," *Acta Med Scand* Suppl. 196 (1947) : 700–44.

81. W. P. Holbrook, "Evaluation of Therapy in Chronic Atrophic Arthritis," *Ann Intern Med* 7 (1933) : 457–67.

82. E. E. Irons, "The Treatment of Chronic Arthritis: General Principles," *JAMA* 103 (1934) : 1579–83.

83. R. L. Cecil, "The Medical Treatment of Chronic Arthritis," *JAMA* 103 (1934) : 1583–89.

84. A. G. Young, "The Use of Drugs in the Treatment of Atrophic Arthritis," *J Lab Clin Med* 15 (1930) : 1231–46.

85. Holbrook, "Therapy in Chronic Atrophic Arthritis."

86. P. J. Hanzlik, "Actions and Uses of the Salicylates and Cinchophen in Medicine," *Medicine* 5 (1926) : 197–373.

87. P. S. Hench, "Derivatives of Cinchophen and their Toxicity," *N Engl J Med* 207 (1932) : 949–50.

88. P. A. McIlhenny, "Chaulmoogra Oil in the Treatment of Arthritis," *New Orleans Med Surg J* 84 (1931) : 182–87.

89. J. Forestier, "L'Aurotherapie dans les Rhumatismes Chroniques," *Bull Mem Soc Med Hôp Paris* 53 (1929) : 323–29.

90. J. Forestier, "The Treatment of Rheumatoid Arthritis with Gold Salts Injections," *Lancet* 1 (1932) : 441–44.

91. C. Reitter and E. Löwenstein, "Akuter Gelenkrheumatismus und Tuberkelbazillämie," *Münch Med Wchnschr* 77 (1930) : 1522–23.

92. J. Forestier, "Rheumatoid Arthritis and Its Treatment by Gold Salts," *J Lab Clin Med* 20 (1935) : 827–40.

93. L. M. Lockie, B. M. Norcross, and D. J. Riordan, "Gold in the Treatment of Rheumatoid Arthritis," *JAMA* 167 (1958) : 1204–7.

94. R. L. Cecil, W. H. Kammerer, and F. J. DePrume, "Gold Salts in the Treatment of Rheumatoid Arthritis: A Study of 245 Cases," *Ann Intern Med* 16 (1942) : 811–27.

95. Cecil, "Medical Treatment of Chronic Arthritis."

96. W. P. Holbrook and D. F. Hill, "Treatment of Atrophic Arthritis," *JAMA* 107 (1936) : 34–38.

97. S. J. Hartfall, H. G. Garland, and W. Goldie, "Gold Treatment of Arthritis: A Review of 900 Cases," *Lancet* 2 (1937) : 784–88, 838–42.

98. R. G. Snyder, C. Traeger, and L. Kelly, "Gold Therapy in Arthritis: Observations on 100 Cases Treated with Gold Sodium Thiosulfate and Aurocein," *Ann Intern Med* 12 (1939) : 1672–81.

99. C. J. Smyth, R. H. Freyberg, and C. McEwen, *History of Rheumatology* (Atlanta: Arthritis Foundation, 1985), 154.

100. Forestier, "Rheumatoid Arthritis and Gold Salts."

101. Smyth et al., *History of Rheumatology.*

102. C. H. Slocumb, "Philip Showalter Hench, 1896–1965, In Memoriam," *Arthritis Rheum* 8 (1965) : 573–76.

103. Slocumb, "Philip Showalter Hench."

104. C. McEwen, personal communication, 1985.

105. Smyth et al., *History of Rheumatology.*

106. G. Rosen, "Special Medical Societies in the United States After 1860," *Ciba Symposia* 9 (1947) : 785–92.

107. J. van Breemen, R. F. Fox, L. J. Llewellyn, et al., "Disablement from Chronic Rheumatism," *Lancet* 2 (1925) : 100–101.

108. International Committee on Rheumatism, "The Campaign Against Rheumatism," *Arch Med Hydrology* 4 (1926) : 190–93.

109. Various reporters, "The Campaign Against Rheumatism: Reports from Countries," *Arch Med Hydrology* 6 (1928) : 81–87.

110. Smyth et al., *History of Rheumatology.*

111. R. Pemberton, "The Work of the American Committee for the Control of Rheumatism," *Med J Record* 138 (1933): 359–63.

112. R. M. Stecher, "The American Rheumatism Association—Its Origins, Development and Maturity," *Arthritis Rheum* 1 (1958): 4–19.

113. R. Pemberton, "The Control of Rheumatism," (editorial) *JAMA* 91 (1928): 30–31.

114. Anonymous, "Announcement and Description of a Scientific Exhibit Prepared for the Detroit Session of the American Rheumatism Association," *JAMA* 94 (1930): 1689.

115. Anonymous, "Announcement and Description of a Scientific Exhibit Prepared for the Philadelphia Session of the American Medical Association," *JAMA* 96 (1931): 1604.

116. Anonymous, "Announcement and Description of a Scientific Exhibit Prepared for the New Orleans Session of the American Medical Association," *JAMA* 98 (1932): 1288.

117. Anonymous, "Announcement and Description of a Scientific Exhibit Prepared for the Milwaukee Session of the American Medical Association," *JAMA* 100 (1933): 1534.

118. Anonymous, "Third Conference on Rheumatic Diseases: Cleveland, June 11, 1934," *JAMA* 103 (1934): 1732–34, 1801–4, 1883–84.

119. Anonymous, "Third Conference on Rheumatic Diseases."

120. Anonymous, "Conference on Rheumatic Diseases: New Orleans, May 9, 1932," *JAMA* 99 (1932): 1020–22.

121. Anonymous, "Second Conference on Rheumatic Diseases: Milwaukee, June 12, 1933," *JAMA* 101 (1933): 1182–84, 1264–66.

122. Smyth et al., *History of Rheumatology,* 29–34.

123. B. I. Comroe, *Arthritis and Allied Conditions* (Philadelphia: Lea & Febiger, 1940), 752, 730.

124. W. A. N. Dorland, *The American Illustrated Medical Dictionary,* ed. 19 (Philadelphia: W. B. Saunders, 1941), 1248.

125. H. L. Wehrbein, "Gonococcus Arthritis—A Study of Six Hundred Ten Cases," *Surg Gynecol Obstet* 49 (1929): 105–13.

126. H. H. Young, J. H. Hill, and W. W. Scott, "The Treatment of Infections and Infectious Diseases with Mercurochrome-220 Soluble," *Arch Surg* 10 (1925): 885–924.

127. C. S. Keefer and W. W. Spink, "Gonococci Arthritis: Pathogenesis, Mechanism of Recovery and Treatment," *JAMA* 109 (1937): 1448–53.

128. J. A. Colston, J. E. Dees, and H. C. Harrill, "The Treatment of Gonococci Infections with Sulfanilamide," *South Med J* 30 (1937): 1165–70.

129. C. S. Keefer and L. A. Rantz, "Sulphanilamide in the Treatment of Gonococcal Arthritis," *Am J Med Sci* 197 (1939): 168–81.

130. O. S. Culp, "Treatment of Gonorrheal Arthritis," *J Urology* 43 (1940): 737–65.

131. J. A. Robinson, H. L. Hirsh, W. W. Zeller, et al., "Gonococcal Arthritis: A Study of 202 Patients Treated with Penicillin, Sulfonamides or Fever Therapy," *Ann Intern Med* 30 (1949): 1212–23.

132. P. S. Hench and E. W. Boland, "The Management of Chronic Arthritis and Other Rheumatic Disorders Among Soldiers of the United States Army," *Ann Intern Med* 24 (1946): 808–25.

133. Smyth et al., *History of Rheumatology*, 17–18.
134. R. T. Smith, "Rheumatic Diseases," in *Internal Medicine in World War II*, W. P. Havens, ed., vol. 3 (Washington, D.C.: 1968), 477–97.
135. Hench and Boland, "Management of Chronic Arthritis."
136. Smith, "Rheumatic Diseases."
137. Smyth et al., *History of Rheumatology*, 17–18.
138. H. F. Swift, J. K. Moen, and G. K. Hirst, "The Action of Sulfanilamide in Rheumatic Fever," *JAMA* 110 (1938): 426–34.
139. C. B. Thomas and R. France, "A Preliminary Report of the Prophylactic Use of Sulfanilamide in Patients Susceptible to Rheumatic Fever," *Bull J Hopkins Hosp* 64 (1939): 67–77.
140. W. W. Spink, L. A. Rantz, P. J. Boisvert, et al., "Sulfadiazine and Penicillin for Hemolytic Streptococcus Infections of the Upper Respiratory Tract," *Arch Intern Med* 77 (1946): 260–94.
141. R. W. Quinn, "Epidemiologic Study of Seven Hundred and Fifty-Seven Cases of Rheumatic Fever," *Arch Intern Med* 80 (1947): 709–27.
142. T. D. Jones, "The Diagnosis of Rheumatic Fever," *JAMA* 126 (1944): 481–84.
143. D. D. Rutstein, W. Bauer, A. Dorfman, et al., "Jones Criteria (Modified) for Guidance in the Diagnosis of Rheumatic Fever," *Mod Conc Cardiovasc Dis* 24 (1955): 291–93.
144. G. H. Stollerman, M. Markowitz, A. Taranta, et al., "Jones Criteria (Revised) for Guidance in the Diagnosis of Rheumatic Fever," *Circulation* 32 (1965): 664–68.
145. W. Bauer and E. P. Engleman, "A Syndrome of Unknown Etiology Characterized by Urethritis, Conjunctivitis and Arthritis (So-called Reiter's Disease)," *Trans Assoc Am Physicians* 57 (1942): 307–13.
146. Simpson, "Keratodermie Blennorrhagique."
147. J. L. Hollander, C. W. Fogarty, N. R. Abrams, et al., "Arthritis Resembling Reiter's Syndrome: Observations on Twenty-Five Cases," *JAMA* 129 (1945): 593–95.
148. Hench and Boland, "Management of Chronic Arthritis Among Soldiers."
149. P. S. Hench, ed., "Ninth Rheumatism Review," *Ann Intern Med* 28 (1948): 74, 125.
150. P. Klemperer, W. D. Pollack, and G. Baehr, "Diffuse Collagen Disease," *JAMA* 119 (1942): 331–32.
151. J. G. Adami, *The Principles of Pathology*, vol. 1 (Philadelphia: Lea & Febiger, 1908), 920–21.
152. H. Schade, "Untersuchungen zur Organfunction des Bindegewebes," *Ztschr Exper Pathol* 11 (1912): 369–99.
153. F. Klinge and N. Grzimek, "Das Gewebsbild des fieberhaften Rheumatismus: VI. Der chronische Gelenkrheumatismus (Infektarthritis, Polyarthritis lenta) und über 'rheumatische Stigmata,'" *Virchow's Arch Pathol Anat* 284 (1932): 646–712.
154. T. G. Benedek, "Subcutaneous Nodules and the Differentiation of Rheumatoid Arthritis from Rheumatic Fever," *Semin Arthritis Rheum* 13 (1984): 305–21.
155. Klemperer et al., "Diffuse Collagen Disease."
156. A. R. Rich, "Hypersensitivity in Disease with Special Reference to Per-

iarteritis Nodosa, Rheumatic Fever, Disseminated Lupus Erythematosus and Rheumatoid Arthritis," *Harvey Lectures* 42 (1947): 106–47.

157. P. Klemperer, "The Concept of Collagen Diseases," *Am J Pathol* 26 (1950): 505–19.

158. W. E. Ehrich, "Nature of Collagen Diseases," *Am Heart J* 43 (1952): 121–56.

159. A. D. Wallis, "Rheumatoid Arthritis: I. Introduction to a Study of its Pathogenesis," *Am J Med Sci* 212 (1946): 713–15; "II. Non-specific Serologic Reactions," ibid., 212: 716–17; "III. The Pneumococcus Antibodies," ibid., 212: 718–22; "IV. Hemolytic Streptococcus Precipitin Reactions," ibid., 213 (1947): 87–93; "V. The Agglutination of Hemolytic Streptococci," ibid., 213: 94–96.

160. E. Waaler, "On the Occurrence of a Factor in Human Serum Activating the Specific Agglutination of Sheep Red Corpuscles," *Acta Pathol Microbiol Scand* 17 (1940): 172–88.

161. H. M. Rose, C. Ragan, and E. Pearce, et al., "Differential Agglutination of Normal and Sensitized Sheep Erythrocytes by Sera of Patients with Rheumatoid Arthritis," *Proc Soc Exp Biol Med* 68 (1948): 1–6.

162. C. Ragan, "The History of the Rheumatoid Factor," *Arthritis Rheum* 4 (1961): 571–73.

163. M. Ziff, "The Agglutination Reaction in Rheumatoid Arthritis," *J Chronic Dis* 5 (1957): 644–67.

164. J. M. Singer and C. M. Plotz, "The Latex Fixation Test: I. Application to the Serologic Diagnosis of Rheumatoid Arthritis," *Am J Med* 21 (1956): 888–92; "II. Results in Rheumatoid Arthritis," ibid., 21: 893–96.

165. E. S. Mongan, R. M. Cass, R. F. Jacox, et al., "Study of the Relation of Seronegative and Seropositive Rheumatoid Arthritis to Each Other and to Necrotizing Vasculitis," *Am J Med* 47 (1969): 23–35.

166. M. M. Hargraves, H. Richmond, and R. Morton, "Presentation of Two Bone Marrow Elements: The 'Tart' Cell and the 'L.E.' Cell," *Proc Staff Mayo Clin* 23 (1948): 25–28.

167. M. M. Hargraves, "Discovery of the LE Cell and its Morphology," *Mayo Clin Proc* 44 (1969): 579–99.

168. J. R. Haserick and R. D. Sundberg, "The Bone Marrow as a Diagnostic Aid in Acute Disseminated Lupus Erythematosus: Report on the Hargraves' 'L.E.' Cell," *J Invest Derm* 11 (1948): 209–13.

169. J. R. Haserick and D. W. Bortz, "A New Diagnostic Test for Acute Disseminated Lupus Erythematosus," *Cleve Clin Q* 16 (1949): 158–61.

170. P. Klemperer, B. Gueft, S. L. Lee, et al., "Cytochemical Changes of Acute Lupus Erythematosus," *Arch Pathol* 49 (1950): 503–16.

171. J. R. Haserick, "Blood Factor in Acute Disseminated Lupus Erythematosus," *Arch Derm Syph* 61 (1950): 889–91.

172. M. M. Hargraves and F. E. Zimmer, "The L.E. Cell Phenomenon," *Proc Staff Mayo Clin* 27 (1952): 419–23.

173. P. Miescher and M. Fauconnet, "L'Absorption du Facteur 'L.E.' par des Noyaux Cellulaires Isolés," *Experientia* 10 (1954): 252–54.

174. H. Holman and H. R. Deicher, "The Reaction of the Lupus Erythematosus (L.E.) Cell Factor with Deoxyribonucleoprotein of the Cell Nucleus," *J Clin Invest* 38 (1959): 2059–72.

175. G. J. Friou, S. C. Finch, and K. D. Detre, "Interaction of Nuclei and Globulin from Lupus Erythematosus Serum Demonstrated by Fluorescent Antibody," *J Immunol* 80 (1958): 324–29.

176. J. S. Beck, "Variations in the Morphological Patterns of 'Autoimmune' Nuclear Fluorescence," *Lancet* 1 (1961) : 1203–5.

177. J. S. Beck, "Antinuclear Antibodies: Methods of Detection and Significance," *Mayo Clin Proc* 44 (1969) : 600–19.

178. J. B. Collip, E. M. Anderson, and D. L. Thomson, "The Adrenotropic Hormone of the Anterior Pituitary Lobe," *Lancet* 2 (1933) : 347–48.

179. K. J. Anselmino, F. Hoffman, and L. Herold, "Das corticotrope Hormon des Hypophysenvorderlappens," *Arch f Gynäk* 157 (1934) : 86–102.

180. C. H. Li, H. M. Evans, and M. E. Simpson, "Adrenocorticotropic Hormone," *J Biol Chem* 149 (1943) : 413–24.

181. G. Sayers, A. White, and C. N. H. Long, "Preparation and Properties of Pituitary Adrenotropic Hormone," *J Biol Chem* 149 (1943) : 425–36.

182. P. S. Hench, "Analgesia Accompanying Hepatitis and Jaundice in Cases of Chronic Arthritis, Fibrositis and Sciatic Pain," *Proc Staff Mayo Clin* 8 (1933) : 430–36.

183. P. S. Hench, "Effect of Jaundice on Chronic Infectious (Atrophic) Arthritis and on Primary Fibrositis," *Arch Intern Med* 61 (1938) : 451–80.

184. P. S. Hench, "The Potential Reversibility of Rheumatoid Arthritis," *Proc Staff Mayo Clin* 24 (1949) : 167–78.

185. P. Hanssen, "The Effect of lactophenin-Icterus on Chronic Infectious Arthritis," *Acta Med Scand* 109 (1942) : 494–506.

186. C. H. Moore, "Periodical Inflammation of the Knee Joint," *Lancet* 1 (1864) : 485–86.

187. P. S. Hench, "The Ameliorating Effect of Pregnancy on Chronic Atrophic (Infectious Rheumatoid) Arthritis, Fibrositis, and Intermittent Hydrarthrosis." *Proc Staff Mayo Clin* 13 (1938) : 161–67.

188. W. P. Holbrook, "Recent Advances in the Management of Patients with Rheumatoid Arthritis," *NY Med* 4 (1948) : 17ff.

189. Hench, "Ameliorating Effect of Pregnancy."

190. E. C. Kendall, "The Development of Cortisone as a Therapeutic Agent," *Antibiot Chemother* 1 (1951) : 7–15.

191. P. S. Hench, "The Reversibility of Certain Rheumatic and Nonrheumatic Conditions by the Use of Cortisone or of the Pituitary Adrenocorticotropic Hormone," *Ann Intern Med* 36 (1952) : 1–38.

192. H. F. Polley and C. H. Slocumb, "Behind the Scenes with Cortisone and ACTH," *Mayo Clin Proc* 51 (1976) : 471–77.

193. P. S. Hench, E. C. Kendall, C. H. Slocumb, et al., "The Effect of a Hormone of the Adrenal Cortex (17-hydroxy-11-dehydrocorticosterone: Compound E) and of Pituitary Adrenocorticotropic Hormone on Rheumatoid Arthritis," *Proc Staff Mayo Clin* 24 (1949) : 181–97.

194. Polley and Slocumb, "Behind the Scenes with Cortisone and ACTH."

195. R. H. Freyberg, C. T. Traeger, C. H. Adams, et al., "Effectiveness of Cortisone Administered Orally," *Science* 112 (1950) : 429.

196. H. F. Polley and H. L. Mason, "Rheumatoid Arthritis: Effects of Certain Steroids Other Than Cortisone and of Some Adrenal Cortex Extracts," *JAMA* 143 (1950) : 1474–81.

197. Polley and Mason, "Rheumatoid Arthritis: Effects of Certain Steroids Other than Cortisone."

198. J. L. Hollander, E. M. Brown, R. E. Jessar, et al.: Hydrocortisone and Cortisone Injected into Arthritic Joints," *JAMA* 147 (1951) : 1629–35.

199. I. F. Duff, W. D. Robinson, W. M. Mikkelsen, et al., "Intra-articular Hy-

drocortisone in Rheumatoid Arthritis: Clinical and Laboratory Studies," *Med Clin North Am* 39 (1955) : 412–37.

200. E. W. Boland, "Clinical Comparison of the Newer Anti-inflammatory Corticosteroids," *Ann Rheum Dis* 21 (1962) : 176–87.

201. P. S. Hench, F. R. Vanzant, and R. Nomland, "Basis for the Early Differential Diagnosis of Gout," *Trans Assoc Am Physicians* 43 (1928) : 217–29.

202. J. P. McCracken, P. S. Owen, and J. H. Pratt, "Gout: Still a Forgotten Disease," *JAMA* 131 (1946) : 367–72.

203. Editorial, "Goutiness," *Med J Record* 135 (1932) : 454.

204. P. S. Hench, W. Bauer, A. A. Fletcher, et al., "The Problem of Rheumatism and Arthritis (Third Rheumatism Review)," *Ann Intern Med* 10 (1936) : 860–61.

205. B. M. Jacobson, "The Uric Acid in the Serum of Gouty and of Non-gouty Individuals: Its Determination by Folin's Recent Method and its Significance in the Diagnosis of Gout," *Ann Intern Med* 11 (1938) : 1277–95.

206. P. S. Hench, "A Clinic on Some Diseases of Joints," *Med Clin North Am* 19 (1935) : 551–83.

207. J. Kinell and R. L. Haden, "Gout: A Review of 62 Cases," *Med Clin North Am* 24 (1940) : 429–41.

208. Hanzlik, "Uses of the Salicylates and Cinchophen in Medicine."

209. Hench, "Derivatives of Cinchophen and their Toxicity."

210. T. G. Benedek, "The Gout of Desiderius Erasmus and Willibald Pirckheimer: Medical Autobiography and its Literary Reflections," *Bull Hist Med* 57 (1983) : 526–44.

211. Comroe, *Arthritis and Allied Conditions*, 502.

212. M. B. Blauch and F. C. Koch, "A New Method for the Determination of Uric Acid in Blood, with Uricase," *J Biol Chem* 130 (1939) : 443–54.

213. E. Praetorius and H. Poulsen, "Enzymatic Determination of Uric Acid, with Detailed Directions," *Scand J Lab Invest* 5 (1953) : 273–80.

214. F. W. Barnes and R. Schoenheimer, "On Biological Synthesis of Purines and Pyrimidines," *J Biol Chem* 151 (1943) : 123–39.

215. J. B. Wyngaarden, "Intermediary Purine Metabolism and the Metabolic Defects of Gout," *Metabolism* 6 (1957) : 244–67.

216. J. D. Benedict, P. H. Forsham, and D. Stetten, "The Metabolism of Uric Acid in the Normal and Gouty Human Studied with the Aid of Isotopic Uric Acid," *J Biol Chem* 181 (1949) : 183–93.

217. W. Q. Wolfson, C. Cohn, R. Levine, et al., "Transport and Excretion of Uric Acid in Man, Physiologic Significance of the Uricosuric Effect of Carinamide," *Am J Med* 4 (1948) : 774.

218. A. B. Gutman and T.-F. Yu, "Benemid ((p-di-n-propylsulfamyl)-benzoic acid) as Uricosuric Agent in Chronic Gouty Arthritis," *Trans Assoc Am Physicians* 64 (1951) : 279–88.

219. W. C. Kuzell and R. W. Schaffarzick, "Phenylbutazone (Butazolidin) and Butapyrin: A Study of Clinical Effects in Arthritis and Gout," *Cal Med* 77 (1952) : 319–25.

220. R. W. Rundles, J. B. Wyngaarden, G. H. Hitchings, et al., "Effects of a Xanthine Oxidase Inhibitor on Thiopurine Metabolism, Hyperuricemia and Gout," *Trans Assoc Am Physicians* 76 (1963) : 126–40.

221. McCracken et al., "Gout: Still a Forgotten Disease."

222. J. D. O'Duffy, G. G. Hunder, and P. J. Kelly, "Decreasing Prevalence of Tophaceous Gout," *Mayo Clin Proc* 50 (1975) : 227–28.

223. P. S. Hench, W. Bauer, E. W. Boland, et al., "Rheumatism and Arthritis (Ninth Rheumatism Review)," *Ann Intern Med* 28 (1948) : 68.

224. E. P. Jordan, W. Bauer, R. H. Boots, et al., "Primer on Arthritis," *JAMA* 119 (1942) : 1090–91.

225. G. P. Rodnan and H. R. Schumacher, eds., *Primer on the Rheumatic Diseases*, ed. 8 (Atlanta: Arthritis Foundation, 1983), 36–37.

226. Jones, "The Diagnosis of Rheumatic Fever."

227. M. W. Ropes, chairman, "Proposed Diagnostic Criteria for Rheumatoid Arthritis," *Bull Rheum Dis* 7 (1956) : 121–24.

228. M. W. Ropes, chairman, "1958 Revision of Diagnostic Criteria for Rheumatoid Arthritis," *Bull Rheum Dis* 9 (1958) : 175–76.

229. A. S. Cohen, chairman, "Preliminary Criteria for the Classification of Systemic Lupus Erythematosus," *Bull Rheum Dis* 21 (1971) : 643–48.

230. E. M. Tan, chairman, "The 1982 Revised Criteria for the Classification of Systemic Lupus Erythematosus," *Arthritis Rheum* 25 (1982) : 1271–77.

231. E. J. Brewer, chairman, "Criteria for the Classification of Juvenile Rheumatoid Arthritis," *Bull Rheum Dis* 23 (1972) : 712–19.

232. E. J. Brewer, chairman, "Revised Criteria for the Classification of Juvenile Rheumatoid Arthritis," *Arthritis Rheum* 20 (1977) (Suppl.) : 195–99.

233. S. L. Wallace, chairman, "Preliminary Criteria for the Classification of the Acute Arthritis of Primary Gout," *Arthritis Rheum* 20 (1977) : 895–900.

234. A. T. Masi, chairman, "Preliminary Criteria for the Classification of Progressive Systemic Sclerosis (Scleroderma)," *Arthritis Rheum* 23 (1980) : 581–90.

235. R. S. Pinals, chairman, "Preliminary Criteria for the Clinical Remission of Rheumatoid Arthritis," *Arthritis Rheum* 24 (1981) : 1308–15.

236. Ropes, "Proposed Diagnostic Criteria for Rheumatoid Arthritis."

237. Ropes, "1958 Revision of Diagnostic Criteria for Rheumatoid Arthritis."

238. Tan, "1982 Revised Criteria for Systemic Lupus Erythematosus."

239. Brewer, "Revised Criteria for Juvenile Rheumatoid Arthritis."

240. H. F. Polley and W. H. Bickel, "Punch Biopsy of Synovial Membrane," *Ann Rheum Dis* 10 (1951) : 277–87.

241. R. H. Parker and C. M. Pearson, "A Simplified Synovial Biopsy Needle," *Arthritis Rheum* 6 (1963) : 172–76.

242. M. S. Burman, H. Finkelstein, and L. Mayer, "Arthroscopy of the Knee Joint," *J Bone Joint Surg* 32 (1934) : 255–68.

243. R. L. O'Connor, "The Arthroscope in the Management of Crystal-Induced Synovitis of the Knee," *J Bone Joint Surg* 55A (1973) : 1443–49.

244. T. E. Weiss, W. S. Maxfield, P. J. Murison, et al., "Iodinated Human Serum Albumin (I^{131}) Localization Studies of Rheumatoid Arthritis Joints by Scintilation Scanning," *Arthritis Rheum* 8 (1965) : 976–87.

245. K. Whaley, A. J. Pack, J. A. Boyle, et al., "The Articular Scan in Patients with Rheumatoid Arthritis: A Possible Method of Quantitating Joint Inflammation Using Radio-technetium," *Clin Sci* 35 (1968) : 547–52.

246. D. J. McCarty, R. E. Polcyn, and P. A. Collins, "^{99m}Technetium Scintiphotography in Arthritis: II. Its Nonspecificity and Clinical and Roentgenographic Correlations in Rheumatoid Arthritis," *Arthritis Rheum* 13 (1970) : 21–32.

247. E. H. Lambert, S. Beckett, C. J. Chen, et al., "Unipolar Electromyograms of Patients with Dermatomyositis," *Fed Proc* 9 (1950) : 73.

248. R. G. Siekert and G. A. Fleisher, "Serum Glutamic Oxalacetic Transaminase in Certain Neurologic and Neuromuscular Diseases," *Proc Staff Mayo Clin* 31 (1956) : 459–64.

249. R. A. Thompson and P. J. Vignos, "Serum Aldolase in Muscle Disease," *Arch Intern Med* 103 (1959) : 551–64.

250. S. Okinaka, H. Kumagai, S. Ebashi, et al., "Serum Creatine Phosphokinase: Activity in Progressive Muscular Dystrophy and Neuromuscular Diseases," *Arch Neurol* 4 (1961) : 64–69.

251. Smyth et al., *History of Rheumatology*, 37–44.

252. Anonymous, "Medical News: The Arthritis and Rheumatism Foundation," *JAMA* 137 (1948) : 1142.

253. Smyth et al., *History of Rheumatology*, 37–44.

254. G. J. Faucher, "History of the Arthritis Foundation Research Fellowship Program 1951–1976," *Arthritis Rheum* 20 (1977) : S249–52.

255. Smyth et al., *History of Rheumatology*, 51–52, 84–85.

256. Stecher, "The American Rheumatism Association."

257. Stecher, "The American Rheumatism Association."

258. Rodnan and Schumacher, *Primer on the Rheumatic Diseases*.

259. P. S. Hench, chairman, "The Present Status of the Problem of 'Rheumatism'; A Review of Recent American and English Literature on 'Rheumatism' and Arthritis," *Ann Intern Med* 8 (1935) : 1315–74.

260. Hench et al., "Rheumatism: Recent Literature," 755.

261. C. J. Smyth, R. L. Black, F. E. Demartini, et al., "Rheumatism and Arthritis (Thirteenth Rheumatism Review)," *Ann Intern Med* 53 (1960) : (Suppl.) 1–365.

262. T. A. Medsger, ed., "25th Rheumatism Review," *Arthritis Rheum* 26 (1983) : 241–456.

263. J. J. Bunim, "Introduction," *Bull Rheum Dis* 1 (1950) : iii.

264. R. M. Stecher, "World List of Periodical Literature in Arthritis and Rheumatism," *Arthritis Rheum* 4 (1961) : 378–88.

265. Smyth et al., *History of Rheumatology*, 106–9.

266. G. P. Rodnan, "Growth and Development of Rheumatology in the United States—A Bicentennial Report," *Arthritis Rheum* 20 (1977) : 1149–68.

267. Smyth et al., *History of Rheumatology*, 37–44.

268. H. C. Coggeshall, in *Arthritis and Allied Conditions*, J. L. Hollander, ed., ed. 6 (Philadelphia: Lea & Febiger, 1960), 76.

269. Hollander, *Arthritis and Allied Conditions*, 77–78.

270. D. J. McCarty and J. L. Hollander, "Identification of Urate Crystals in Gouty Synovial Fluid," *Ann Intern Med* 54 (1961) : 452–54.

271. J. E. Seegmiller, R. R. Howell, and S. E. Malawista, "The Inflammatory Reaction to Sodium Urate: Its Possible Relationship to the Genesis of Acute Gouty Arthritis," *JAMA* 180 (1962) : 469–74.

272. D. J. McCarty, N. N. Kohn, and J. S. Faires, "The Significance of Calcium Phosphate Crystals in the Synovial Fluid of Arthritic Patients: The 'Pseudogout Syndrome:' I. Clinical Aspects," *Ann Intern Med* 56 (1962) : 711–17.

273. D. J. McCarty and R. A. Gatter, "Recurrent Acute Inflammation Associated with Focal Apatite Crystal Deposition," *Arthritis Rheum* 9 (1966) : 804–19.

274. M. Lesch and W. L. Nyhan, "A Familial Disorder of Uric Acid Metabolism and Central Nervous System Function," *Am J Med* 36 (1964) : 561–70.

275. J. E. Seegmiller, F. M. Rosenbloom, and W. N. Kelley, "Enzyme Defect Associated with a Sex-linked Human Neurological Disorder and Excessive Purine Synthesis," *Science* 155 (1967) : 1682–84.

276. S. B. Moore, "HLA," *Mayo Clin Proc* 54 (1979) : 385–93.

277. P. I. Terasaki and J. D. McClelland, "Microdroplet Assay of Human Serum Cytotoxins," *Nature* 204 (1964) : 998–1000.

278. F. H. Bach and K. Hirschhorn, "Lymphocyte Interaction: A Potential Histocompatibility Test in Vitro," *Science* 143 (1964) : 813–14.

279. F. C. Grumet, A. Coukell, M. A. Bodmer, et al., "Histocompatibility (HL-A) Antigens Associated with Systemic Lupus Erythematosus," *N Engl J Med* 285 (1971) : 193–96.

280. L. Schlosstein, P. I. Terasaki, R. Bluestone, et al., "High Association of an HL-A Antigen, W27, with Ankylosing Spondylitis," *N Engl J Med* 288 (1973) : 704–6.

281. D. A. Brewerton, F. D. Hart, A. Nicholls, et al., "Ankylosing Spondylitis and HL-A27," *Lancet* 1 (1973) : 904–7.

282. D. A. Brewerton, A. Nicholls, J. K. Oates, et al., "Reiter's Disease and HL-27," *Lancet* 2 (1973) : 996–98.

283. P. Stastny, "Association of the B-cell Alloantigen DRw4 with Rheumatoid Arthritis," *N Engl J Med* 298 (1978) : 869–71.

284. Rodnan, "Development of Rheumatology in the United States."

285. Arthritis Foundation, *1984–85 ARA/AHPA Membership Directory* (Atlanta: Arthritis Foundation, 1985).

286. Smyth et al., *History of Rheumatology*, 95–100.

287. Smyth et al., *History of Rheumatology*, 109–14.

288. L. B. Salans, *Third Annual Report of the Director, National Institute of Arthritis, Diabetes, and Digestive and Kidney Diseases* (Washington, D.C.: National Institutes of Health, Publication No. 84-2493, 1984), 15.

289. Rodnan, "Development of Rheumatology in the United States."

290. M. W. Cox, L. A. Aday, G. S. Levey, et al., "National Study of Internal Medicine Manpower: X. Internal Medicine Residency and Fellowship Training: 1985 Update," *Ann Intern Med* 104 (1986) : 241–45.

291. Smyth et al., *History of Rheumatology*, 71–73.

292. B. Hopkins, for American Board of Internal Medicine: Personal communications, 1984, 1985.

293. Ragan, "History of the Rheumatoid Factor."

294. Hargraves et al., "Presentation of the 'Tart' Cell and the 'L.E.' Cell."

295. W. H. Bickel, H. H. Young, K. H. Pfuetze, et al., "Streptomycin in Tuberculosis of Bone and Joint," *JAMA* 137 (1948) : 682–87.

296. Smyth et al., *History of Rheumatology*, 37–44.

297. Hench et al., "Effect of a Hormone of the Adrenal Cortex."

298. Smyth et al., *History of Rheumatology*, 106–9.

299. Gutman and Yu, "Benemid in Chronic Gouty Arthritis."

300. Kuzell and Schaffarzick, "Phenylbutazone and Butapyrin."

301. Hollander et al., "Hydrocortisone and Cortisone."

302. Polley and Bickel, "Punch Biopsy of Synovial Membrane."

303. Faucher, "History of the Arthritis Foundation Research Fellowship Program."

304. Smyth et al., *History of Rheumatology*, 106–9.

7

Nephrology in America from Thomas Addis to the Artificial Kidney

STEVEN J. PEITZMAN

Among subspecialties of internal medicine in America, nephrology seems an infant. Not until 1965 did the *Directory* of the American College of Physicians even recognize a renal designation.[1] The American Society of Nephrology was not founded until 1966, and the nephrology subspecialty board first offered a certifying examination in 1972. Indeed, when considered as a practice specialty nephrology is surely a post-World War II baby. And, of course, its growth hormone was secreted by the dialysis machine. But as an *academic* specialty, to use Paul Beeson's helpful distinction,[2] nephrology goes back very far. And the source of nephrology's split structure today lies clearly in the story of those men and women who created the esoteric knowledge base of renal physiology and medicine during the first half of the twentieth century. So this account will not begin with the inception of hemodialysis, but rather will conclude there.

The story must begin with Bright's Disease. Before Richard Bright's monumental work and its first publication in 1827, almost nothing was known of renal diseases other than stones. Bright associated the findings of dropsy, albuminous urine (as detected by heat or acid), and the uremic symptom complex with each other and with the discovery of morphologically deranged kidneys at autopsy. He described the granular kidney, the acute nephritic kidney, and the "large white kidney," but with restraint chose not to conclude whether these were separate diseases or merely stages of one process. Bright's way of investigating the disease that he discovered strikes the present-day nephrologist as remarkably "modern." Interested in learning more about the albuminuria and other chemical changes in his patients, but lacking chemical skills himself, he obtained the help of physician-chemists William Prout, John Bostock, and George Owen Rees. These colleagues not only quantified—albeit crudely—the alterations in blood and urine albumin, but also were able to detect retention of urea in the blood of patients with "renal dropsy." A landmark in the history of clinical investigation occurred in 1842. Bright received permission from the managers of Guy's Hospital to assign for the summer the "clinical wards" (i.e., teaching wards of the Hospital) to an orderly study of renal disease. Two young colleagues were assigned the basic clinical chores, a small laboratory was set up adjacent to the wards, and Owen Rees was given the task of performing the chemical determinations. Only cases of renal disease were entered into the two wards during the summer, and the clinical, chemical, and pathological findings were prospectively studied and later published.[3]

For our purposes, several elements of Bright's work are critical. One, obviously, is the established recognition of a medical category of renal disease—Bright's Disease, or nephritis. From the 1820s it was clear that the kidneys get sick in two important ways—wasting albumin, and causing uremia, a toxic devastation of the whole organism. The second, almost equally obvious point, is that the kidneys are chemical organs, the "great depurators" as physicians of Bright's time would label the pair of them, and therefore the investigation of renal disease must be at least in great part a chemical investigation. The remainder of the nineteenth century saw little added to the chemical work of Bright's friends. Further advance awaited the invention of analytical techniques quicker and far more sophisticated than those available to Bostock, Prout, and Rees.

How renal disease was understood in the early twentieth century may be seen in Osler's *Principles and Practice of Medicine,* the seventh edition of 1909.[4] Osler discussed "acute Bright's Disease" and "chronic Bright's Disease." Exactly like Richard Bright in 1827, Osler believed the acute form to be caused mainly by cold: "Exposure to cold and wet is one of the most common causes. It is particularly prone to follow exposure after a drinking bout."[5] The chronic forms of Bright's Disease Osler divided into "chronic parenchymatous nephritis" and "chronic interstitial nephritis," the latter term not meaning what it does today. But the distinctions were less impor-

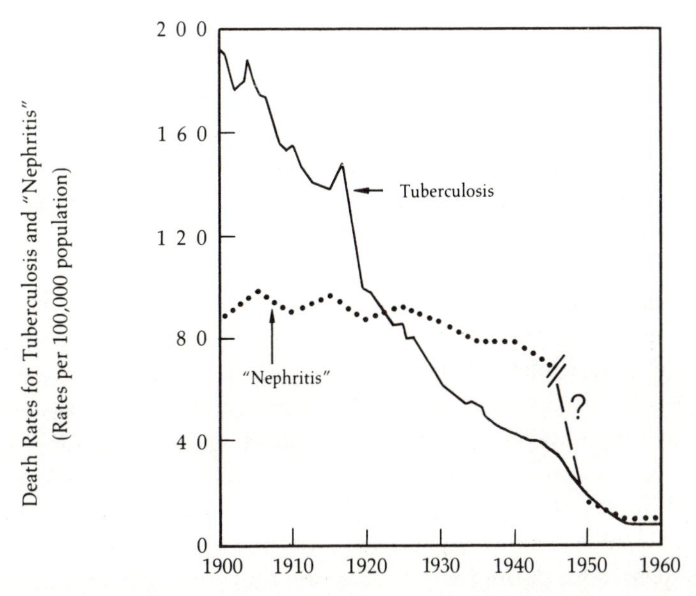

Figure 7.1. Death rates from "nephritis" compared with tuberculosis from 1900 to 1940. Redrawn from graphs in Grove and Hetzel, Vital Statistics *(note 6).*

tant than the whole: "Bright's Disease" retained its meaning as the way early twentieth-century physicians thought of sickness in the kidneys.

And Bright's Disease (or nephritis) was not a rare medical problem: vital statistics data show it as the sixth most frequent cause of death in 1900 and the fourth in 1940.[6] Although disease classification changed, as did the methods of gathering vital statistics, it appears that renal disease broadly defined remained steadily prevalent as the decades of the twentieth century advanced, while previously important infections such as tuberculosis and typhoid fever retreated (*Figure 7.1*).

Building a Knowledge Base: 1915–1940

Two post-Oslerian internists appear as transition figures in the history of American nephrology—Henry A. Christian (1874–1956) and Warfield T. Longcope (1877–1953). Both added newer modes of investigation to the bedrock of pathology, and both did important work on nephritis. Early in his career, Christian and colleagues performed studies in which they created animal models of Bright's Disease, using uranium nitrate as a toxin; they published results in the *Archives of Internal Medicine* beginning in 1911. They attempted to correlate the renal histological changes, fluid retention, and secondary cardiac effects with the "functional" disturbances, such as a deficit in the widely used phenolsulfonphthalein (phenol red) test. In his Harvey Lecture of 1915, Christian endorsed the prognostic and to some extent the diagnostic utility of the new renal function tests, but doubted they would succeed in predicting the histologic findings, still of primary importance in his mind.[7]

Coming early under the influence of William Henry Welch, William Osler, and Simon Flexner, Warfield T. Longcope also saw pathology, particularly experimental pathology, as an essential process for the advance of medicine.[8] His important experimental work, again with animal models of renal disease, and his clinical studies pointed to the immunologic basis of certain types of nephritis. In 1933 he published a valuable paper on the contracted kidneys of so-called chronic pyelonephritis. This paper was in the form of traditional clinical-pathological correlation. But Christian and Longcope studied other diseases as well; these were new-style investigating internists with a special interest in the kidneys, not renal specialists.

Descriptive and experimental pathology would never vanish from the repertory of renal investigation, but both entered a period of decline after about 1910. In their place appeared a fervid conversion to "functional diagnosis" and to the analysis of disease in the laboratory.[9] This shift was obviously influenced by the German school and impelled by remarkable new techniques devised by American chemists Otto Folin (1867–1934) and Donald D. Van Slyke (1883–1971). These methods proved most fully applicable to the study of renal physiology and Bright's Disease. The kidneys are chemical machines and the guardians of the electrolytes; they demand chemical study. Among the new and practicable techniques were assays for blood urea, total carbon dioxide, and creatinine. As American academic internists beginning in about 1915 felt a growing compulsion to measure, much of what they could measure concerned the kidney.

Otto Folin and his co-workers at Harvard ingeniously developed colorometric determinations for urea, creatinine, uric acid, and many other substances. His methods were rapid and required only a few milliliters of blood—these were crucial advances. As Folin pointed out in a 1917 lecture, "it is only when we come down to the very shortest of biochemical methods that we begin to appeal to clinicians." Folin promptly offered his skill to the clinic, including Henry Christian's group, and collaborated on several investigations of renal insufficiency.[10]

With a Ph.D. in organic chemistry from the University of Michigan, Donald D. Van Slyke entered the Rockefeller Institute as a research chemist with Phoebus A. Levene in 1907.[11] In 1914 he was moved from his "quiet corner in Levene's laboratory" to the new Rockefeller Institute Hospital. Van Slyke applied his inventiveness first to diabetic ketoacidosis. He devised a suitable gasometric method to measure the carbon dioxide content of a small blood sample. Building on the formulations of Lawrence J. Henderson,[12] Van Slyke and co-workers subsequently generated much of the current theory of acid-base balance in health and disease, including the importance of buffers, bicarbonate measurement, and associated electrolyte shifts. Van Slyke also devised a practical gasometric assay for urea which became widely adopted. With his new techniques, he "decided to take on the renal problem because there was a chance for quantitative chemistry there—measurement of function and the metabolic things that the kidney did."[13] In 1923, Rufus Cole listed nephritis as a disease to be formally studied by the Rockefeller Institute Hospital, a decision reminiscent of that made by the managers of Guy's Hospital for Richard Bright nearly a hundred years earlier. Van Slyke "worked-up" and followed a growing group of nephritic patients, aided by a series of hospital residents. Although not an M.D., "I became a pretty good clinician on Bright's Disease," he would later recall. "I made the rounds regularly."[14] A massive article in *Medicine* in 1930 described the clinical, chemical, and available pathological findings for the series of patients. It emphasized the usefulness of Van Slyke's "urea clearance" as a test for renal function.[15]

Two physicians who spent time with Van Slyke and helped build the knowledge base of nephrology were John P. Peters and Thomas Addis.

John Punnett Peters (1887–1956) (*Figure 7.2*) became interested in the kidney while he was a research fellow under Longcope at Columbia and Presbyterian Hospital in New York.[16] Peters then joined Van Slyke for one year (1920–21) at the Rockefeller Institute and helped his chief begin a series of studies concerning electrolyte equilibria. The friendship and collaboration begun in that year would last over decades. One of the products of the association was *Quantitative Clinical Chemistry* (1931–32), two monumental volumes of interpretation and methods.[17] Peters spent the remainder of his career in the Department of Medicine at Yale. He retained interest in nephritis, but his focus drifted outward from the kidneys, so that the complex and interacting balances of bodily water and electrolytes acquired a sort of primacy in his mind and in his program.[18] This expansion of domain would powerfully influence the future of nephrology through Peters' train-

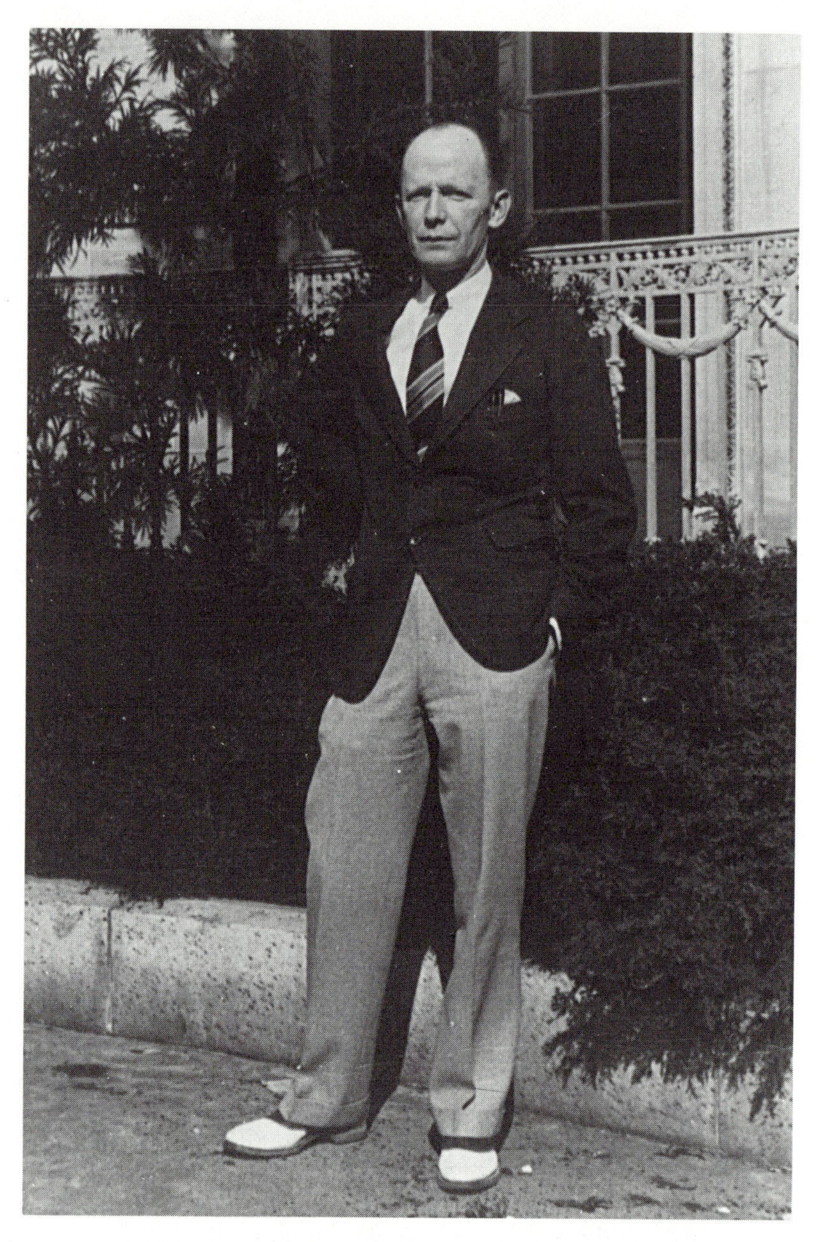

Figure 7.2. John Punnett Peters (1887–1956) of the Yale School of Medicine. His work in acid-base and fluid metabolism molded academic nephrology as his trainees developed renal sections at other prestigious medical schools. (Photograph courtesy of Diana E. Long.)

ees and associates such as Thaddeus Danowski, Maurice B. Strauss, Louis G. Welt, Jack Orloff, J. Russell Elkinton, and Donald Seldin. Peters, Yale, and this group of colleagues engendered the "metabolic" wing of nephrology, which came to dominate the field, at least academically. Here is not the place to discuss, though one ought at least to recall, John P. Peters' courageous concern for free speech, social justice, and access to medical care; he seemed to cherish balance and equilibria both as scientist and citizen.[19]

Seven years later, in 1928, Thomas Addis (*Figure 7.3*) was a visiting fellow in Van Slyke's lab at the Rockefeller Institute Hospital. Addis was "full of his own excellent ideas, which grow and change from day to day as do the ideas of any thinking man," Van Slyke wrote of Addis in 1930 to Rufus Cole, who wished to (and did) invite Addis to join the permanent staff of the Rockefeller Institute Hospital.[20] But Addis declined. "For one thing," he wrote to Cole, "I have [at Stanford] collected a group of nephritics which I have nursed along and watched over for the past ten years. You know that twenty years at least are needed to get anywhere with prognosis."[21]

Addis remained at Stanford, where he advanced the use of the urea ratio, which really was the urea clearance, as an indicator of functioning renal mass.[22] He combined renal ablation experiments in the laboratory with clinical work to refine this functional concept of the "lesion in Bright's Disease." In collaboration with the pathologist Jean Oliver, Addis also put forth what became a generally accepted categorization of Bright's Disease, which was in use almost until the era of renal biopsy in the 1950s.[23] He is remembered perhaps most for the "Addis count," his method of standardizing and quantifying the examination of urine sediment. In later writings he deplored the separation of physician and laboratory worker, and advocated direct and simple estimates of renal function that the physician himself might carry out as an integral part of the patient examination. Addis' second book, *Glomerular Nephritis: Diagnosis and Treatment*, published in 1948, one year before his death, summarized a lifetime of work and stressed his dietary "rest" treatment for Bright's Disease, an approach again in vogue in the 1980s with perhaps a transformed theoretical underpinning.[24]

In the laboratory and at the bedside, Addis was the complete student of Bright's Disease: he watched over nephritics. Fluid balance and acid-base physiology seemed to concern him much less. Although intellectually influential in his day, Addis' idiosyncratic personality perhaps was not the sort to build a "program." He had pupils and collaborators, but did not foster a dynasty, as did Peters and Homer Smith. The geographical separation of Stanford from the eastern clinical centers may have been a factor in this

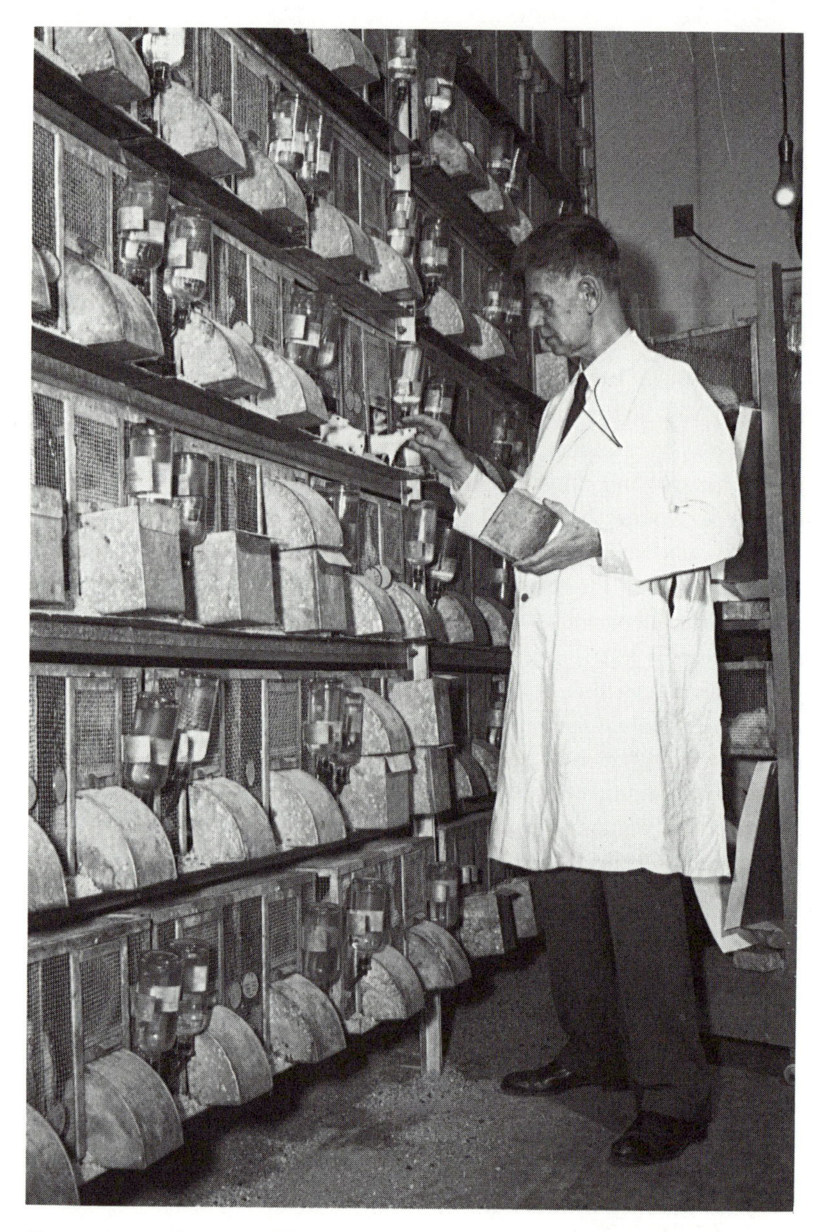

Figure 7.3. *Thomas Addis (1881–1949) with some of his white rats at Stanford University. Addis promoted the notion of functioning nephron mass, provided a working nosology of Bright's Disease, and described a standardized method for viewing the urinary sediment. (Photograph courtesy of the Lane Medical Library, Stanford University Medical Center.)*

genealogic failure. Certainly another was Addis' difficult struggle to win outside grant support for his program (see below, p. 222). Whatever may be the reasons, Addis' small place in the collective memory of internal medicine hardly corresponds with the breadth and richness of his work.

Although few young nephrologists today know anything of Thomas Addis, a lingering mystique still surrounds the name of Homer W. Smith (1895–1962) (*Figure 7.4*).[25] In the minds of many, *he* stands as the progenitor of modern American nephrology. Yet Smith held a doctorate of science, not an M.D., and began his career as a physiologist of fish. He became professor of physiology at New York University School of Medicine in 1928. There he began a fruitful collaboration with clinicians William Goldring, Herbert Chasis, Norman Jolliffe, James Shannon, and many others. Their dominant cumulative contribution was the refinement and utilization of the idea of clearance. With suitably chosen solutes they learned to measure and clarify glomerular filtration and tubular transport. These workers built much of the language of renal physiology, so they guided the way subsequent physicians and physiologists would think and talk about kidney function.

The collaboration was intimate and symmetric: Smith the physiologist took a lively interest in clinical questions and published important critical reviews on renal hypertension and volume receptors.[26] The internists, in turn, contributed substantively to knowledge of renal physiology. Smith's laboratory at New York University and its close affiliation with the Department of Medicine emerged as a nuclear center for the preparation of internists who would pursue academic clinical careers in nephrology.[27] Indeed many nephrologists who never spent time at New York University, or were born too late to have even met Smith, still like to think of themselves as somehow his children. Smith's book *The Kidney: Structure and Function in Health and Disease* (New York: Oxford University Press, 1951), with its massive list of references, became the renal bible for students and clinicians. Erudite and commanding, at times distant yet cherished by his friends, Homer W. Smith, Sc.D., was and remains the American legend of renal medicine.

Yet Smith's work with whole-kidney clearances depended for its very meaning on the masterful accomplishments of Alfred Newton Richards (1876–1966), another nonphysician, who worked in the pharmacology department of the University of Pennsylvania during the 1920s and 1930s.[28] It is a small exaggeration, if any, to assert that Richards and his team achieved for the kidney what Harvey had for the heart about three hundred years

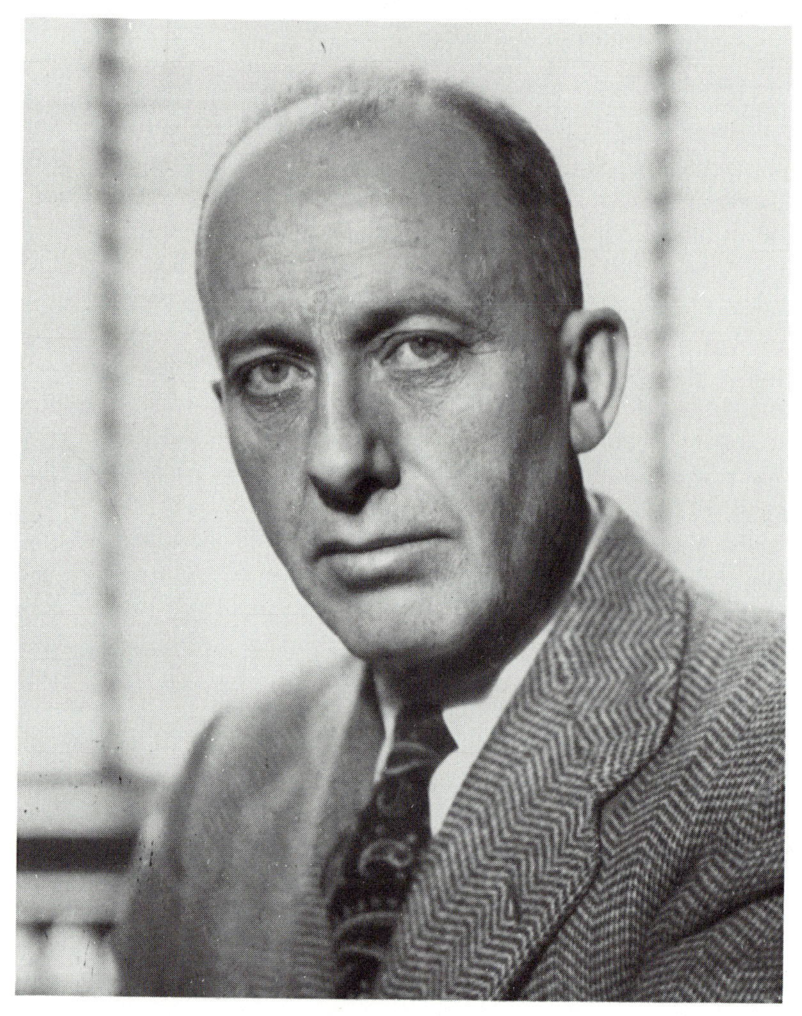

Figure 7.4. Homer W. Smith (1895–1962), a physiologist, expanded the concept of clearance, helped make physiology useful at the bedside, and, through his collaborators and trainees at New York University, powerfully influenced future nephrology. (Photograph courtesy of the Archives, New York University School of Medicine.)

earlier: they presented the first demonstration of how the organ did its job that was persuasively satisfying within the science of the day. Using techniques which still amaze, Richards, Joseph Wearn (who provided a key initial suggestion), the chemist Phyllis Bott, Arthur M. Walker, and others punctured living frog nephrons with micropipettes and carried out chemical assays on the tiny samples obtained. They confirmed the filtration-reabsorption model of Carl Ludwig and Arthur Cushny, and settled the fundamental question: How does the kidney make urine? Richards and his colleagues then expanded the new understanding of tubular reabsorption and secretion with a series of further experiments. They also studied with micropuncture the mechanism of oliguria in toxic acute renal failure. Richards' legacy was not only new knowledge[29] but also a set of methods—micropuncture—that could be taught and transferred (albeit with difficulty). It would become an important vehicle providing work and publication for many future nephrologists as they mapped tubular function with ever-increasing refinement.

Like Van Slyke and Smith, Richards reached out to the clinic. As part of his proposal in 1931 to a receptive Commonwealth Fund, Richards called for a "small section of the hospital . . . devoted to the scientific care and study of human patients with renal disease . . . in charge of a skilled physician, highly trained in fundamental science."[30] Richards won what was then the Commonwealth Fund's largest single grant in medicine or public health, $100,000 over three years, to support his laboratory and its small clinical appendage.[31] The University of Pennsylvania Hospital's renal clinic opened in 1932 under Eugene M. Landis (who also mastered the micropipette and worked at the bench). In its first year, this clinic studied urea and creatinine clearance in normal humans as well as renal function in toxemia of pregnancy and in hypertensive nephrosclerosis.[32]

So these were the influentials in renal physiology and medicine in the period between the World Wars: Donald Van Slyke, Thomas Addis, John P. Peters, Homer W. Smith, and A. Newton Richards. Lawrence J. Henderson (1878–1942) and James L. Gamble (1883–1959) of Harvard must also be added for their work on acid-base chemistry and the composition of extracellular fluid.[33] Only three of these seven were physicians. And of these three, Peters was as much chemist as doctor, and Addis nearly so.[34] It is hardly surprising that a preferred attention to metabolic and physiologic problems and discourse would infuse the profession—when there eventually grew up a profession. Many of the internists who would become renal division chiefs in the medical schools of the 1950s and 1960s were first or second generation products of Homer Smith at New York University or Peters at Yale. But this strange process, the fathering of nearly an entire subspecialty of internal medicine by chemists and physiologists, could occur because of the successful integration of the bedside and bench fostered by Van Slyke, Addis, Smith, Peters, and to a lesser extent by Richards and even Otto Folin. By the very nature of what the kidney is and does, laboratory workers had to lead, because they provided the needed probes.

Another important generalization concerning this group is the central role of the foundations—the Rockefeller Institute (nurturing Van Slyke, and briefly Addis and Peters); and the Commonwealth Fund (which supported Richards and later Smith). Clinical scientists of recent decades may not appreciate the importance of such support in the period before the explosion of federally financed research. Thomas Addis in San Francisco seems to have had poor luck with the begging bowl and struggled along with modest support from Stanford.[35]

Surviving correspondence[36] readily documents that Addis, Peters, Van Slyke, Smith, and Richards not only knew each other but paid frequent visits to each others' laboratories and homes. All but Addis were geographically proximate. They exchanged data, galleys, ideas, reagents, and even their underlings: in 1935 Smith and Richards arranged a temporary trade of James Shannon for Phyllis Bott, in order to work out some differences concerning inulin measurement.[37] That no clinical renal society grew up in the 1930s or 1940s is hardly surprising: the renal influentials were largely nonphysicians and could not have very well founded an organization within internal medicine. And they seemed not to need one to share ideas.

The Emergence of Acute Renal Failure

Here it will prove helpful to summarize the status of renal medicine in America as World War II approached.

Two levels of renal knowledge existed by 1940. The first was a general basis for the diagnosis, classification, and treatment of Bright's Disease accessible to most physicians. Acute glomerulonephritis (as we would now call it) was managed symptomatically and sometimes with sedatives and phlebotomy. The term comprised postinfectious glomerulonephritis as now understood but must have counted many other types not yet categorized by 1940. Much of Bright's Disease was chronic and simply treated at home with rest, encouragement, and dietary measures.[38] The chemical work-up of the nephritic patient might include at most the Addis count (quantified urinary sediment examination), perhaps some urea or creatinine measurements in sophisticated renal clinics, and the phenylsulfonphthalein (PSP) test.

The second level of knowledge was a sophisticated comprehension of pathophysiology open only to those who cultivated it. This latter level, the *esoteric knowledge base,* included the languages of clearance, water and electrolyte balance, and acid-base disorders. It was created largely by the laboratory workers and collaborations already discussed.

But even for the internist with special interest in disease of the kidney, there existed no basis for in-hospital renal consultation until a remarkable event, the rediscovery and definition of acute renal failure in the early 1940s. Acute renal failure called for the display of special expertise in the ward and would provide impetus for two special techniques—renal biopsy and dialysis.

Curiously, acute renal failure ("acute tubular necrosis") nearly vanished from the minds of English-speaking clinicians after World War I.[39] Sudden renal shutdown as part of mercuric chloride toxicity—a frequent suicidal manifestation of the Depression—occasionally was reported. But not until 1941 did E. G. Bywaters and D. Beale newly make clear the syndrome of ultimately reversible acute cessation of renal filtration.[40] They described acute renal failure as a sad consequence of crush injuries incurred by Londoners during the Battle of Britain. At the same time, shock-induced acute renal failure, with or without rhabdomyolysis, increasingly challenged military surgeons.[41] Coincidentally, a new and vigorous source of nephrotoxic acute renal failure, the early sulfonamide antimicrobials, had entered widespread use in the late 1930s.

From about 1946 through 1955 acute renal failure increasingly captured the attention of internists interested in renal disease, as evidenced by journal articles and a cluster of monographs in English appearing during this decade.[42] The diagnosis and treatment of acute renal failure (then called "lower nephron nephrosis") required consultative expertise in the hospital, and the expert might make a difference. Careful attention to management of electrolyte and acid-base disorders might help the patient survive into the "diuretic phase." Two specialty procedures, renal biopsy and renal dialysis, could be offered in some circumstances. Thus the appearance of acute renal failure (ARF) as a new entity exercised the practical arm of the renal specialist as nothing else had before.

From here a chronological narrative becomes difficult to maintain, and two of the developments noted, biopsy and dialysis, will be discussed now.

Renal Biopsy and a Return to Pathology

Percutaneous biopsy of the kidney using a needle was a European invention stimulated by a desire to establish diagnosis in the patient with ARF. Soon, however, on both sides of the Atlantic clinicians expanded the indications for renal biopsy.[43]

Alvin E. Parrish of George Washington University was among the first

Americans to report a large series of patients evaluated with renal biopsy, most of whom showed glomerulonephritis or nephrosclerosis.[44] But Robert M. Kark of Chicago receives the credit for establishing the clinical and investigational worth of renal biopsy in the United States. Beginning in the early 1950s, Kark and co-workers published one major paper after another, clarifying and redefining glomerular disease.[45] This group was, of course, joined by many others as the method proved safe and, as Kark stresses, suitable to be "generally applied to the sick."[46]

There were several effects of renal biopsy on the developing subspecialty of nephrology. The technique represented a "procedure" requiring the skilled hand and eye of the subspecialist, and thus added another reason for a "renal consult." Biopsy could be taught; learning to do it soon formed a part of renal "fellowships" as these sprang up, and eventually it would guide the treatment of nephrotic patients.

For the intellectual content of the discipline, biopsy accomplished two seemingly contradictory tasks: it drew attention back to Bright's Disease, but also destroyed it. The Vim-Silverman needle helped point some nephrologists away from the numerical allure of electrolytes and equilibria and bring them back to pathology, back to the deranged kidney itself, the original problem. Biopsy provided a way to see the renal lesion before death, while the patient might benefit from the information and while subtle histologic characteristics might still shine through, undistorted by chronic degeneration. As biopsy rebuilt the nosology of diffuse renal disease, subdividing nephritis and nephrosis into an intimidating menu of new entities, "Bright's Disease" finally lost any meaning, and even the useful old classification of Addis gave way to the current cloud of glomerular lesions.[47] Renal biopsy added many bricks to the structure of esoteric knowledge which could house a renal subspecialty. The point is worth belaboring: general physicians could comfortably know Bright's Disease, but "mesangiocapillary glomerulonephritis, Type II" belongs to the specialist.

The Beginning of Clinical Hemodialysis

Dialysis was another largely European invention induced by the new awareness of acute renal failure.[48] Sporadic attempts at clinical dialysis occurred in the 1920s and 1930s, but those that proved fruitful began in the 1940s, when war and sulfa made acute renal failure plentiful. Four individuals or groups, working almost simultaneously, rightly may claim credit: Willem Kolff in the Netherlands, Nils Alwall in Sweden, Gordon Murray in Canada, and Leonard Skeggs and Jack Leonards in America (Cleveland).

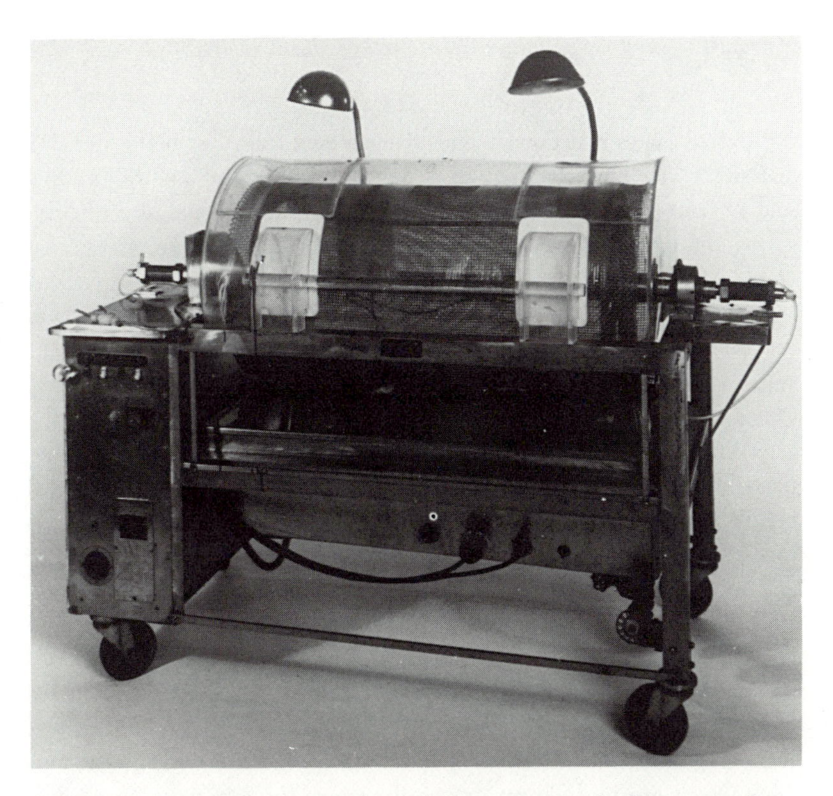

Figure 7.5. An early rotating drum dialysis machine built using Willem Kolff's device as its model and used at the Peter Bent Brigham Hospital in Boston in the late 1940s. (Photograph courtesy of the National Museum of American History, The Smithsonian Institutions.)

Kolff achieved the earliest success (after fifteen deaths) in 1945, reviving a comatose uremic woman who went on to regain renal function. A key event for American nephrology seems to have been Kolff's demonstration in early 1948 of his "rotating drum" kidney by invitation at Mount Sinai Hospital in New York City. Several physicians came to see the Dutch investigator's awkward but promising contraption. Among them were George Thorn and John P. Merrill from the Peter Bent Brigham Hospital in Boston and George Schreiner, later of Georgetown University. (Some accounts indicate that Thorn and Merrill started work on their replica of the Kolff kidney in 1947.) Subsequently, the "Kolff-Brigham" refinement of the rotating drum established Boston as a center of dialysis (*Figure 7.5*), and Schreiner developed an active program in Washington. Merrill was an entirely Harvard-bred internist with a strong leaning toward pathophysiology and chemistry. Schreiner had been a fellow of Homer Smith.

By 1952, Merrill reported that about forty-five dialyzers were in use in the United States and Canada and that his own team had performed 210 dialyses.[49] The most frequent use was for acute renal failure. By the mid-1950s commercial manufacture of dialysis machines and filters helped spread the technique, although some machines purchased in that period were undoubtedly destined to gather dust in a hospital closet.

Probably the most crucial invention after the dialysis device itself was the first "permanent" access to the circulation, the indwelling arterial-venous shunt created by physician Belding Scribner and engineer Wayne Quinton at the University of Washington in 1960.[50] This technique and the arterialized venous fistula which followed in 1964 made repeated "maintenance" dialysis feasible for the large number of persons with chronic renal failure. During the 1960s and beyond, following Scribner's lead, dialysis centers sprang up as units of medical school renal divisions, within community and Veterans Administration hospitals, and eventually as commercial free-standing entities. Again emulating the pioneering direction of Scribner's team in Seattle, some centers began to teach persons with chronic renal failure (CRF) to perform their dialytic treatments at home. A survey conducted in 1971 found 312 chronic dialysis facilities in forty-four states.[51] This was two years before the implementation of PL92-603, the famous act of Congress which provided almost universal support for Americans in need of chronic dialysis.[52]

The implications of dialysis for nephrology as a subspecialty have been staggering. Dialysis, with its opaque technical language, represented another component of the cumulating esoteric knowledge base of the discipline. And the increasing number of chronic dialysis patients soon demonstrated a set of new diseases and derangements, both unmasked effects of chronic renal failure and unexpected complications of an imperfect therapy. Hemodialysis is also, of course, a procedure and one not viewed as part of the required skills of the general internist. Rarely does someone other than a nephrologist write dialysis orders, although many sorts of physicians supervise respirators.

Dialysis, like renal biopsy, became an intrinsic part of new, structured nephrology training programs beginning in the 1950s. Most chiefs of nephrology in medical schools saw research and teaching as their job, not the direct supervision of often troublesome dialysis treatments; fellows were needed to do this work. In turn, the advent of federally supported chronic dialysis eventually expanded opportunity for practice for those fellows not choosing an academic career after training.

Through hemodialysis internists such as Belding Scribner, John P. Merrill and George Schreiner initiated a new model of renal physician—what Eli Friedman (himself one of them) has called the "craftsmen" of nephrology. That is, soundly based in physiology and pathophysiology, they mastered in addition the practical elements of dialysis, renal biopsy (especially Schreiner), and transplantation (Merrill). Although few would contribute as much as these pioneers, all subsequent "boarded" nephrologists could presumably claim functional expertise in all parts of the discipline. But even as a sort of unity of training and expected skills increasingly defined the subspecies "nephrologist," an almost inevitable division arose between "dialyzers" (the men, not the membranes), and "the fluid-electrolyte" people.

The Decades After World War II: Growth and Division

Nephrology from the 1950s into the 1970s blossomed within academic medicine and advanced more slowly outside it. Most departments of medicine in medical schools grew immensely and adopted the now familiar divisional structure by subspecialty. Exponential increase in funding from the National Institutes of Health nourished this growth.[53] Renal divisions (sometimes called the "electrolyte division" or even "chemical section") proliferated under the new compartmentalization. Often their chiefs were drawn from the trainees of John P. Peters or Homer W. Smith, and their research favored electrolyte transport, mineral metabolism, fluid and acid-base balance, and experimental acute renal failure. The flame photometer, which entered research and clinical laboratories in the late 1940s and 1950s, markedly simplified and quickened the measurement of serum sodium and potassium, and further stimulated interest in extracellular solute balance. Micropuncture was revived and taught by such masters as Phyllis Bott, Carl Gottschalk, and Gerhard Giebisch. Renal fellows became plentiful by the 1960s; seemingly untired by their clinical chores, they learned micropipette methods or grappled with the vagaries of toad bladders and frog skins. The less steady of hand perhaps chose studies based on classic clearance methods. Everyone seemed happy and published lavishly.

The primary reason for calling the nephrologist to the bedside remained acute renal failure. More and more patients survived shock, surgery, trauma, and other calamities, but caught acute tubular necrosis (ATN) along the way. New nephrotoxic agents displaced mercury and the sulfa drugs as tormentors of kidneys—aminoglycoside antibiotics, amphotericin, and radiographic contrast, for example.

But a too steady diet of renal failure tires the nephrologist, and the progeny of Smith and Peters sought clinical problems more aligned with their research interests and their physiologic fascination with the numerology of electrolytes and acid-base balance. Possibly this hope would have been only occasionally satisfied had not a remarkable event occurred in the clinical laboratory. In 1957 Leonard T. Skeggs, who had also helped construct an early hemodialysis system, reported his new invention, a string of pumps, timers, and a colorimeter, which would become the famous "AutoAnalyzer" of Technicon Instruments Company.[54] This was a leap in laboratory speed and convenience equal to that achieved by Folin and Van Slyke in the early part of the century. Desired and even unwanted values for sodium, potassium, chloride, total carbon dioxide, calcium, and other chemistries spewed forth from the multichannel autoanalyzer with amazing quickness and in unprecedented abundance. Undoubtedly, after the flame photometer was incorporated into the autoanalyzer, cases of hyponatremia, hyperkalemia, and metabolic acidosis surfaced in patients in whom no such disorder was suspected.[55] Such findings invited explanation, and sometimes required treatment; the nephrologist was prepared and eager to explore and teach about them. It was in good part the automated laboratory that allowed this daily display of virtuosity. The cult of the "anion gap"[56] derives as much from the "SMA-6" machine as it does from Van Slyke and Gamble.[57]

Hemodialysis in the 1960s and early 1970s grew up within medical school renal divisions at such centers as the University of Washington, Georgetown University, and the Peter Bent Brigham Hospital. In some schools a renal division member interested in the process would develop a suitable research program in hemodialysis. But elsewhere its accommodation into the academic program could prove problematic. In its natal period, dialysis had seemed to some of the then senior protonephrologists as a dubious flash in the pan, cherished by neophytes. Sometimes dialysis research depended as much on engineering as it did on renal physiology, and its language of discourse became increasingly opaque to other nephrologists in a division. (That dialysis investigators occasionally used goats for their experiments added little to their popularity.)

Not infrequently, but regrettably, a division chief raised in the metabolic-physiology tradition viewed the increasing clinical demands of hemodialysis care with derision and dealt with them functionally by delegation. A junior faculty member would be hired as the "dialyzer"; or the growing burden of chronic hemodialysis care was assigned almost entirely to the first-year fellows. This latter solution sometimes impaired continuity of care, and probably sent unspoken messages about priorities. So while in some medical school renal divisions dialysis was intellectually and functionally well integrated, in others a bipartite reality evolved.[58]

Outside the medical schools during the 1960s, only a small number of practitioners, usually in large communities, became identified as renal specialists. In some cities several community hospitals opened small dialysis units, and these required someone with expertise to supervise them. Some such practitioners were self-taught in dialysis, while others had trained with someone like George Schreiner or Belding Scribner. Often they would mix nephrology and general internal medicine in their practice.

The growing group of renal specialists and trainees could not forever rely only on Homer Smith's 1951 one-man "bible" of kidney function and disease. The first two American renal texts of the "modern period" appeared in the early 1960s: *Clinical Disorders of Fluid and Electrolyte Metabolism* (1962) by Morton H. Maxwell and Charles R. Kleeman and *Diseases of the Kidney* (1963) by Maurice B. Strauss and Louis G. Welt. Both of these were multiauthored volumes. These four authors (really editors) and almost all authors of subsequent major American renal texts came out of the physiology-metabolism tradition.

The establishment of organizations and of a certifying board marked further steps in the consolidation of nephrology. Founded in 1954, the American Society for Artificial Internal Organs (ASAIO) from its inception included as active members and officers such leaders in dialysis as Willem Kolff, John P. Merrill, George Schreiner, and Belding Scribner.[59] The ASAIO was, and has remained, a forum for the presentation of research in dialysis and chronic renal failure. Its provision of such a forum may have allowed the eventual American Society of Nephrology to perhaps favor physiology and pathophysiology in its meetings.

The first national nephrology organization in America seems to have been the Renal Section of the Circulation Council of the American Heart Association (AHA), first proposed in 1961 and founded in 1963 as one of the professional subunits of the AHA.[60] How this curiosity arose is not entirely clear. Certainly the relationships of renal disease and heart disease—particularly through hypertension—grew increasingly apparent during the 1940s and beyond. A so-called cardiorenal syndrome was much discussed in the 1930s and 1940s. And by 1960 the AHA had become a major source of support for research into renal disease and function. For example, John P. Merrill was an early AHA Career Investigator, and Homer W. Smith enjoyed support of the AHA New York affiliate. What most urgently prompted the genesis of the new body was the need to represent the American nephrology community to the already established International Society of Nephrology (ISN). The Renal Section also ran several seminars, advised the parent body on research grants, and published a directory of nephrology training programs. It proved reluctant to commit itself to the guidance of community renal programs, and the minutes of the Renal Section almost from the start reveal a vagueness of purpose and debate over its need.[61] As candidate for *the* national renal society, the Renal Section of the AHA was doomed from the beginning: there were more than a few invested renal specialists by 1964, and most would not suffer remaining a section of a council of an association devoted to a muscle that pumps.

Growing sentiment in favor of a separate scientific renal group was sounded by some leaders in the field as early as 1964.[62] The American Society of Nephrology (ASN) was founded on 26 June 1966 at a meeting of influential renal specialists at the Gramercy Park Hotel in New York.[63] Active at the founding meeting were Neal Bricker, John Merrill, George Schreiner, Donald Seldin, David Earle, and Louis Welt. The start-up was supported by a grant from the National Kidney Foundation. Also in 1966, the ISN held a successful Congress in Washington, D.C., with the Renal Section of the AHA serving as host society. About 400 Americans registered. These two events in 1966—the ISN Congress and the founding of the ASN—indicated considerable maturity of the subspecialty in America by that year.

The ASN has proved robust, reaching over 3,800 members by 1985.[64] Its primary activity has been an annual scientific meeting conducted traditionally. Registration at the annual meeting has exceeded 2,500 since 1977—the halls of the meeting hotel fill impressively with a vast sea of nephrologists and their trainees, men and women of every size, age, and color.

Although renal enthusiasts of all interests do gather together agreeably at the annual ASN meeting, the Society's leadership has come largely from the academic community, and particularly (although not entirely) from those favoring physiologic research and "electrolyte nephrology." In recent years, occasional complaints were heard that the ASN meetings offered too little that was accessible to the renal clinician. The Society has made some adjustments to address this perception and now seems a strong and stable body.

Another indicator of maturity was subspecialty certification in nephrology. The first examination in nephrology in 1972 was passed by 212 physicians. By 1984, 2,594 certifications in nephrology had been issued.[65] Nineteen nephrologists have served on the subspecialty board or committee from its inception in 1972 through 1985 (Thomas Andreoli, Neal Bricker,

Jordan Cohen, Vincent Dennis, Franklin Epstein, Thomas Ferris, Richard Glassock, Martin Goldberg, Charles Kleeman, Norman Levinsky, Manuel Martinez-Maldonado, Arnold Relman, Roscoe Robinson, Robert Schrier, William Schwartz, Donald Seldin, Jay Stein, Wadi Suki, and Louis Welt). Most of these men represent (like most of the ASN presidents) the metabolic-physiologic school. While all are or were broadly knowedgeable, it is striking that not a single of the names is recognizably associated with hemodialysis.

With the establishment of a subspecialty board, an independent society, strong representation in medicine departments, a basis for consultative practice, and a source of sustained outpatient practice, nephrology by the mid-1970s had more than met criteria for a stable subspecialty. The implementation of the federal end-stage renal failure program in 1973 greatly expanded the opportunities for practicing nephrologists and for training programs.

Nephrology in the 1980s

The subspecialty of nephrology today comprises two segments: academicians, many of old lineage and prestige; and an army of private practitioners, many of whom are the former trainees of the academicians. Ironically, how these numerous new private practitioners spend their days has relatively little to do with renal tubular acidosis, Bartter's Syndrome, or other such intriguing puzzles of which they heard so much in fellowship. Indeed these practitioners mainly look after Bright's Disease—Bright's Disease arrived at its burnt-out form, when better labels matter little. That is, they attend the approximately 80,000 end-stage renal failure patients receiving dialytic care in the United States through the federal and state programs. This activity accounts for about 60 to 70 percent of their working time. Acute renal failure remains the second most frequent problem nephrologists in private practice treat, but consultations for acid-base or electrolyte problems consume far less than 10 percent of their time.[66]

At the other extreme, the traditional renal investigator at a medical school passes many hours at the bench, working with micropipettes, Ussing chambers, hydrogen electrodes, or more recently, with assays for prostaglandins, leukotrienes, or atrial natriuretic factor. Perhaps for two or three months this nephrologist emerges from the laboratory to perform teaching rounds, during which most emphasis might be placed on pathophysiology. He or she may only occasionally enter the dialysis unit.

Both of these subspecies of subspecialist deal frequently with acute renal failure, and both will usually perform biopsies for cases of nephrotic syndrome. Both remain familiar with the causes and natural history of chronic renal failure, stay alert to new ideas, such as the currently popular "hyperfiltration" hypothesis, and seek the welfare of patients with acute and chronic renal disease. Both will very likely hold nephrology boards and membership in the American Society of Nephrology, although some private practitioners rarely attend the annual meeting.

Summary and Conclusions: Nephrology and the History of Internal Medicine

The history of nephrology, both as a body of esoteric knowledge and as a subspecialty, has retraced in microcosm the recent history of what has come to be known as internal medicine. This history reveals increasingly refined science and increasingly specialized and subspecialized practice: a pathway from the general and the broad, to the highly defined and the restricted. Bright's Disease was born in the classic period of whole-organ correlative pathology; the patient's symptoms were assigned to a visible category of lesion ("granulated kidney") seen after death through autopsy. This pathology base and the simple unity of Bright's Disease may be said to have retained at least some vigor from Bright to Henry Christian. Within this period and tradition the physicians studying renal disease would have pointedly denied the label "specialist." Both kidney disease and those doctors taking an interest in it formed parts of a larger general community of knowledge and practice.

American academic physicians in the early twentieth century shared the growing fervor for "functional diagnosis" and physiological exploration of disease, products mainly of German medicine of the late nineteenth century. The kidney lent itself to chemical investigation, and American practitioners studying renal disorders were helpfully joined by members of new professional disciplines—trained chemists and physiologists such as Otto Folin, Lawrence J. Henderson, Donald D. Van Slyke, and Homer W. Smith. Such collaboration proved unusually fruitful and amiable among students of the kidney. An immense growth in knowledge of renal physiology and body fluids resulted. More recently, expanding understanding of immunology has invigorated the investigation of glomerulonephritis.

Assembled before World War II by metabolic-physiology workers such as John P. Peters and James Gamble, an ordered knowledge of extracellular fluid balance was crucial for the development of clinical dialysis. But this technique entered American nephrology largely from outside of its existing centers, and in fact, largely from outside the country. With the successful refinement of hemodialysis, nephrology in the decades after World War II in the United States spawned a practice wing fully in step with the "procedure-based" internal medicine that began to dominate cardiology and gastroenterology. Renal biopsy played a similar but smaller role in this genesis. Medical school renal divisions, although training both future academicians and practitioners, mainly continued to nurture and champion physiology and pathophysiological investigation. Boards, a society, and a shared knowledge base permitted the now bipartite discipline of nephrology to add itself to the list of internal medicine subspecialties of the 1970s and 1980s.

Intellectual, ideologic, and financial considerations all influence the way in which a contemporary nephrologist sees himself or herself within the discipline. Certainly not all locate readily at one of the poles emphasized in this review, academics/physiology or practice/dialysis. These individual considerations and national trends in American medicine will shape the future of nephrology. Possibly the next decade will show whether the specialty will experience further subdivision, gradual dominance by the ranks of dialysis practitioners, or, one may hope, a salutary solidification with new forms of collaboration, generating fresh knowledge and unforeseen therapies helpful to all persons with Bright's Disease and its successors.

I am grateful to George Schreiner for his generous willingness to discuss the earlier years of clinical nephrology. Nancy Taylor of the National Center of the American Heart Association discovered and provided important primary materials. All opinions and interpretations in this chapter are, however, my responsibility.

NOTES

1. The author reviewed directories from the 1930s until the present. Before the mid-1960s, internists with strong association with renal disease or physiology identified their area usually as "metabolic diseases."

2. Paul Beeson, "The Natural History of Medical Subspecialties," *Ann Intern Med* 93 (1980): 624–26.

3. For the work of Bright and his colleagues, see Steven J. Peitzman, "Bright's Disease and Bright's Generation—Toward Exact Medicine at Guy's Hospital," *Bull Hist Med* 55 (1981): 307–21; Lester King, "Richard Bright," in *Dictionary of Scientific Biography*, Charles Gillispie, ed. (New York: Scribners, 1981) (hereafter referred to as *DSB*), vol. 2, 463–65; Noel G. Coley, "George Owen Rees, M.D.,

F.R.S. (1813–89): Pioneer of Medical Chemistry," *Med Hist* 30 (1986): 173–90. Pamela Bright's *Dr. Richard Bright, 1789–1885* (London: The Bodley Head, 1984) gives details of Bright's family life but is weak on his medical and pathological accomplishments. Important primary sources include Bright's magnificent *Reports of Medical Cases* (London: Longman, 1827–31) and "Cases and Observations Illustrative of Renal Disease Accompanied with the Secretion of Albuminous Urine," *Guy's Hosp Rep* 1 (1836): 338–79; and George H. Barlow, "Account of Observations Made Under the Superintendence of Dr. Bright on Patients Whose Urine Was Albuminous, with a Chemical Analysis of the Blood and Secretions by G. O. Rees, M.D." *Guy's Hosp Rep* ser. II, 1 (1843): 189–330.

4. A. McGehee Harvey and Victor McKusick, eds., *Osler's Textbook Revisited* (New York: Appleton-Century-Crofts, 1967), 246–62. This is a volume of excerpted chapters from Osler's 1909 edition, with commentary by recent authorities.

5. By maintaining the notion that acute nephritis is caused most often by a chill, Osler reaches back, through Bright, to Galen and the ancient theory of suppressed perspiration and sympathy—in his 1909 edition!

6. Robert D. Grove and Alice M. Hetzel, *Vital Statistic Rates in the United States 1940–1960* (Washington: National Center for Health Statistics, 1968), 79, 82.

7. For the work of Christian, see A. McGehee Harvey, *Science at the Bedside: Clinical Research in American Medicine, 1905–1945* (Baltimore: Johns Hopkins University Press, 1981), 260–61 and Henry Christian, "Some Phases of the Nephritis Problem," *Harvey Lectures* 11 (1915–16):303–25.

8. For the life and work of Longcope, see Harvey, *Science at the Bedside*, 172–74, 192–94, 642–63 (lists his major publications); idem, "Science at the Bedside: the Story of Warfield Theobald Longcope," *Trans Stud Coll Physicians Phila* 3 (1981):161–73; W. Longcope, "The Pathogenesis of Glomerular Nephritis," *Bull J Hopkins Hosp* 45 (1929):335–60.

9. See Knud Faber, *Nosography in Internal Medicine* (New York: Paul Hoeber, 1923), 112–71 and Harvey, *Science at the Bedside*, 18–30.

10. The quote is from Folin's Mellon Lecture, "Recent Biochemical Investigations on Blood and Urine: Their Bearing on Clinical and Experimental Medicine" (Pittsburgh: University of Pittsburgh, 1917). The importance of Folin's colorometric micromethods in opening up immense possibilities in clinical medicine and in research of all types has been scarcely appreciated in historical writing. For brief reviews of Folin's life and work, see the article by Henry Leicester in *DSB*, vol. 5, 53 and Samuel Meites, "Otto Folin's Medical Legacy," *Clin Chem* 31 (1985):1402–4. I refer to Folin as an American biochemist, although he was born in Sweden.

11. For Van Slyke's work at the Rockefeller Institute, see his oral history memoir, conducted by Peter Olch, 27–28 May 1969, the transcript of which is on file at the National Library of Medicine and at the Rockefeller University Archives; D. Van Slyke, "Acceptance of the Kober Medal Award," *Trans Assoc Am Physicians* 57 (1942):42–43; idem, "Studies of Normal and Pathological Physiology of the Kidney," the thirtieth Mellon Lecture (Pittsburgh: University of Pittsburgh, 1947); George W. Corner, *A History of the Rockefeller Institute* (New York: Rockefeller Institute Press, 1964), 276–77; and the article by John Parascandola in *DSB*, vol. 14, 574–75.

12. For a synopsis of the work of Henderson, see the article by John Parascandola in *DSB*, vol. 6, 260–62.

13. Van Slyke oral history memoir, 25.

14. Van Slyke oral history memoir, 55. Tom Rivers supported this claim of the usually modest Van Slyke: "Although Van Slyke was a Ph.D. he had charge of all the kidney cases in the hospital, and over the years I must say that he was a better physician as far as handling of nephritis and nephrosis was concerned than most M.D.'s. . . . As far as I am concerned, no one in the United States has done as much as Donald Van Slyke to unravel the riddles regarding the physiology and diseases of the kidney." Saul Benison, *Tom Rivers: Reflections on a Life in Medicine and Science, An Oral History Memoir* (Cambridge, MA: The M.I.T. Press, 1967), 199–200.

15. Donald Van Slyke, Edgar Stillman, et al., "Observations on the Courses of Different Types of Bright's Disease and on the Resultant Changes in Renal Anatomy," *Medicine* 9 (1930):257–392. "Clearance" is not an actual observable function of the kidney, such as filtration, reabsorption, or concentration, but rather is a conceptual term applicable to any excretory organ. It designates the rate of excretion of a given substance in relation to the concentration of that substance in the blood. The idea of renal clearance grew incrementally. Addis' "urea ratio" was really the urea clearance, but the latter term is credited to Van Slyke. Addis and Van Slyke both arrived at the ratio or clearance in their search for an empirical laboratory indicator of functioning renal mass. Later, Homer W. Smith took "clearance" from the clinic to the physiology department. By finding suitable substances, he used the idea of clearance to measure "real" physiologic variables of the kidneys, such as plasma flow, maximal secretion, and, most importantly, glomerular filtration rate. But the clinical notion of clearance, or the earlier urea ratio, was empiric, and presupposed no reductionist knowledge of how the kidney actually "cleared" urea. For a brief discussion of the generation of clearance as a conceptual tool, see Harvey, *Science at the Bedside*, 522–23. See also the references cited with the discussion of Addis in this paper; to understand why some sort of ratio is suitable, rather than the simple excretory rate (substance appearing in the urine per unit time), see the first three chapters of Addis' *Glomerular Nephritis: Diagnosis and Treatment* (New York: Macmillan, 1948). For a recent review of the use of clearance measurement in contemporary renal research, see Thomas Maack, "Renal Clearance and Isolated Kidney Perfusion Techniques," *Kidney International* 30 (1986): 142–51.

16. For biographical information on Peters, see Donald D. Van Slyke, "John P. Peters," *Clin Chem* 3 (1957):287–93 and Paul H. Lavietes, "John Punnett Peters: An Appreciation," *Yale J Biol Med* 29 (1957):175–90 (contains a bibliography of Peters' publications).

17. John P. Peters and Donald D. Van Slyke, *Quantitative Clinical Chemistry*, 2 vols. (Baltimore: Williams & Wilkins, 1931–32).

18. Another landmark publication was Peters' *Body Water: The Exchange of Fluids in Man* (Springfield, IL: Charles C. Thomas, 1935).

19. Peters supported national health insurance, improved relations with the Soviet Union, and other progressive causes. He was active in the Physicians' Forum. By 1949 his membership in the endocrinology study section of the NIH was challenged by the Loyalty Review Board of the US Civil Service Commission. In 1953 his appointment was terminated because of alleged disloyalty to the government of the United States. "At great physical and emotional cost," according to Lavietes, Peters carried the case to the Supreme Court, hoping to set a precedent for freedom of speech. The Court did rule in Peters' favor, but the ruling was based on a technicality, and did not fulfill Peters' hope for a repudiation of anonymous ac-

cusations. A large collection of Peters' papers at the Yale University Library documents his social and political activities and beliefs.

20. Donald Van Slyke to Rufus Cole, 9 July 1930, in Cole Papers, Library of the American Philosophical Society, Philadelphia, PA (hereafter APS).

21. Thomas Addis to Cole, 19 January 1930, Cole Papers, APS.

22. See Thomas Addis, "The Renal Lesion in Bright's Disease," *Harvey Lectures* 23 (1927–28):222–50; idem, "The Rate of Urea Excretion," *J Biol Chem* 24 (1916):203–20; and the first three chapters of Addis' *Glomerular Nephritis.*

23. See Addis, "Renal Lesion." A fuller treatment in collaboration with pathologist Jean Oliver is the handsome monograph also titled *The Renal Lesion in Bright's Disease* (New York: Paul Hoeber, 1931). It appeared almost at the same time as Van Slyke's similar treatise in the 1930 volume of *Medicine* (note 15). One cannot resist designating these two major contributions in the clinical-pathological-chemical correlation of Bright's Disease as the twentieth-century continuation of Bright's similar work conducted exactly one hundred years earlier. In some ways these were the last such heroic works in that tradition: clinical and chemical derangements recorded during life, the morphologic renal lesion revealed at necropsy.

24. Addis saw the main "work" of the kidney as nitrogen (urea) excretion and knew that in animals renal weight and creatinine clearance increase with the amount of protein in the diet. Thus he urged low-protein diets to provide renal "rest" for his nephritic patients. Recently Barry Brenner, of the Harvard Medical School, and others have rediscovered some of this earlier work, and related work of others. Based on their own new observations in the clinic and the laboratory, they have elaborated a synthetic hypothesis for the progression of chronic renal failure. It is based on the belief that hyperfiltration in remaining functioning nephrons of a diseased kidney will eventually destroy such nephrons. Renal blood flow and filtration pressures rise with increased dietary protein load. See Barry Brenner, Timothy Meyer, and Thomas Hostetter, "Dietary Protein Intake and the Progressive Nature of Renal Disease," *N Engl J Med* 307 (1982):652–59.

25. For the life and work of Smith, see the article by William Bynum in *DSB,* vol. 12, 470–71; Herbert Chasis and William Goldring, eds., *Homer William Smith, Sc.D.: His Scientific and Literary Achievements* (New York: New York University Press, 1965); and Herbert Chasis, "History of Collaboration by Department of Physiology at New York University School of Medicine," *The Physiologist* 26 (1983):64–70.

26. Homer W. Smith, "Unilateral Nephrectomy in Hypertensive Disease," *J Urol* 76 (1956):685–701; idem, "Salt and Water Volume Receptors: An Exercise in Physiologic Apologetics," *Am J Med* 23 (1957):623–52. A full bibliography of Smith's physiologic, medical, philosophical, and historical writings forms appendix A of Chasis and Goldring, *Homer W. Smith.*

27. A partial list of Smith's fellows and associates is appendix D of Chasis and Goldring, *Homer W. Smith.*

28. See David Cooper, "Alfred N. Richards and the Discovery of the Mechanism of Urine Formation," *Trans Stud Coll Physicians Phila* 6 (1984):63–73; Carl Gottschalk, "Dr. A. N. Richards and Kidney Micropuncture," *Ann Intern Med* 71 (1969):28–37; and Harvey, *Science at the Bedside,* 211–14, 472–73.

29. Alfred Newton Richards, *Methods and Results of Direct Investigations of the Function of the Kidney: The Beaumont Foundation Lectures* (Baltimore: Williams & Wilkins, 1929).

30. Proposal to Commonwealth Fund by Alfred Newton Richards, 16 January

1931, typescript copy in Richards Papers, Archives of the University of Pennsylvania, Philadelphia, 12.

31. Commonwealth Fund, *Thirteenth Annual Report*, 1931, 58–59. The grant was renewed generously in 1934 and again in 1937. Subsequently, the Commonwealth Fund expanded its support of renal research to other centers.

32. "Second Annual Progress Report of Investigation of the Function of the Kidney at the University of Pennsylvania, 1932" typescript, Richards Papers, Archives of the University of Pennsylvania.

33. See article about Henderson by John Parascandola in *DSB*, vol. 6, 260–62.

34. Addis was perhaps the most "clinical" of these, and in his later writings self-consciously dwelled on "doctoring" and the needs of plain doctors, while he wrote almost apologetically about his scientific work (see his *Glomerular Nephritis*). But, as pointed out earlier in this essay, his lasting influence and ability to generate a succession of leaders in nephrology seem to have been less than the others discussed.

35. Declining Rufus Cole's offer of a permanent position at the Rockefeller Institute, Addis in 1930 wrote: "And then, of course, here I am kept anxious all the time about money, and though it never yet has happened, I may at any time be forced to stop my work for lack of funds. You see the school really is hard up and though they do the best they can for the laboratory they really can't keep it going" (Addis to Cole, 19 January 1930, Cole Papers, APS). As noted earlier, he elected to stick it out at Stanford. The following year, reading of the Commonwealth Fund's large grant to A. N. Richards, Addis wrote to the Philadelphian: "I am hard up. I get $3000.00 a year from the University and have to beg for $5000.00 a year from various funds and individuals. And this year it is harder than ever and I am growing tired of asking committees and writing long letters about 'plans and purposes'" (Addis to Richards, 30 September 1931, Richards Papers, University of Pennsylvania Archives). Addis goes on to ask Richards for help to support Addis' work on compensatory renal hypertrophy. By the time these pathetic letters were written, Addis was already widely published and was indeed among the leading authorities on the kidney and its diseases. I again suggest that his lack of foundation support may have retarded Addis' ability to develop his laboratory and clinic into a "program" and training center (should he have wished to do so, which I believe doubtful). Thus the more physiologically and "metabolically" oriented Peters and Smith seeded the future field of academic nephrology more widely than Addis—the doctor who did his own chemistry and gazed carefully at urine sediments.

36. In addition to letters already cited there are letters between Richards and Smith in the Richards Papers (University of Pennsylvania Archives) from 1935 through 1937, mostly dealing with inulin methods; between Van Slyke and Richards in the Richards papers; between Van Slyke and Peters, and Richards and Peters, in the John P. Peters Papers, Yale University Library. I have not found any large collections of correspondence of Homer Smith or Donald Van Slyke. While the content of those letters I have discovered is sometimes trivial, casual closing comments often refer to visits and the pleasure gained from them.

37. Smith to Richards, 16 March 1935; James A. Shannon (a co-worker of Smith) to Richards, 3 April 1935; and Richards to Shannon 5 April 1935 (all in Richards Papers, University of Pennsylvania Archives). The scientists hoped the exchange could work out certain differences concerning the relationship between measurement of creatinine clearance and inulin clearance, as indicators of glomerular filtration rate.

38. Russell L. Cecil, *A Textbook of Medicine by American Authors,* ed. 5, (Philadelphia: W. B. Saunders, 1941).

39. Claus Brun, *Acute Anuria: A Study Based on Renal Function Tests and Aspiration Biopsy of the Kidney* (Copenhagen: Munksgaard, 1954), 15–32.

40. Eric Bywaters and D. Beall, "Crush Injuries with Impairment of Renal Function," *Med J* 1 (1941):427–32.

41. Balduin Lucké, "Lower Nephron Nephrosis," *Milit Surgeon* 99 (1946): 371–96.

42. Although acute renal failure (ARF) was "discovered" in the early 1940s, a publishing lag phase is predictably evident. Together the *Annals of Internal Medicine* and *Archives of Internal Medicine* published during 1945–47 only three papers dealing in some way with ARF; but from 1948 through 1951, sixteen such papers may be found (author's review of contents). Monographs also showed a lag, appearing in the early 1950s. These included: Roy C. Swan and John P. Merrill, "The Clinical Course of Acute Renal Failure," *Medicine* 32 (1953):215–92; John T. MacLean, *Acute Renal Failure Including the Use of the Artificial Kidney* (Springfield, IL: Charles C. Thomas, 1952); Claus Brun, *Acute Anuria,* 1953; Arthur Grollman, *Acute Renal Failure* (Springfield, IL: Charles C. Thomas, 1954); and John P. Merrill, *The Treatment of Renal Failure* (New York: Grune and Stratton, 1955).

43. See Robert M. Kark, "The Nephrotic Syndrome, Renal Biopsy, and the Modern Era," in *Nephrotic Syndrome,* John S. Cameron and Richard Glassock, eds. (Marcel Dekker, forthcoming); Poul Iverson and Claus Brun, "Aspiration Biopsy of the Kidney," *Am J Med* 11 (1951):324–30; and Claus Brun, *Acute Anuria.*

44. Alvin E. Parrish and John Howe, "Kidney Biopsy: A Review of One Hundred Successful Needle Biopsies," *Arch Intern Med* 96 (1955):712–16.

45. These papers have appeared mostly in the *New England Journal of Medicine, Annals of Internal Medicine, Journal of Clinical Investigation,* and *Medicine;* a bibliography is found in Kark, "The Nephrotic Syndrome."

46. Kark, "The Nephrotic Syndrome."

47. For a recent review of the current categorization of nephrotic syndrome based on renal biopsy, see Keith E. Holley, James V. Donadio, Richard D. Wagoner, et al., "Renal Biopsy in the Adult Nephrotic Syndrome," *Semin Nephrol* 5 (1985):274–93.

48. There is as yet no book-length history of dialysis. For a brief overview see Patrick McBride, "The Development of Hemodialysis and Peritoneal Dialysis," in *Clinical Dialysis,* Allen Nissenson, Richard N. Fine, and Dominick E. Gentile, eds. (Norwalk, CT: Appleton-Century-Crofts, 1985), 1–22. For its early clinical history see Willem Kolff, "First Clinical Experience with the Artificial Kidney," *Ann Intern Med* 62 (1965):608–19; George Schreiner, "Personalized History of Artificial Organ Development," *Trans Am Soc Artif Intern Organs* 30 (1984):1–10; John P. Merrill, "Early Days of the Artificial Kidney and Transplantation," *Transplant Proc* 13 (1981) (Suppl. 1):4–8. The first important monograph in English was certainly the little paperback volume of Willem Kolff, *New Ways of Treating Uremia* (London: Churchill, 1946), now a scarce classic.

49. John P. Merrill, "The Artificial Kidney," *N Engl J Med* 246 (1952):17–27.

50. Wayne Quinton, David Dillard, and Belding Scribner, "Cannulation of Blood Vessels for Prolonged Hemodialysis," *Trans Am Soc Artif Intern Organs* 6 (1960):104–13; Belding Scribner, et al., "The Treatment of Chronic Uremia by Means of Intermittent Hemodialysis: A Preliminary Report," *Trans Am Soc Artif*

Intern Organs 6 (1960):114–22. Scribner's group in Seattle developed the first outpatient dialysis "center" and also undertook to train patients to perform their treatments at home. An account of the many difficulties and perplexing questions accompanying these unprecedented efforts may be found in Renée C. Fox and Judith P. Swazey, *The Courage to Fail,* ed. 2 (Chicago: University of Chicago Press, 1978), 201–25.

51. Department of Health, Education, and Welfare, Regional Program Service, Kidney Disease Control Program, and the National Kidney Foundation, *Kidney Disease Services, Facilities and Programs in the United States,* rev. 2 (Rockville, MD and New York City: 1971).

52. For a brief account of PL92-603, see Fox and Swazey, *Courage to Fail,* 345–75. I have chosen not to investigate the detailed history of the complex and politically tumultuous events leading up to the passage of this landmark legislation. Never before had Congress singled out one disease for a program of nearly universal support of a "halfway" technique for a large number of patients. Estimates over the years have consistently failed to predict the expanding number of end-stage renal failure patients and the cost of the program.

53. The National Institute for Arthritis, Diabetes and Digestive and Kidney Diseases and its predecessors showed a quadrupling of grant support, from about 46 million to 167 million dollars from 1960 to 1973. See National Institutes of Health, *1984 NIH Almanac* (Rockville, MD: Department of Health and Human Services, 1984), 129–49.

54. Skeggs constructed his first "breadboard" model in 1951; it measured blood or serum urea. Several subsequent models built by Skeggs were used by him in clinical laboratories in Cleveland. He signed a contract with Technicon in 1954 and saw the first production models appear in 1957. See Leonard T. Skeggs, "A Brief Summary of the Early Development of the Autoanalyzer," typescript dated 20 June 1984, deposited with artifacts by Dr. Skeggs at the Medical Sciences Division, National Museum of American History, Smithsonian Institutions, Washington, D.C.; idem, "New Dimensions in Medical Diagnosis," *Anal Chem* 38 (1966):31A–44A; idem, "An Automatic Method for Colorimetric Analysis," *Am J Clin Pathol* 28 (1957):311–22; Walton H. Marsh, *Automation in Clinical Chemistry* (Springfield, IL: Charles C. Thomas, 1963), 3–12; Leon A. Lewis, "Leonard Tucker Skeggs—a Multifaceted Diamond," *Clin Chem* 27 (1981):1465–68.

55. In an interesting paper Stan N. Finkelstein challenges the assumption that increased automation in the clinical laboratory increased the volume of tests ordered by physicians. His survey of test use over an eight-year period showed "no definitive correlation between technological change and growth in volume of well-established clinical laboratory tests" ("Technological Change and Clinical Laboratory Utilization," *Medical Care* 18 [1980]:1048–56). Even if Finkelstein's conclusion is valid, it is still striking that his survey of the years 1970–77 showed that serum sodium, potassium, chloride, urea, and carbon dioxide were five of the six tests showing the greatest volume increase (the other was cholesterol). This may well reflect at least in part their "linkage" in the multichannel autoanalyzer, so that a physician mainly interested in, say, urea might obtain the full "panel" and discover an unsuspected electrolyte or acid-base abnormality. It is, of course, possible that an increased interest in such disorders among the medical profession drove the increasing requests for serum electrolyte surveys. Still, all present-day internists and medical residents will admit the frequency with which abnormalities in a multichannel analysis appear as surprises, the test having been ordered as an admission

"routine" or for some purpose unrelated to the unsuspected derangement that was found.

56. The "anion gap" is the difference of the serum sodium and the sum of the chloride and bicarbonate (or total carbon dioxide). The gap reveals the presence of an "unmeasured" anion, usually that of a strong acid present in excess. Most often, then, the elevated anion gap—also called a "delta"—indicates metabolic acidosis.

57. James Lawder Gamble (1883–1959) was a physician and pediatrician at Johns Hopkins and Harvard. He was influenced early in his training by Henderson. He became one of the major contributors to the understanding of the relationships of water and mineral distribution within the body's "compartments." He devised clear graphic displays of his data and concepts, later called "Gamblegrams." See Harvey, *Science at the Bedside,* 163–65. Gamble is one of many important contributors not discussed in this essay because of the usual need for at least some restraint on length.

58. The skeptical reader will be aware of dwindling documentation amidst these last paragraphs, a sort of oliguria of footnote flow. Obviously the statements made cannot be secured by the usual citation of printed sources. Many of the conclusions emerge from the author's experience in academic nephrology and his conversations with both senior and junior nephrologists and with nephrology fellows from programs in several cities. But the emergence of a sometimes disquieting craft-versus-science dichotomy within nephrology should not surprise the student of medical specialties. Other examples are found in this volume.

59. For a brief historical account of the ASAIO see Peter F. Salisbury, "History: The American Society for Artificial Internal Organs," *Trans Am Soc Artif Intern Organs* 6 (1960):ii–vi.

60. For my sources concerning the early history of the Renal Section, I am indebted to Nancy Taylor of the American Heart Association National Center in Dallas, Texas, for supplying me with copies of typescripts of "Brief Review of History of Renal Section," 1967; "Rules of Incorporation of Renal Section," 19 April 1963; and various minutes of the executive committees of the Renal Section from 1961 to 1970.

61. Minutes, Executive Committee of the Renal Section, 18 January 1964, 30 September 1966, 27 February 1967, 16 June 1967, and 8 September 1967, provided by American Heart Association, National Center, Dallas.

62. The minutes of the 18 January 1964 meeting of the Executive Committee of the Renal Section refer to "discussion of the informal proposal made at the recent NKDF (National Kidney Disease Foundation) meeting that consideration be given to the formation of an American Renal Disease Society." The Renal Section moved its opposition to such a "separate American Nephrological Society." I am excluding from my account organizations which existed largely for purposes of public service or fund-raising, such as the National Kidney Foundation and its predecessors, although some renal physicians were of course active in these.

63. My main source for the founding of the ASN is: Minutes of Meeting, Founders Committee, American Society of Nephrology, 26 June 1966 (copy of typescript provided by American Heart Association, National Center, Dallas). The figure for Americans registering for the ISN Congress is from these minutes. The ASN maintains no archives and has not appointed a historian.

64. Data on ASN membership and meeting attendance were provided by its National Office, Thorofare, NJ.

65. Data supplied by American Board of Internal Medicine, Philadelphia, PA. I thank its Vice-president for Evaluation and Research, George D. Webster, MD, for his help.

66. These figures are derived from a survey of nephrologists in private practice in the Philadelphia area which I conducted while preparing this paper. I found a surprising uniformity in the self-reported estimates of percent of time devoted to chronic renal failure care, acute renal failure, renal biopsy and nephrotic syndrome, and acid-base or electrolyte consultation.

8

Hearts and Minds: The Invention and Transformation of American Cardiology

JOEL D. HOWELL

Today, the heart is usually considered the central organ of the body. American physicians diagnose diseases of the heart as the cause of death more often than they diagnose diseases of any other organ. Moreover, the heart can be easily studied by a wide variety of scientific technologies and sophisticated tools. It hardly appears surprising that late twentieth-century American cardiology is the largest and most powerful subspecialty within the specialty of internal medicine.[1]

To write the history of American cardiology might seem, at first glance, a relatively straightforward task of chronicling advances in the field. However, such a perspective, although it makes sense in the late 1980s, may be misleading when used to analyze other historical periods. For both the term "cardiology" and the concept of specialization have had different meanings at different times. Merely to summarize the scientific and technologic history of what we now define as cardiology would be arbitrary at best, superficial at worst, and ultimately, from a historical point of view, not particularly interesting.

Instead, I shall examine in this chapter how Americans, primarily physicians, have conceptualized the specialty of cardiology during the twentieth century. I shall discuss how the definition of cardiology has changed, from public health to physiology, from model clinics to molecular biology. Physicians have institutionalized various definitions of cardiology by forming organizations, publishing journals, and awarding certificates of specialization. But at the same time, those physicians have had to negotiate relationships with other interest groups, both medical and nonmedical. The word "cardiology" has no meaning save its definition within a web of organizations, relationships, and ideas. That definition has changed, and has been shaped by social and historical events. The transformation of the definition of cardiology is the subject of this chapter.[2]

Tuberculosis and Heart Disease: The Conception and Birth of the American Heart Association

The most useful way to identify medical specialty formation is probably through the formation of specialized societies. By the act of forming such organizations, physicians indicated their desire to separate themselves based on a goal, technique, or body of knowledge. By analyzing how and why physicians formed specialty societies, historians can gain insight into how people at that time defined the meaning of the specialty.

Although we now think of cardiology in terms of physiology and the natural sciences, the formation of the first national society devoted to heart disease, the American Heart Association (AHA), must be understood within the context of early twentieth-century voluntary health societies.[3] Voluntary health societies were founded on two basic concepts: that education could improve public health and that the physician—by seeing individual patients—could be an effective force in disease prevention.[4] On the basis of these ideas, several national health societies were formed early in the century. The first, founded in 1904, was the National Association for the Study and Prevention of Tuberculosis, which was renamed the National Tuberculosis Association in 1918. It was soon followed by, among others, the National Committee for Mental Hygiene and the American Association for the Study and Prevention of Infant Mortality in 1909, the American Federation for Sex Hygiene in 1910, the American Society for the Control of Cancer in 1913, and the American Social Hygiene Association in 1914.[5] The antituberculosis movement, having achieved the greatest visibility, served as the model for many that followed. Some have argued that its success was based not on any particular success in combating disease, but more on an affinity with Progressive era desires to use social control to improve public health.[6]

Whatever the reason, the number of tuberculosis clinics where individual patients could be educated and examined by a physician rose from twenty in 1905 to more than 500 in 1915.[7]

Like other voluntary societies of the day, and unlike most present-day scientific societies, early cardiac societies emphasized the importance of social work. A social worker at Bellevue Hospital described the situation in 1911: "scores of cardiacs discharged from the wards were referred to Social Service for convalescent care and for assistance in finding suitable employment. This we could do, but continued medical oversight was obtainable only in the day clinics, and day clinics and jobs were incompatible."[8] In 1915 there were four cardiac clinics in New York City; a year later there were twenty-four. Eight, including the Bellevue Clinic, held evening sessions, which working class patients could attend.[9] The New York-based Association for the Prevention and Relief of Heart Disease was founded in 1916.[10] By 1921 there were thirty-one cardiac clinics in New York City, fourteen for children and seventeen for adults, altogether following over 4,500 patients. The movement had spread beyond New York, and there were at least twenty-eight clinics in other cities as well.[11]

Many of the members of the New York Association for the Prevention and Relief of Heart Disease gathered in St. Louis at the 1922 annual meeting of the American Medical Association. There forty-one prominent physicians decided to form an organization "of continental scope," to "develop sound public opinion as to the true meaning and seriousness of the problem."[12] That new organization, the AHA, was formally incorporated in 1924. The antituberculosis movement served explicitly as a conceptual and organizational model. In one of its early publications, the Association outlined how it perceived the similarities between tuberculosis and cardiac disease (*Figure 8.1*).[13] The outline listed four categories in which tuberculosis and heart disease were seen as similar: Medical Aspects, Social Aspects, Public Education, and Equipment and Facilities. Consistent with the public health movement, the outline emphasized social approaches to the disease, such as improving economic conditions, utilizing publicity channels, and training the public in health habits. The AHA also promoted the creation of weekend and evening clinics for working class cardiac patients.[14] Lists of new clinics are found throughout early numbers of the *American Heart Association Bulletin*, many of them designated as an "Industrial Cardiac Clinic" or as one for children.[15]

Although it emphasized issues of public concern, the AHA of the 1920s and 1930s was controlled by physicians, not lay people. In 1923, in response

Similarity of Tuberculosis and Heart Disease

The following outline shows some of the parallels that may be drawn between tuberculosis and heart disease. This outline should prove of interest to those who are considering the organization of cardiac work with the cooperation of tuberculosis associations.

TUBERCULOSIS	HEART DISEASE
Medical Aspects	*Medical Aspects*
1. Communicable disease	1. Ditto (Rheumatic & Syphilitic)
2. Involves childhood chiefly	2. Ditto (Rheumatic & Congenital)
3. Chronic infection	3. Ditto
4. May become active	4. Exacerbations occur
5. Handicaps physical efficiency	5. Ditto
6. Treatment chiefly hygienic with emphasis on rest	6. Ditto (except for Syphilitic)
Social Aspects	*Social Aspects*
1. Influenced profoundly by economic conditions	1. Probably influenced by economic conditions
2. Requires guidance of P.H. nurse and social worker	2. Ditto
3. Handicaps but does not necessarily destroy efficiency	3. Ditto
4. Usual methods of quarantine useless	4. Ditto
5. Control of carrier through hospitalization and education important	5. Ditto (communicable types)
Public Education	*Public Education*
1. Accomplished through all publicity channels reaching individuals, home, school	1. Ditto
2. Channels of reaching people well developed	2. Channels not yet developed
3. Training in health habits important	3. Ditto
4. Both knowledge and motivation necessary	4. Ditto
Equipment and Facilities	*Equipment and Facilities*
1. Sanatoria necessary and well developed	1. No Sanatoria. Heart cases need similar facilities
2. Preventoria growing in popularity	2. Preventoria needed but not now generally available
3. Preventorium class rooms being established	3. Heart cases would profit by similar equipment
4. Health camps, especially when regarded as training camps, are valuable and popular	4. Similar opportunities valuable for heart cases
5. Tuberculosis clinics universally accepted	5. Chest clinics easily care for tuberculosis and heart cases

Figure 8.1. Outline article from Bulletin of the American Heart Association *2(1927):22.*

to fears expressed by the Chicago Medical Society about "some form of state medicine," the Chicago Association for the Prevention and Relief of Heart Disease changed its bylaws so that the majority of the Board of Governors would always be physicians.[16] The tension between lay and physician participation extended into debates over how clinics should be operated and what information should be gathered. For example, the early AHA collected statistical data on patients with heart disease, distributing detailed charts for data collection. Some medical observers objected that "a form of record like this is more complicated and requires greater expenditure of time and labor than is at the disposal of physicians in the clinics at the present time."[17] According to the AHA, however, this criticism merely indicated that the clinic was poorly run, failing to use secretarial and volunteer staffs adequately. In order to share what it had learned about organizing care, the AHA published a set of guidelines for running cardiac clinics.[18] These documents set forth minimum requirements and outlined what an ideal clinic would be like in seven different respects: (1) medical organization, (2) social service, (3) space, equipment and facilities, (4) records, (5) admission and distribution of patients, (6) standards for physical examination, and (7) standards for treatment.

Many AHA forms were designed to be filled out by nonphysicians. Because the data were obtained for use in public health research, traditional diagnostic information such as findings on percussion and auscultation was not included. This shift did not go unquestioned, and some criticized the AHA's records for failing to portray an accurate clinical picture of the patient.[19] However, the AHA's detailed attention to standardization of clinics and their record keeping was very much in line with Progressive ideology.

These detailed records helped to draw attention to the growing importance of chronic disease, a problem caused by both tuberculosis and heart disease. Although tuberculosis had a single etiology, heart disease could by the 1920s be separated into two groups. The first type was acute heart disease, common in those less than forty years of age and caused by a variety of agents. Some were understood to be infectious, others—such as "rheumatism"—had etiologies not yet determined. The second type of heart disease, typically found in patients older than forty years of age, was chronic heart disease, thought to be caused by degenerative diseases and senescence. Interestingly, despite the perceived differences in etiology, tuberculosis sanitariums and convalescent homes were still seen as the ideal model for treating chronic heart disease.[20]

One of the most striking changes in the ideology of American medicine during the early twentieth century was an increasing belief that medicine should be based largely on science.[21] Ernest Starling's bold pronouncement that "the physiology of today is the medicine of tomorrow" no doubt rang true to many of his contemporaries,[22] and physiologists made significant inroads into the newly scientific early twentieth-century American medical school. Much of their physiology was focused on the heart; much of the physiology used new medical technology, such as the electrocardiogram. However, the formation of American cardiology was based on neither natural science nor medical technology. It was based on public health, not physiology. Although some electrocardiography researchers were associated with the AHA, they saw their laboratory research as more relevant to basic science than to the AHA; a few attempted to relate laboratory science to the once popular but ill-fated concept of "experimental medicine."[23]

Journals

A characteristic feature of almost any organized medical specialty is a regular journal. Journals serve as another way to define the intellectual area of a specialty, as well as providing a place for members of that specialty to publish their own work and to read about that of others.

In 1925, only one year after its incorporation, the AHA founded the *American Heart Journal* as its official journal, a journal not only published but also financially sponsored by the C. V. Mosby Publishing House.[24] The decision to establish a separate specialty journal did not meet with unanimous approval. Alfred Cohn of the Rockefeller Institute, a distinguished physician most highly regarded for his work on the heart, commented bitterly on this decision in a letter to Canby Robinson, Professor of Medicine at Vanderbilt and editor of the *Journal of Clinical Investigation* (*JCI*). Robinson had written Cohn a letter suggesting that two manuscripts submitted to the *JCI* ought to be published in the more specialized *American Heart Journal*. Cohn replied:

> I am quite frankly opposed to the founding of journals devoted to the study of specific viscera. It seems to me that the study of heart disease from 1909 onward lost a great deal in significance on account of its divorce from the main current of clinical medicine while the study of medicine itself was deprived of proper contact with the development of knowledge in this field by publishing good things in separate journals. In a sense the tendency is created for fellows who work on heart disease to study no other journals and for the fellows who do not work on heart

disease not to study the heart journals so that an isolated specialty, lacking a good deal in meaning arose.[25]

Despite opposition by those such as Cohn, the specialty journal survived, and even prospered. Circulation of the *American Heart Journal* rapidly reached 4,000.[26]

The AHA did not content itself with a single publication. The *American Heart Journal* was a forum for scientific papers. For Association news, announcements of meetings, and other general matters, the AHA published the *American Heart Association Bulletin*, a monthly magazine of which 17,000 copies were published per month in 1932.[27] Also in 1932, the AHA started publishing its *Modern Concepts in Cardiovascular Disease*, a monthly publication designed to present discussions of cardiovascular disease that were "simple and useful and of such a type that they may be of help in ordinary general practice."[28] The AHA distributed a total of 125,000 copies of this new publication in 1932.

For its first several decades, the AHA operated on a limited budget and depended on the larger and better established National Tuberculosis Association (NTA) for office space and secretarial help.[29] The AHA moved into its own quarters in 1929 but kept its offices in the same building as the NTA until 1934. Without the NTA's financial support, the AHA might not have survived the 1930s.[30] The two voluntary organizations seriously considered a merger at least twice. In 1927 a memorandum entitled *Mutual Advantages of Amalgamation of American Heart Association and National Tuberculosis Association* concluded that "unification . . . of public health effort is the trend of the time."[31] The outline shown in Figure 1 may have been designed to encourage such a unification. For reasons that remain unclear, no merger took place. Early in the 1950s, the two organizations again seriously considered merging.[32] However, the merger again failed to occur, in part because of administrative difficulties and in part because the two groups shared few specific diseases to combat. In addition, and perhaps most importantly, the AHA's financial dependence was no longer an issue by the 1950s.

Who Is a Cardiologist? Specialization and Certification

Although it meant one thing for a physician to join a society such as the AHA, it meant something quite different for that physician to consider himself or herself a specialist. In fact, most of the AHA founders would not have wished to be considered specialists.[33] They would have agreed with Sir James Mackenzie, who wrote in the lead article for a special issue of the *New York Medical Journal,* that specialization was "an affront to the essential unity of medicine."[34] It was "almost always a hindrance to progress." Mackenzie thought that although men "devoting themselves entirely to the study of affectations of the heart" might appeal to the general public, this approach showed a "complete misconception of the principles of medical practice." Physicians trying to become cardiac specialists were attacked on not only theoretical but also economic grounds from other practitioners fearing competition.[35]

By the mid-1920s it was apparent to at least one prominent heart physician that "specialism is here and is bound to stay, if not permanently, at least for a long season."[36] In 1928 the American College of Physicians heard an address on "The Practice of Cardiology" by a prominent New York practitioner who dared to use that term.[37] Louis Bishop thought modern cardiology differed from earlier practice because it was based more on the heart's function and less on its structure.[38] He stressed that heart specialists should act not as consultants, but as physicians primarily responsible for the care of a patient with heart disease. However, the word "cardiologist" was avoided before the mid-1930s, and even then many prominent heart physicians nursed misgivings about whether specialism was wise.[39] Samuel Levine, later a prominent cardiologist at the Peter Bent Brigham Hospital, noted with "regret" that "whether we wish it or not, specialization in medicine is here." He emphasized that a cardiologist should remain well trained in general medical practice.[40]

Cardiology became formally established as a subspecialty of internal medicine in 1940, when the newly formed American Board of Internal Medicine (ABIM) voted to certify internists as subspecialists in four areas: allergy, gastroenterology, pulmonary disease, and cardiovascular disease.[41] In so doing, the ABIM, which had started to certify candidates in internal medicine only four years earlier, made a critical decision very much in keeping with Levine's feelings: candidates could be certified as cardiologists only after demonstrating expertise in the broader area of internal medicine. In 1940 there was little opposition to the Board's perspective; such a decision might provoke more debate today, however. For assistance in judging the qualifications of candidates in the area of cardiovascular disease, the ABIM asked the AHA to provide suitable examiners.

Expansion and Conflict

The AHA had hoped to provide funds for research in cardiac disease. Such support was difficult to find early in the twentieth century. Alfred Cohn was funded by the Rockefeller Institute, and occasional foundation support existed elsewhere, but at very low levels. In 1919 Fred Smith, who with James Herrick first described the characteristic electrocardiographic (ECG) changes of myocardial infarction, received $600 per year for cardiac research—research that occupied half of his time.[42] These funds came from private sources, as did almost all pre-World War II research support. But in its early decades, the AHA was not in a position to be of much help financially. From 1936 to 1944 its budget remained below $15,000 per year.[43]

Through the 1930s and 1940s, the AHA became a larger and more complex organization. In 1935 the first of several separate groups was formed within the AHA, the Council on Circulation.[44] In 1944, when physical examinations on potential military recruits during World War II revealed an appalling prevalence of rheumatic fever, the Council on Rheumatic Diseases was formed. Unfortunately, at that time the directors of the AHA had very limited resources for public health concerns.[45] The financial situation improved somewhat when the American Legion donated $50,000 in 1946. In 1947 the AHA became the beneficiary of a radio contest sponsored by Proctor and Gamble. During that contest, thousands of people tried to guess the identity of the "Walking Man," a mystery man who would walk back and forth in front of the microphone with a slow and heavy step. Each week a new clue was given and, for a $1.00 contribution to the AHA, listeners could try to guess who was filling the "Walking Man's" shoes. Before the "Walking Man" was identified as Jack Benny, more than two million letters had been received, and the AHA was $1,472,000 richer.[46]

Also in 1947 the Association was reorganized to allow lay people to be members and to serve on the Board of Directors. Not surprisingly, introducing nonphysicians into the power structure of the AHA produced some tension, particularly because a substantial sum of money was now available. This tension was stated explicitly by a prominent physician, who remarked, in reference to the Council on High Blood Pressure Research, "We are not interested in public health nursing, cardiac clinics, care of patients, or propaganda. Our sole purpose is to see that research in arteriosclerosis and hypertension is carried out."[47]

The AHA started to support research at significant levels. Through public donations it raised over $4,000,000 in 1950 and $5,500,000 in 1951. By the early 1960s the AHA was *awarding* over $10,000,000 per year[48] and funding, among other projects, early studies on replacing cardiac valves.[49] At the same time, the nonmedical membership became increasingly active in the AHA, as the AHA tried to strike a "democratic" balance between the medical and nonmedical membership.[50]

A New Society: The American College of Cardiology

When specialties enlarge, as did cardiology, not all members of a single specialty organization may feel equally well served. Some may feel that the organization's aims and goals should be changed, or they may feel that they are being personally discriminated against on a social or religious basis. Both of these factors contributed to the decision to form what has become the second major national cardiology society in the United States, the American College of Cardiology (ACC). Although the AHA and the ACC now enjoy reasonably cordial relations and board-certified cardiologists are very likely to join both societies, at one time the two groups had different goals, different members, and a different vision of what cardiology was and should be.

The ACC was composed exclusively of physicians and concerned largely with postgraduate education. It grew out of the New York Cardiological Society, a group informally constituted in 1927 and formally established in 1934 because of the perceived need for a group of physicians to spread the "technical knowledge of cardiology."[51] Those who formed this new group believed the existing societies expended too much time with the social aspects of health care for the poor and underprivileged and too little time helping to teach physicians about the technical specialty's newest features, features which had reached their most advanced stage in Germany. All members of the New York Cardiological Society were physicians; most were from New York City. Many had been forced to leave Germany in the 1930s.[52]

The New York Cardiological Society became a national society largely through the efforts of Franz Maximilian Groedel, who fled Germany for the United States in 1934 following Hitler's rise to power. When Groedel became president of the New York Cardiological Society in 1949, he worked to have the local society become a national one. The ACC was formed in 1950 and held its first national meeting in 1951. Unlike the AHA, the College was designed as a purely professional society—almost a guild—with no lay members and no salaries for officers or lecturers. It decided at the outset to emphasize postgraduate education of physicians and not to support research projects.[53]

There were tensions between the ACC and AHA. In response to formation of the ACC, the AHA in 1952 formed the Council on Clinical Cardiology, which is now responsible for the AHA's Scientific Sessions. Many of the recent European immigrants who formed the ACC found the AHA inhospitable and believed that they were denied access to positions of responsibility in the AHA.[54] Some academic cardiologists were told by their superiors not to join the ACC in the 1950s, and those who did were considered disloyal to the AHA.[55] Although there was at first little overlap in membership between the two organizations, eventually the leaders of one started to become the leaders of the other.[56] Probably highly symbolic at the time was Paul Dudley White's presentation of the Gold Medal Lecture to the ACC in 1963. White, a member of the "old guard" of the AHA, had opposed formation of the ACC. The ACC's decision to invite him, and his decision to accept, reflected a distinct thaw in relations between the two groups. In his address, White called for a "practical liaison" between the two organizations, but one without "any loss of identity."[57]

For a time there was even talk of a merger, although neither group ever produced a formal proposal.[58] Three-member delegations from the two societies met around 1960. They reached agreement on almost every detail of a proposed merger, except for the ACC's practice of awarding members a plaque and calling them "fellows" of the ACC. The AHA representatives insisted that the ACC discontinue both practices as a condition of a merger. After protracted debate, the ACC agreed to stop giving out plaques, but it felt that it could not retract the already awarded designation of "fellow." On this latter issue, the merger foundered. A few years later, the AHA started calling its members of the Council on Clinical Cardiology "fellows."[59]

More Journals

By midcentury a second national cardiology journal had been established. In 1950, the AHA cancelled its association with the *American Heart Journal* and began publishing a new journal, *Circulation*. The decision was primarily financial.[60] During the three years before the schism, the AHA tried to acquire more advertising revenue, but C. V. Mosby would not cooperate. Eventually, the entire editorial staff of the *American Heart Journal* moved to *Circulation*. Although H. M. Marvin, AHA President, wrote in the lead issue of *Circulation* that the name of this new journal reflected a broadening of subject matter beyond the heart alone, he was actually unhappy with the choice of title.[61] The AHA wanted to keep the title "American Heart Journal" for its new publication, but C. V. Mosby would not consider selling it.[62]

Both the new and the old journal were successful. The number of subscriptions to *Circulation* was initially over 7,000; it reached 10,000 by 1968 and 24,368 by 1985. The *American Heart Journal* may have suffered by losing its AHA affiliation, or perhaps the AHA correctly perceived that a cardiology journal could be more effectively marketed. The *American Heart Journal's* circulation dropped from 9,443 in 1951 to a low of 5,638 in 1956, not reaching 10,000 until 1977. In 1985 its circulation was 11,310. In 1953 the AHA formed a sister journal devoted to more basic research, *Circulation Research.* Not surprisingly, its circulation has remained quite a bit lower, never exceeding 4,500.

The ACC experience with cardiology journals resembled that of the AHA. After publishing seven volumes of its *Transactions* between 1952 and 1957, in 1958 the ACC started publishing a new journal, the *American Journal of Cardiology.* In keeping with the ACC's primary mission, the *American Journal of Cardiology* was intended to be "a teaching journal, dedicated to practicing clinicians and cardiologists."[63] This new journal started with an initial circulation of 5,470, which reached 10,000 by 1969 and 23,169 in 1985. The similarity of these benchmarks to those of *Circulation* suggests that the two journals may frequently travel to the same address. The ACC broke off its relationship with the *American Journal of Cardiology* much as the AHA had done with its first journal. The ACC wanted a greater share of the profits; the publisher did not concur.[64] Reluctantly, the ACC broke off its association with the *American Journal of Cardiology* and in 1983 formed its own *Journal of the American College of Cardiology,* which had reached a circulation of 19,227 by the end of 1985.[65] There seems to have been no problem with adding an additional cardiology journal; the *American Journal of Cardiology* received 1,100 manuscripts in 1982, the year before a new journal was formed, and 1,750 manuscripts in 1985, a jump suggesting that the new journal has filled a need (or at least a desire) for more cardiology papers rather than depleting a small pool of potential articles for publication.[66]

Expansion and Coexistence

After World War II, scientific research became increasingly important for academic departments of medicine, and it was in these departments of medicine, not in departments of public health, that most cardiology investigations were carried out. Departments of medicine expanded rapidly, fueled by an unprecedented infusion of federal funds through the National Institutes of Health, an infusion that far outstripped the support given by the AHA.[67] During that expansion, the research mission of academic departments of medicine started to become more self-consciously scientific, and less focused on such tasks as opening health clinics for the poor working class. Heart disease was one of many biomedical beneficiaries of increased federal support of research after World War II. In 1948 the National Heart Institute, now called the National Heart, Lung and Blood Institute (NHLBI), was formed as the second categorical research institute of the National Institutes of Health. Its annual budget was $16 million in 1950, a sum similar to that of the AHA. By 1978, the NHLBI's annual budget was $450 million.[68] In the interim, the NHLBI had expended almost $4 billion, supporting both intramural and extramural programs and developing specialized centers of research in atherosclerosis, hypertension, and ischemic heart disease.[69] Academic cardiologists increasingly moved their research from the outpatient clinic to the laboratory workbench, a move that paralleled a general transformation in academic medicine.

Some of these federal funds went to provide specialty training. There had been little opportunity for formal training in cardiology before World War II, although the *Bulletin of the American Heart Association* did occasionally note postgraduate courses, often designed to train physicians to use "instruments of precision."[70] Starting in 1949, Carl Wiggers offered a formal twelve-month training course for cardiovascular researchers at Case Western Reserve University. This course was jointly sponsored by the AHA and the U.S. Public Health Service.[71] The National Heart Institute soon began to sponsor training programs as well, a decision that fostered closer ties between cardiovascular research and the basic sciences.[72]

Those training programs helped to produce more board-certified cardiologists who could apply for grants. Physicians' initial response to subspecialty certification had been modest. After an initial 223 candidates were certified in 1941, the yearly number of cardiologists certified remained fewer than thirty-four until 1965 and did not reach three digit figures until 1972 (*Figure 8.2*). Subspecialization in any field was relatively uncommon through the 1960s, though, and the number of board-certified subspecialists in cardiology remained comfortably ahead of those in allergy, gastroenterology, and pulmonary medicine. In the 1970s and 1980s, certification of all subspecialists, including cardiologists, has increased rapidly. The total number

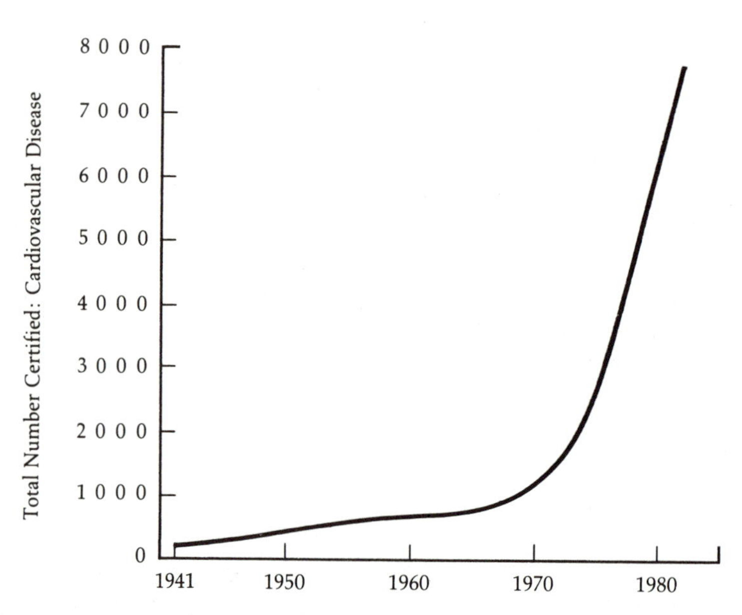

Figure 8.2. Cumulative number of physicians certified by the American Board of Internal Medicine in Cardiovascular Disease.

of physicians certified as cardiologists by the ABIM did not reach 1,000 until 1969, twenty-eight years after such certification was started. It took only five years for the next 1,000 physicians to receive the right to call themselves "Board Certified Cardiologists," and since 1975 over 1,000 physicians have passed each examination. The total number of cardiologists stood at 9,066 in 1986, almost twice as many as the next largest field, gastroenterology, with 4,754. Pulmonary medicine had certified 5,174, medical oncology (a rapidly rising late entrant) 3,659, and nephrology, 3,163.

The increased number of subspecialty training programs has led recent observers to be concerned that American medicine is training too many subspecialists.[73] Cardiology, in particular, has been identified as an overcrowded subspecialty.[74] There are now about 2,000 trainees in the 273 United States adult cardiology programs, more than twice the number in either of the two next most popular subspecialties, gastroenterology and pulmonary disease.[75] There have been several responses to the perceived surplus of cardiologists. In 1977, "short tracking," a policy allowing the first year of subspecialty training to count as the required third year of training in internal medicine, was eliminated. This change has not, as intended, reduced the number of people choosing to subspecialize. A recent ACC conference recommended lengthening the cardiology fellowship from two to three years; most future academicians already spend three years.[76] Hoping that the longer training program will produce fewer, better trained cardiologists, some propose making the required training program four years.[77] The additional year might lead to separate certification in two of the most highly technical areas of cardiology: angioplasty and electrophysiology.[78]

The two major cardiology societies have continued to serve somewhat different roles. The AHA has lay members, mounts a fund-raising drive each year, and contributes a significant amount to cardiac research—$52.9 million in 1985–1986.[79] In 1986, it had 130,000 members and a staff of 240. The ACC is a much smaller, purely professional society, supported mainly by membership dues. It had 13,000 members and staff of 65 in 1986.[80] The AHA, in keeping with its origins as a voluntary health society, is deeply involved in educating the lay public about heart disease; the ACC directs its educational efforts exclusively to physicians, although not exclusively to cardiologists. The ACC also acts as the primary spokesman for cardiologists on legislative and regulatory issues, in areas ranging from economics to health care delivery.[81] The move of the ACC in the late 1970s from New York offices to the Heart House in Bethesda, Maryland, close to Congress and to the National Institutes of Health, has no doubt encouraged even closer contact with the federal government.[82]

Both groups mount impressive national meetings. Most academicians still see the AHA meetings as more prestigious, the place where leading scientific advances are presented. The ACC is seen more as a place to learn, a place for the practicing physician to keep up with innovations. However, differences between the meetings are becoming smaller, not larger.

Relationships

Cardiology and its organizations have always existed within a larger context. Cardiology has not been the only specialty or organization to develop during the past century of American medicine. Other specialties have also been created, and those specialties' members have revised the meaning of their own specialty. The site of medical care has changed as well, and cardiologists have had to define and defend their position, both physical and intellectual, within the hospital. In this second section of the paper, I shall explore the interactions of cardiology with several of these groups. In each instance, decisions had to be made about what cardiology was to be, who it was to care for, and where and how that care was to be performed. At every stage, those negotiations have defined the meaning of "cardiology."

Surgery By midcentury other specialties and subspecialties within American medicine had created powerful organizations. One of the strongest was surgery, a specialty that had been a particularly prominent symbol of American medicine since the start of the twentieth century. Attempts to deal surgically with heart disease early in the century had been tentative.[83] Internists held all the cards and turned to surgeons only rarely; cardiology had very little to do with surgery. But something remarkable happened to heart disease during the 1950s and 1960s: it became susceptible to routine surgical treatment.[84] This change resulted in part from advances by cardiologists in preoperative diagnosis and postoperative care and in part from improvements in surgical technique and intraoperative support. The first stage in the development of cardiac surgery came from 1946 to 1953, when mechanical problems were paramount and the problems of a heart-lung machine were slowly overcome.[85] From 1953 to 1960, early attempts were made at treating coronary disease as surgeons, perhaps emboldened by recent advances in mechanical circulatory support, attempted to intervene in atherosclerotic heart disease. These attempts subjected the heart to "cauterization, abrasion, implantation, denervation, epilation, and acupuncture perforation" and, if nothing else, demonstrated "the amazing capacity of the human heart to tolerate surgical trauma."[86] Shortly after 1960, surgical treatment for coronary artery disease entered a new era, as coronary arteriography allowed physicians to visualize the site of obstruction to coronary blood flow and to bypass that obstruction with grafts of either arteries or veins.[87] Coronary artery bypass surgery underwent a dramatic, and according to some, lamentable, rise in popularity during the 1970s. By 1980, the operation accounted for 1 percent of total health care costs in the United States.[88] Questions were raised about the rapid dissemination of a therapeutic technique which, unlike drugs, required no formal governmental approval. Cardiac surgeons went from single to multiple bypasses, with four, five, or even six grafts no longer considered remarkable in a single operation.

But more changed during the 1960s and 1970s than merely the developments of new techniques and treatments. Cardiology was becoming more scientific, more technical. As a result of this change in the nature of cardiology, cardiologists first acquired and then maintained control of the catheterization laboratories, the space through which all patients undergoing coronary bypass surgery must pass.[89] Their ability to control this area meant that cardiology remained in the foreground, although not at the center, of the heart disease picture. And now in the 1980s, the cardiologists are moving back into the center. Balloon angioplasty and intravenous clot-dissolving agents, the latter now manufactured using recombinant DNA technology, may make coronary bypass far less attractive as a therapeutic modality. A new set of imaging techniques are being evaluated in the late 1980s. Some of these techniques, such as positron emission tomography scanning or thallium scanning, evaluate the heart's physiological functioning. Others, such as echocardiography, computerized axial tomography, or magnetic resonance imaging, can detect proximal lesions of the coronary arteries. But these techniques cannot now provide adequate detail of the distal portion of the coronary arteries. Cardiac catheterization appears likely to remain for some time central to cardiology and to the treatment of heart disease.

One might speculate on how cardiology has been influenced through its relationship with surgery and compare that relationship with other medical subspecialties. Consider gastroenterology.[90] Both cardiology and gastroenterology have become highly technical fields, using invasive techniques for both diagnosis and therapy. Yet until the 1950s surgery had very little to offer the cardiologist, whereas abdominal surgeons were removing appendices and oversewing ulcers with abandon in the 1920s. Understanding internists' relationships with surgeons may help us understand the different histories of their subspecialties.

As cardiac surgery developed, cardiology became much more device-oriented, a transformation with implications for everything from practice to payment. Machines have become important mediators in the relationships between internists and patients.[91] Two high technology devices, the pacemaker and the defibrillator, have become in some ways symbolic of late twentieth-century cardiology. Once a heart-lung machine allowed surgeons inside the heart, they quickly started to replace damaged valves with substitutes—an idea a good deal more problematic than it first appeared.[92] And, if end-stage myocardial disease has left the patient a "cardiac cripple," why not just go ahead and replace the whole thing? The 1980s have seen a highly publicized series of implantations of the total artificial heart.[93] William DeVries' move to a for-profit chain of hospitals has raised a series of questions about the cost (for whom?) and benefit (to whom?) of such high technology ventures. At the same time as these artificial heart implants have been making headlines, a diagnosis-related group system for prospective payment has been applied to more and more groups of patients. Under this new system, cardiologists—now doing "surgical" procedures in the catheterization laboratory—may drastically increase their reimbursement if they are reimbursed at rates consistent with surgery rather than internal medicine.[94]

Hospitals With the advent of high technology cardiology, cardiologists started to behave more and more like surgeons. In order to do so, they needed a place to work. Of all the subspecialties of internal medicine, probably none has moved into the hospital as vigorously as cardiology, particularly in the form known as "invasive cardiology." This move started with the advent of coronary care units (CCUs) in the 1960s.[95] These units, developed to save "hearts too young to die," were specialized areas of the hospital with highly technical electrical equipment for around-the-clock monitoring. Perhaps most important, these units defined areas of the hospital as the natural domain of the cardiologist, much as the surgeon had long claimed implicit dominance over the operating theater. While other practitioners, particularly in smaller hospitals, often cared for patients in coronary care units, such units were specialized areas of the hospital within which the cardiologist could, and did, claim special expertise. CCUs also drastically altered the work environment. Nurses' responsibilities were shaped by the need for continuous care. They became responsible for learning and implementing protocols for immediate response to a heart which had stopped. The tempo of care increased. CCUs were the first of a wide range of intensive care units—surgical, neonatal, neurosurgical, and medical.

Cardiologists in CCUs soon did more than merely monitor electrical phenomena susceptible to surface measurement. They also started to insert tubes into the central circulation and measure physiological parameters at the bedside.[96] Recently, cardiologists have gone beyond watching patients with acute myocardial infarction and have started to intervene actively; "invasive cardiology" has been followed by "interventional cardiology."[97] The early 1980s have seen an interesting collaboration between physiologically based catheterization investigators and laboratory-based molecular biologists, with the former using specific factors made by the latter to open clogged arteries within the heart.[98] Because this technique is valuable only if begun in the first few hours after a myocardial infarction, before damage is irreversible, rapid transportation to a medical facility capable of performing such therapy is essential. For the small but rapidly increasing number of patients treated by such therapy, this means of transportation has often been the helicopter. In such instances, physiology, molecular biology, and aviation have all helped strengthen the link between cardiology and the hospital.

Hence, Charles Rosenberg has astutely observed that not only did twentieth-century hospitals become medicalized, but medicine became hospitalized.[99] Cardiologists now train in hospitals, spend their time in intensive care units, see their patients in hospital clinics. How has this changed physicians' response to heart disease? It would be instructive to compare the definitions of subspecialties that are often practiced in intensive care units, such as cardiology and pulmonary medicine, with those of subspecialties such as rheumatology or endocrinology, which are sometimes hospital-based but less attuned to acute intervention.

Pediatrics Another transformation of cardiology took place when cardiologists restricted the age range of patients that they wanted to treat. Comparing the development of cardiology within pediatrics with its development within internal medicine allows a kind of "ecology of subspecialization" and provides some insight into differences between attitudes towards and encouragement of subspecialty fields within two specialties.

Internal medicine and pediatrics have not always been clearly differentiated. Many founders of the American Pediatrics Society were well known as internists.[100] Physicians particularly interested in heart disease focused a substantial portion of their attention on heart disease in children, and cardiac clinics had care for children as a major role.[101] Many of those children suffered from rheumatic fever, and this disease was initially the focus for the subspecialty of pediatric cardiology. In 1925 James Herrick considered rheumatic fever the most deserving target for the AHA's scarce research funds.[102]

By the 1940s, fears about many other infectious diseases had abated. The prevalence of tuberculosis was declining, albeit not from any specific therapy, and new sulfa drugs were proving effective against many infections. But rheumatic fever remained, according to some in the popular press, the most dangerous disease of school years.[103] The AHA, concerned that many draftees had been rejected because of rheumatic heart disease, formed the Council on Rheumatic Fever in 1944. Although the Council was sponsored in part by the American Academy of Pediatrics, not until 1952 did a pediatrician, Helen B. Taussig, become a member of the Executive Committee of the Council. The Council played an active role in educational programs in the 1950s and 1960s, although its members continued to fear, probably correctly, that the AHA was concerned primarily with cardiac disease in adults.[104]

Rheumatic fever also provided the impetus for the American Academy of Pediatrics to recognize the subspecialty of pediatric cardiology. In 1954 the Committee on Rheumatic Fever and Cardiac Disease of the Academy of Pediatrics recommended creating a Section on Cardiology.[105] This section was formally organized in 1957, the Sub-Board of Pediatric Cardiology in 1961.

But pediatric cardiology has changed since rheumatic fever prompted formation of these first organizations, and it is now something quite different than it was in the 1940s. The incidence of rheumatic fever has decreased dramatically, in part because of penicillin therapy for streptococcal infections and in part because of improved living conditions.[106] Even two decades ago, the appearance of a patient with rheumatic carditis was "sufficiently uncommon to warrant full-scale clinics and visits by all and sundry to the ward."[107]

In place of rheumatic fever, pediatric cardiologists now mainly concern themselves with congenital heart disease, a problem little studied or diagnosed until the middle of the twentieth century. In the early part of the century Maude Abbott made a detailed pathological study of congenital heart disease, first published as a section in William Osler's *System of Medicine*, later in a 1936 monograph analyzing 1,000 cases.[108] However, many clinicians paid little attention to the study of the cardiac malformations because "they were hopeless finalities in which the function of the physician was limited to matters of general advice and prognosis."[109] But such lesions started to attract more attention from clinicians after 1939, when Gross and Hubbard reported the first operation to correct surgically a congenital heart lesion.[110] Soon thereafter investigators developed palliative procedures to increase blood flow to the lungs, improved diagnostic techniques, and, by the mid-1950s, invented a heart-lung machine that allowed cardiopulmonary bypass.[111] As rheumatic fever has decreased, pediatric cardiology has become practically defined by congenital heart disease.

Pediatric cardiologists now use many of the ideas and techniques of their cardiologist colleagues in internal medicine. Yet, pediatric and adult cardiology have drifted far apart indeed. Only 8.3 percent of the articles in the four major U.S. cardiology journals during 1983 were devoted to congenital heart disease, and even these were primarily articles about congenital heart disease in adults.[112] Within pediatrics, pediatric cardiology has remained relatively unpopular. By 1981, academic pediatric cardiologists perceived a shortage of qualified applicants for available positions.[113] This is in sharp contrast to cardiology's dominant position in internal medicine.

Pediatric cardiology was once a central feature of American cardiology. That it is no longer is partly a result of changing epidemiology—rheumatic fever is a far less common disease than it once was. However, one cannot explain the difference between how cardiology has fared in pediatrics and internal medicine only on the basis of disease prevalence. General internists see more patients with diseases of the cardiovascular system than with diseases of any other organ system.[114] Cardiologists, like most subspecialists in internal medicine, spend the majority of their time delivering primary care to patients who could be cared for by a general internist. Only 29.8 percent of visits to cardiologists are for consultations or for specialized care. The prevalence of cardiac disease in the adult population is not a sufficient explanation for the strong subspecialist orientation of internal medicine; there is no epidemiological reason why internal medicine could not have developed with fewer cardiologists doing primarily consultations, while general internists delivered most of the primary care. Conversely, the fact that pediatrics has not developed a dominant subspecialty system and remains a specialty in which most care is delivered by general pediatricians suggests that pediatrics has been less hospitable to the growth of subspecialties in general, including cardiology, than has been internal medicine.[115]

Internal Medicine But, if pediatrics has not been particularly hospitable to cardiology, internal medicine has; cardiologists now comprise about one third of the members of academic medical departments. However, cardiology's success may eventually threaten the relationship between cardiology and internal medicine, a relationship that already appears strained to some observers. Only 5 percent of recently elected members of the American Society for Clinical Investigation—arguably the leading American academic medical society—have been cardiologists.[116] The chief of a leading section of cardiology relates that his section's clinical and research interests are much closer to organ-related sections of other specialties, such as radiology, pathology, and surgery, than to other subspecialties in internal medicine.[117] The Cardiology Section of the Marshfield Clinic split off from the Department of Internal Medicine to form its own department in 1979, and the process continues elsewhere.[118]

Some reasons for this schism are easy to see. Academic sections of cardiology are usually the largest in departments of internal medicine, and often the richest as well. As these sections see disproportionate amounts of their resources siphoned off to support less wealthy sections, they naturally tend to consider "seceding" to form departments of cardiology, as many European medical schools have done.[119] Medical residents already view cardiology differently from the other medical subspecialties.[120] However, sentiments favoring a divorce of cardiology from internal medicine may falter if, as many within cardiology fear, research funds and patient-care income both fall.[121]

For practitioners as well as for academicians, the relationship between cardiology and internal medicine has not been a stable one, and it is one that may continue to change. Cardiac disease is common, and diseases classified as those of the circulatory system are the most common reason for visits to general internists.[122] These general internists, along with family practitioners and subspecialists in areas other than cardiovascular disease, deliver the vast majority of care to patients with heart disease.

On the other hand, as more and more cardiologists are trained, their practice, like that of other subspecialists, will become less and less subspecialty oriented. Most major urban areas are already saturated with cardiologists. National trends toward cost containment will make it difficult for cardiologists simply to increase the number of procedures per capita in order to continue practicing high technology medicine. As a result, recent trainees will be forced to deliver increasingly more primary care. Already, well over half (58.2 percent) of all cardiologists' patient encounters are to deliver primary care, only 21.7 percent of all cardiologists' encounters are for consultations, and 8.1 percent are for specialized care.[123] Cardiologists do more than deliver ongoing care to patients with cardiac disease. Almost one third of the patients seen by cardiologists have a primary diagnosis outside of the circulatory system.[124] Thus, cardiology fellowships are training physicians who will spend the majority of their time practicing primary care medicine, often caring for patients with diseases unrelated to the circulatory system. One hopes that these trainees will emerge from their fellowships as facile with preventive medicine as with percutaneous transluminal angioplasty, as concerned about reducing smoking behavior as they are about reducing pulmonary capillary wedge pressure. Such an orientation would fit well with the original goals that motivated the formation of the AHA: prevention of disease and improved public health.

Conclusion

The history of twentieth-century American cardiology reflects the history of American society and American medicine, influenced by the nature of the heart and by the changing epidemiology of cardiac disease. From Harvey's classic seventeenth-century study of the heart to the present, the heart has been widely perceived as the central organ of the body. The nature of its physiologic functioning made the heart's functions easily susceptible to measurement by late nineteenth- and early twentieth-century inventions, such as the sphygmograph and the electrocardiogram.

However, the early twentieth-century Americans who founded organizations for heart disease were primarily influenced not by instrumental intervention, which they saw as most closely linked to physiology, but by the apparent success of the public health movement against tuberculosis. Born in the Progressive era, the early AHA saw its mission in terms of public health and public clinics.

Starting near midcentury, medicine changed and moved away from public health, and so did cardiology. Medicine was transformed into a more specialized profession, a more scientific profession, a more procedure-oriented profession, a more technological profession. All of these changes were faintly visible in the background before World War II but came clearly into the foreground after that conflict.

Before World War II, few physicians who cared for patients with heart disease were AHA members or specialists. General practitioners provided medical care to most Americans. However, after the war specialization and board certification rapidly became the norm. At the same time, the dramatic rise in research funding provided through the National Institutes of Health, using mechanisms devised during World War II, encouraged research—based in the natural sciences. These same funds encouraged subspecialization in many areas of medicine, including cardiology, and helped to support faculty salaries as well as fellowship training programs.[125] The AHA, once one of the leading sources of support for research in cardiac disease, found itself following a road hewn by a far larger organization. The rise of widespread health insurance and a fee-for-service reimbursement structure encouraged procedure-based, technology-centered medical practice. This trend influenced American medicine in general, but cardiologists, with their dramatic procedures and instruments, were particularly well positioned to benefit from the shift in public attitudes and health policy.

Part of the reason for cardiology's rise to a dominant position in internal medicine has also been the prevalence of cardiac disease. Yet one should not overstate the importance of epidemiology or lose sight of the ways in which many factors may interact to encourage the strengthening of a discipline. Partially because cardiac diseases are common, cardiology has received the benefit of substantial amounts of post-World War II federal funds. And strong disciplines tend to become stronger, perhaps following an institutional version of the Matthew effect in science as described by the sociologist Robert Merton.[126] Merton observed that the reward structure in science tends to follow the Gospel According to St. Matthew, "For unto every one that hath shall be given." Because cardiology has been a successful subspecialty, researchers from a wide range of basic disciplines have chosen to base their work in cardiology, and to call themselves cardiologists. Epidemiology, too, may reflect cardiology's dominant position. Diseases may be perceived as originating in several different organ systems and sometimes can be coded in a variety of different ways; the choice is often arbitrary.[127]

The meaning of cardiology has changed throughout the past century. That change has been mediated in part through various organizations, ranging from Progressive public health movements to the American Board of Internal Medicine, and in part by political and social occurrences, such as war and transatlantic migration. The meaning of cardiology has also been mediated by a series of relationships with other groups, such as pediatricians, and broader social issues, such as how to pay for health care. Both American cardiology and cardiologists have always been heterogeneous, and tensions within the field have always existed.

Nothing is inevitable about either the intellectual content of cardiology or its placement in American medicine. Cardiologists could have continued to see children, or could have been based in schools of public health. Surgeons or radiologists might have taken control of cardiac catheterization laboratories. At every stage, it could have been different.

The current shape of cardiology, therefore, reflects continued tensions about who cardiologists are and what they should do. Are cardiologists scientists or sanitarians? Is their goal greater knowledge or improved public health? Are they consultants or primary care physicians? Molecular biologists? Technicians? The answers to these questions and to similar ones faced by many other subspecialties have been, and continue to be, negotiated. There is a natural tendency to look to the past to define and defend the present state of an organization, to "invent" a tradition of what cardiology was like before.[128] Doing so is misleading. Cardiology has not always been physiological, or even scientific, as we now define the term. Nor has it always been instrumentally based. Although cardiology now shares some of the "seductive images" of surgery, this development is relatively new, as is cardiology's move into the hospital. The system of American medicine is changing. Cardiology will change, too. But the questions will remain the same: Who are cardiologists? What do cardiologists do? What is cardiology? The theme of this chapter is that the answers to these questions, and the answers to similar questions for any area of medicine, are complex, historically mediated, and constantly changing.

I would like to thank Daniel Fox, Barbara Gastel, Laurence McMahon, Russell Maulitz, Jeoffrey Stross, and an anonymous reviewer for their insightful comments.

NOTES

1. In 1985, over 21,000 people attended the annual meetings of the American Heart Association, and around 18,500 attended those of the American College of Cardiology. The two programs included over 3,000 original papers on topics ranging from the molecular biology of specific clot-dissolving agents to how best to set up a program for training lay people to perform cardiac resuscitation. In 1984 alone, the four major American cardiology journals—the *American Heart Journal, American Journal of Cardiology, Circulation,* and the most recent addition to the field, the *Journal of the American College of Cardiology*—together published 1,878 articles on over 11,377 pages. William C. Roberts, "Analysis of Page Utilization and Types of Articles Published in Four Major American Cardiology Journals in 1984," *Int J Cardiol* 8 (1985):353–60.

2. The best starting point for a history of cardiology is W. Bruce Fye's bibliography, "History of Cardiology," *Circulation* 64 (1981):434–36. See also James Herrick, *A Short History of Cardiology* (Springfield, IL: Charles C. Thomas, 1942); Fredrick A. Willius and Thomas J. Dry, *A History of the Heart and Circulation* (Philadelphia: W. B. Saunders, 1948); Alfred P. Fishman and Dickson W. Richards, eds., *Circulation of the Blood-Men and Ideas* (New York: Oxford, 1964); and H. A. Snellen, *History of Cardiology: A Brief Outline of the 350 Years' Prelude to an Explosive Growth* (Rotterdam: Donker Academic Publications, 1984). These books provide some helpful background but do not focus on the process of specialty formation or go far into the twentieth century. Dealing more with the past century are Howard B. Burchell, "Important Events in Cardiology, 1940–1982: A Retrospective View," *JAMA* 249 (1983):1197–1200; H. A. Snellen, A. J. Dunning, and A. C. Arntzenius, eds., *History and Perspectives of Cardiology: Catheterization, Angiography, Surgery, and Concepts of Circular Control* (The Hague: Leiden University Press, 1981); and Julius H. Comroe, Jr., *Exploring the Heart: Discoveries in Heart Disease and High Blood Pressure* (New York: W. W. Norton, 1983).

3. For a comparison with the British definition of cardiology and thoughts on the formation of the British Cardiac Club, see Joel D. Howell, "Soldier's Heart: The

Redefinition of Heart Disease and Speciality Formation in Early Twentieth-Century Great Britain," *Med Hist* (1985) (Suppl. 5):34–52.

4. C. E. A. Winslow, *The Evolution and Significance of the Modern Public Health Campaign* (New Haven: Yale University Press, 1923), 55, 57.

5. George Rosen, *A History of Public Health* (New York: M. D. Publications, 1958), 390–91.

6. John C. Burnham, "Medical Specialists and Movements Toward Social Control in the Progressive Era: Three Examples," in *Building the Organizational Society: Essays on Associational Activities in Modern America*, Jerry Israel, ed. (New York, Free Press, 1972), 19–30.

7. Paul Starr, *The Social Transformation of American Medicine* (New York: Basic Books, 1982), 191–92.

8. Mary E. Wadley to Alfred E. Cohen, 3 February 1938, quoted in William W. Moore, *Fighting for Life: The Story of the American Heart Association 1911–1975* (Dallas: American Heart Association, 1983), 3.

9. Edwin P. Maynard, Jr., "Origin and Development of the Medical Programs," in *The New York Heart Association Origins and Development: 1915–1965*, Clarence E. de la Chapelle, ed. (New York: New York Heart Association, 1966).

10. H. M. Marvin, "The Prevention and Relief of Heart Disease as a Public Health Problem," in *Diagnosis and Treatment of Cardiovascular Disease*, William D. Stroud, ed. (Philadelphia: F. A. Davis, 1940), 1023–47.

11. Haven Emerson, "The Prevention of Heart Disease: A New Practical Problem" (The 1921 Shattuck Lecture), *Boston Med Surg J* 184 (1921):587–607 and in *Selected Papers of Haven Emerson* (Battle Creek, MI: W. F. Kellog Foundation, 1949), 70–108.

12. Moore, *Fighting for Life*, 15.

13. "Similarity of Tuberculosis and Heart Disease," *Bull Am Heart Assoc* 2 (1927): 22.

14. For a typical description see Eleanor Dodge, "Cardiac Clinic of the Michael Reese Dispensary: Definitely Organized to Meet the Needs of Patients with Cardiac Handicap who Require Prolonged Supervision as well as Social Adjustment," *The Nation's Health* 5 (1923):1–3. This clinic, for example, met Saturday mornings.

15. For example, the Westinghouse Electric and Manufacturing Company of Pittsburgh, *Bull Am Heart Assoc* 2 (1927): 28 or ibid., "News Notes," 1 (1926):2.

16. Herrick, and others, to Frank R. Morton, Secretary, Chicago Medical Society (no date, but from context certainly 1923), in Herrick Papers, box 5, folder 2, Special Collections, University of Chicago; see also James B. Herrick, *Memories of Eighty Years* (Chicago: University of Chicago Press, 1949), 202–4.

17. See for example, Alfred E. Cohn, "Clinical Charts Recommended by The Association for the Prevention and Relief of Heart Disease: The Plans for Their Use," *JAMA* 78 (1922):1559–62 and "Clinical Charts Recommended by the Heart Committee of the New York Tuberculosis and Health Association," *Am Heart J* 2 (1927):655–70 and distributed separately "with the compliments of the American Heart Association."

18. "Requirements for an Ideal Cardiac Clinic: By the Committee on Cardiac Clinics of the Heart Committee, New York Tuberculosis and Health Association," *Boston Med Surg J* 189 (1923):762–68 and issued separately by the American Heart Association.

19. Morris H. Kahn, "Principles of Conducting a Cardiac Clinic," *The Modern Hospital* 25 (1925):22–25.

20. Alfred E. Cohn, "Statistical Studies Bearing on Problems In the Classification of Heart Diseases: I. Introduction," *Am Heart J* 1 (1925–26):442–45; Alfred E. Cohn, "Heart Disease From the Point of View of the Public Health," *Am Heart J* 2 (1926–27):275–301, 386–407; and Louis I. Dublin, "The Problem of Heart Disease," *Harpers* 154 (1927):196–204. I am grateful to Daniel M. Fox for bringing this subject to my attention.

21. John Harley Warner, "Science in Medicine," *Osiris* 1 (1985):37–58.

22. Quoted by Eugene F. DuBois in "Fifty Years of Physiology in America—A Letter to the Editor," in *The Excitement and Fascination of Science* (Palo Alto, CA: Annual Reviews, 1965), 86.

23. Gerald Geison, "Divided We Stand: Physiologists and Clinicians in the American Context," in *The Therapeutic Revolution*, Morris J. Vogel and Charles E. Rosenberg, eds. (Philadelphia: University of Pennsylvania Press, 1979), 67–90.

24. "The American Heart Journal," *Bull Am Heart Assoc* 6 (1931):1.

25. Alfred Cohn to Canby Robinson, 8 January 1926. Rockefeller Archive Center, Alfred Cohn Papers. The 1909 event was probably the founding of the journal *Heart* in Great Britain by Thomas Lewis, a key figure in training many American heart doctors, including Cohn.

26. The source for this and subsequent circulation figures is either *Ayre's Directory to Publications* (Fort Washington, PA: IMS Press, 1985 and previous editions) or *Ulrich's International Periodicals Directory*, ed. 24 and previous (New York: R. R. Bowker, 1985). Unfortunately, these sources do not always distinguish paid from unpaid subscriptions. When a distinction is made, I have used figures for paid subscriptions.

27. Moore, *Fighting for Life*, 32.

28. "Foreword," *Modern Concepts of Cardiovascular Disease* 1 (1932):1.

29. Richard Harrison Shryock, *National Tuberculosis Association 1904–1954: A Study of the Voluntary Health Movement in the United States* (New York: National Tuberculosis Association, 1957).

30. Moore, *Fighting for Life*, 30.

31. Moore, *Fighting for Life*, 30.

32. Moore, *Fighting for Life*, 242–43.

33. Rosemary Stevens, *American Medicine and the Public Interest* (New Haven: Yale, 1971). See also Glenn Gritzer and Arnold Arluke, *The Making of Rehabilitation: A Political Economy of Medical Specialization 1890–1980* (Berkeley and Los Angeles: University of California Press, 1985).

34. Sir James Mackenzie, "The Role of Medicine at the Beginning of the Twentieth Century as Illustrated by the State of Cardiology," *NY J Med* 65 (1922):61–66.

35. Herrick, *Memories*, 202–3.

36. James B. Herrick, "The Clinician of the Future," *JAMA* 86 (1926):1–6.

37. Louis Faugeres Bishop, "The Practice of Cardiology: A Consideration of the Continuous Care of Heart Patients by the Prolonged Use of Drugs, Physiotherapy, and Psychotherapy," *Ann Intern Med* 2 (1928):352–66.

38. Christopher Lawrence has explored a similar shift in ideas about heart disease in "Moderns and Ancients: The 'New Cardiology' in Britain 1880–1930," *Med Hist* 1 (1985) (Suppl. 5):1–33. A full study of the American scene remains to be done, but at least Bishop would agree with British ideas.

39. Paul D. White, "Men's Lives are Chains of Chances: Cardiology 1913–1956," *Med Clin North Am* 41 (1957):987–1004.

40. Samuel A. Levine, "Special Fields in Medicine—Cardiology as a Specialty," *Phi Delta Epsilon NEWS* (Oct. 1937):138–40.

41. Joel D. Howell, "Specialties and the American Board of Internal Medicine: A Historical Perspective," in *American Board of Internal Medicine: Fiftieth Anniversary Symposium and Celebration* (Portland, OR: American Board of Internal Medicine, 1987), 9–17.

42. James Herrick to Oliver Ormsby, 21 November 1919. In University of Chicago Special Collections.

43. Moore, *Fighting for Life*, 35. The Life Insurance Medical Research Fund provided several hundred thousand dollars a year for a few years. See Life Insurance Medical Research Fund, *Annual Reports 1–5* (New York: George Grady Press, 1945–1950).

44. *A History of the Scientific Councils of the American Heart Association* (American Heart Association, 1967).

45. "History of the American Heart Association," *J Natl Med Assoc* 48 (1956):59–63, 67.

46. Alfred S. Hartwell, "The American Heart Association," *Straub Clin Proc* 24 (1958):11–15 and Moore, *Fighting for Life*, 51.

47. Irving Page, quoted in Moore, *Fighting for Life*, 145.

48. American Heart Association, *Annual Report*, 1964.

49. Shabudin H. Rahimtoola, "The Twenty-Fifth Anniversary of Valve Replacement: A Time for Reflection," *Circulation* 71 (1985):1–3.

50. Oglesby Paul, "The Heart Association and the Physician," *Circulation* 21 (1969):165–66.

51. P. Reichert, "A History of the Develoment of Cardiology as a Medical Specialty," *Clin Cardiol* 1 (1978):5–15; Louis F. Bishop, "Cardiology as a Specialty," *NY State J Med* 76 (1976):1170–74.

52. Reichert, "Cardiology," 12. In the early twentieth century, most ambitious American physicians who wanted advanced training went to Europe. Many who went on to help define the field of American cardiology first trained in England with Sir James Mackenzie, or with his student, Sir Thomas Lewis. A partial list of people who trained with Lewis reads like a "Who's Who" of midcentury American cardiology: H. C. Bazett, Alfred Cohn, Harold Feil, Eugene Landis, H. M. Marvin, Harold Pardee, W. D. Stroud, Paul Dudley White, Frank Wilson, and Charles Wolferth. World War I gave Americans further opportunity to interact with their British colleagues. Gathering around the problem of "soldiers' heart," as it was originally called in Great Britain (although the disease entity was renamed the "effort syndrome" by the end of the war), and "neurocirculatory aesthenia," as the syndrome was called by the American physicians, they formed lasting friendships. The experiences shared by the relatively small number of Americans who went overseas may have encouraged their postwar association. Most of those who went to England came to be associated with the AHA. It appears that early members of the ACC, by contrast, were more likely to have been recent immigrants to America, and that they saw their European ties as more continental, particularly German. A detailed prosopographical analysis could prove valuable in elucidating different national styles of cardiology. See Medical Research Council Annual Reports and Joel D. Howell, "Early Perceptions of the Electrocardiogram: From Arrhythmia to Infarction," *Bull Hist Med* 58 (1984):83–98.

53. Ashton Graybiel, "Inaugural Address of the New President," *Trans Am Coll Cardiol* 4 (1954):184–86.

54. Howard Burchell, personal communication, 1986.

55. James V. Warren, personal communication, 1986; Richard Judge, personal communication, 1987.

56. From 1950 to 1969 no person had served as an officer of both the AHA and the ACC. In 1969 James V. Warren, who had been President of the AHA during 1962–63, was elected as a Vice-President of the ACC.

57. Paul Dudley White, "Reflections of a Pioneer in Cardiology," *Am J Cardiol*, 1963, 11: 697–702.

58. Louis Faugeres Bishop, *The Birth of a Specialty: The Diary of an American Cardiologist 1926–1972* (New York: Vantage Press, 1977), 156.

59. Stuart Wolf, personal communication, 1986.

60. Howard Burchell, personal communication based on his memories of conversations with Edgar V. Allan, 1986.

61. H. M. Marvin, "Foreword," *Circulation* 1 (1950):1.

62. H. M. Marvin to James Herrick, 26 October 1949. In Herrick Papers, Box 5, Folder 1, Special Collections, University of Chicago.

63. Simon Dack, "Looking Ahead," *Am J Cardiol* 1 (1958):1–2.

64. William C. Roberts, personal communication, 1986.

65. Paul O. Weislogel, personal communication, 1987.

66. William C. Roberts, personal communication. For comparisons between the various cardiology journals, see William C. Roberts, "Comparison of 7 English-Language Cardiology Journals for 1983," *Am J Cardiol* 53 (1984):862–69 and idem, "Analysis of Page Utilization."

67. Donald C. Swain, "The Rise of a Research Empire: NIH, 1930 to 1950," *Science* 138 (1962):1233–37; James A. Shannon, "The Advancement of Medical Research: A Twenty-Year View of the Role of the National Institutes of Health," *J Med Ed* 42 (1967):97–108; Stephen P. Strickland, *Politics, Science, and Dread Disease: A Short History of United States Medical Research Policy* (Cambridge, MA: Harvard University Press, 1972); and Elizabeth Brenner Drew, "The Health Syndicate: Washington's Noble Conspirators," *Atlantic Monthly* 221 (1967):75–82.

68. Robert I. Levy, "Progress Towards Prevention of Cardiovascular Disease: A 30-year Retrospective," *Circulation* 60 (1979):1555–59; Strickland, *Politics, Science, and Dread Disease*, 51–53.

69. Eugene Braunwald, "Thirty-Five Years of Progress in Cardiovascular Research," *Circulation* 70 (1984) (Suppl. III):8–25.

70. For example, the course at the University of California noted in the *Bull Am Heart Assoc* 3 (1928):12.

71. Notice in the first volume of *Circulation*, also see Carl J. Wiggers, *Reminiscences and Adventures in Circulation Research* (New York: Grune and Stratton, 1958), 171–73.

72. "Editorial: A Milestone in Cardiovascular Training," *Circulation* 11 (1960): 321–22.

73. U.S. Department of Health and Human Services, *Summary Report of the Graduate Medical Education National Advisory Committee* (GMENAC) (Washington: Government Printing Office, 1980).

74. Robert A. O'Rourke, "Cardiology at a Precipice," *Circulation* 72 (1985): 258–61.

75. William W. Parmley, "President's Page: The College and Affiliates in Training," *J Am Coll Cardiol* 6 (1985):262–63.

76. William Nelligan, personal communication, 1986; Michael W. Cox, LuAnn

Aday, Gerald S. Levey, et al., "National Study of Internal Medicine Manpower: X. Internal Medicine Residency and Fellowship Training: 1985 Update," *Ann Intern Med* 104 (1986):241–45.

77. Bertram Pitt, personal communication, 1986.

78. William W. Parmley, "President's Page: Certification, Recertification and Continuing Medical Education," *J Am Coll Cardiol* 6 (1985):1180–81.

79. Data from the AHA National Office. Of that $52.9 million, approximately half was awarded by the national office, and half by local and regional affiliates.

80. Katherine Gruber, ed., *Encyclopedia of Associations 1986*, ed. 20 (Detroit: Gale Research Company, 1986).

81. Suzanne B. Knoebel, "President's Page: The Next Challenge: Balancing Individual Quality Care with Community Resources," *J Am Coll Cardiol* 1 (1983): 972–74 and Leonard S. Dreifus, "President's Page: Membership Services," *Am J Cardiol* 42 (1978):336–38.

82. H. Mahr, "Heart House," *Clin Cardiol* 1 (1978):48–49.

83. J. O. Leibowitz, *The History of Coronary Heart Disease* (Berkeley and Los Angeles: University of California Press, 1970) and George H. A. Clowes, Jr., "The Historical Development of the Surgical Treatment of Heart Disease," *Bull Hist Med* 34 (1960):29–51.

84. For a detailed chronology of this process see Comroe and Dripps, *The Top Ten Advances in Cardiopulmonary Medicine and Surgery 1945–1975* (Washington: Government Printing Office, 1977). See also Alfred Blalock, "Cardiovascular Surgery, Past and Present," *J Thorac Cardiovasc Surg* 51 (1966):153–67; Ronald Sandor Liss, *The History of Heart Surgery in the United States (1938–1960) (Zurich: Juris Druck and Verlag, 1967)*; Robert S. Litwak, "The Growth of Cardiac Surgery: Historical Notes," *Cardiovasc Clin* 3 (1967):6–50; and Stephen L. Johnson, *The History of Cardiac Surgery 1896–1955* (Baltimore: Johns Hopkins Press, 1970). For more dramatic accounts see Hugh McLeave, *The Risk Takers* (London: Frederick Muller, 1962) and Rowan Nicks, *Surgeons All: The Story of Cardiothoracic Surgery in Australia and New Zealand* (Sydney: Hale and Iremonger, 1984).

85. Howard B. Burchell, "A Cardiologist's View of Modern Cardiovascular Surgery," *Dis Chest* 55 (1969):323–29.

86. Donald Brian Effler, "Myocardial Revascularization Surgery Since 1945 A.D.: Its Evolution and Impact," *J Thorac Cardiovasc Surg* 72 (1976):823–28 and John E. Connolly, "The History of Coronary Artery Surgery," *J Thorac Cardiovasc Surg* 76 (1978):733–44.

87. T. Doby, "History of Cardiovascular Catheterization," *Clio Medica* 12 (1977):185–88 and W. Bruce Fye, "Coronary Arteriography—It Took a Long Time," *Circulation* 79 (1984):781–87.

88. M. C. Weinstein and W. B. Stason, "Cost Effectiveness of Coronary Bypass Surgery," *Circulation* 66 (1982):56.

89. The fault lines between cardiology and radiology would be well worth a detailed analysis. The right to do cardiac catheterization, nuclear medicine studies, and noninvasive studies such as echocardiography is more than highly symbolic, it is a major source of revenue. In today's hospitals, radiologists routinely do these studies for noncardiac disease—they inject dye into the pulmonary arteries and perform ultrasound examinations of the abdomen. Yet those same studies are done by cardiologists when the organ in question is the heart. Interestingly, radiologists have maintained control of two of the most recent and potentially most valuable imaging devices of recent years, the CAT (computerized axial tomography) scan

and the MRI (magnetic resonance imaging, known as nuclear magnetic resonance until the mid-1980s). The process by which these diagnostic technologies came to lie in radiology or cardiology may tell us a great deal about twentieth-century American medicine.

90. C. C. Booth, "What has Technology Done to Gastroenterology?" *Gut* 26 (1985):1088–94.

91. For an analysis of the influence of medical technology on the doctor-patient relationship, see Stanley Joel Reiser, *Medicine and the Reign of Technology* (Cambridge: Cambridge University Press, 1978). Edward Shorter has also provided useful insights in *Bedside Manners: The Troubled History of Doctors and Patients* (New York: Simon and Schuster, 1985).

92. Charles A. Hufnagel, "Basic Concepts in the Development of Cardiovascular Prostheses," *Am J Surg* 139 (1979):285–300.

93. William C. DeVries, Jeffrey L. Anderson, Lyle D. Joyce, et al., "Clinical Use of the Total Artificial Heart," *N Engl J Med* 310 (1984):273–79 and Pierre M. Galletti, "Replacement of the Heart with a Mechanical Device; The Case of Dr. Barney Clark," *N Engl J Med* 310 (1984):312–14.

94. Helen L. Smits and Rita E. Watson, "DRGs and the Future of Surgical Practice," *N Engl J Med* 311 (1984):1612–15.

95. Hughes W. Day, "An Intensive Coronary Care Area," *Dis Chest* 44 (1963):423–27; J. Edgar Caswell, "A Brief History of Coronary Care Units," *Public Health Rep* 82 (1967):1105–7; Hughes W. Day, "History of Coronary Care Units," *Am J Cardiol* 39 (1972): 405–7; and James H. Maxwell, "The Iron Lung: Halfway Technology or Necessary Step?" *Milback Q* 64 (1986):3–29.

96. H. J. C. Swan and William Ganz, "Hemodynamic Monitoring: A Personal and Historical Perspective," *Can Med Assoc J* 121 (1979):868–71 and William A. Knaus and George E. Thibault, "Intensive Care Units Today," in *Critical Issues in Medical Technology*, Barbara J. McNeil and E. G. Cravalho, eds. (Boston: Auburn House, 1982), 193–215.

97. This new cardiology has been predicated largely on the ability to perform cardiac catheterization; for a readable description of the key developments, told in many instances by the participants themselves, see J. Willis Hurst, "History of Cardiac Catheterization," in *Coronary Arteriography and Angioplasty*, Spencer B. King and John S. Douglas, eds. (New York: McGraw Hill, 1985). For a discussion of newer approaches to interventional cardiology see William O'Neill, Gerald C. Timmis, Patrick D. Bourdillion, et al., "A Prospective Randomized Clinical Trial of Intracoronary Streptokinase Versus Coronary Angioplasty for Acute Myocardial Infarction," *N Engl J Med* 314 (1986):812–18.

98. Diane Pennica, William E. Holmes, William J. Kohr, et al., "Cloning and Expression of Human Tissue-Type Plasminogen Activator cDNA in *E. Coli*," *Nature* 301 (1983):214–21; Desire Collen, Eric J. Topol, Alan J. Tiefenbrunn, et al., "Coronary Thrombolysis with Recombinant Human Tissue-Type Plasminogen Activator: A Prospective, Randomized, Placebo-controlled Trial," *Circulation* 70 (1984):1012–17.

99. Charles E. Rosenberg, presentation at the first Wood Institute Conference, on the history of the hospital (publication forthcoming).

100. Harold Kniest Faber and Rustin McIntosh, *History of the American Pediatric Society, 1887–1965* (New York: McGraw Hill, 1966).

101. For example, see Morris H. Kahn, "Principles of Conducting a Cardiac Clinic," *Mod Hosp* 25 (1925):22–25.

102. James Herrick to W. D. Stroud, 28 November 1928. In Herrick Papers, Box 5, Folder 8, Special Collections, University of Chicago.

103. Metropolitan Life Insurance Company, "What's the Most Dangerous Disease of School Years?" *American Magazine* 132 (1941):51; another dramatic story is Maxine Davis, "Rheumatic Fever," *Good Housekeeping* 35 (1941):199–200.

104. *A History of the Scientific Councils*, 11.

105. Forrest H. Adams, "Development of Pediatric Cardiology," *Am J Cardiol* 22 (1968):452–55.

106. Leon Gordis, "The Virtual Disappearance of Rheumatic Fever in the United States: Lessons in the Rise and Fall of Disease" (The T. Duckett Jones Memorial Lecture), *Circulation* 72 (1985):1155–62.

107. Sir Ian Hill, "The Wind of Change in Cardiology," *Practitioner* 201 (1968):44.

108. Maude Abbott, "Congenital Heart Disease," in *A System of Medicine, by Eminent Authorities in Great Britain, the United States, and the Continent*, William Osler and Thomas McCrae, eds., vol. 4: *Diseases of the Circulatory System* (London: Henry Frowde, Hodder, and Stoughton, 1908), 323–425 and *Atlas of Congenital Heart Disease* (New York: American Heart Association, 1936).

109. Edward A. Park, "Foreword," in *Congenital Malformations of the Heart*, Helen B. Taussig, ed. (New York: The Commonwealth Fund, 1947), vii–ix.

110. R. E. Gross and J. P. Hubbard, "Surgical Ligation of a Patent Ductus Arteriosus. Report of First Successful Case," *JAMA* 112 (1939):729–31.

111. For an early review see Sir Russell Brock, ed., "Guy's Hospital Reports: Special Number Devoted to Cardiovascular Diseases," *Guy's Hosp Rep* 8 (1959): 101–402.

112. Roberts, "Comparison." There was considerable heterogeneity among the four journals. The *American Journal of Cardiology* devoted 12.3 percent of its 643 articles to congenital heart disease; the figures for the other three, including the official journals of the two main societies, were below 7 percent. Of note is that the *British Heart Journal* devoted over 15 percent of its articles to this topic; this may reflect some difference in national styles. Although these differences may reflect a number of factors, including personal editorial decisions, congenital heart disease seems not to be a major concern of the internist/cardiologists who read the major cardiology journals.

113. Thomas P. Graham, "Manpower and Training in Pediatric Cardiology," *J Am Coll Cardiol* 4 (1984):644–45.

114. Roger A. Girard, Robert C. Mendenhall, Alvin R. Tarlov, et al., "A National Study of Internal Medicine and Its Specialties: I. An Overview of the Practice of Internal Medicine," *Ann Intern Med* 90 (1979):965–75.

115. Robert C. Mendenhall, Alvin R. Tarlov, Roger A. Girard, et al., "A National Study of Internal Medicine and Its Specialties: II. Primary Care in Internal Medicine," *Ann Intern Med* 91 (1979):275–87; Joel D. Howell, "Pediatric Cardiology in Perspective" (letter), *Ann Intern Med* 107 (1987):602–3.

116. Raymond D. Pruitt, "The Greying of Academic Cardiology," *Mayo Clin Proc* 53 (1978):411–12.

117. Bertram Pitt, personal communication, 1986.

118. W. Bruce Fye, personal communication, 1986.

119. Eugene Braunwald, "Tensions Between Academic Cardiology and Internal Medicine," *Int J Cardiol* 5 (1984):223–28.

120. Eugene Braunwald, "The Present State and Future of Academic Cardiology," *Circulation* 66 (1982):487–90.

121. Leon Resnekov, "Issues and Challenges for Academic Cardiology: Introduction to Views of the Future Leaders," *Chest* 81 (1982):137–38.

122. Girard, et al., "Internal Medicine and Its Specialties: I."

123. Mendenhall, et al., "Internal Medicine and Its Specialties: II."

124. Girard, et al., "Internal Medicine and Its Specialties: I."

125. Alvin R. Tarlov, Peter A. Weil, and Mary Kay Schleiter, "National Study of Internal Medicine Manpower: III. Subspecialty Fellowship Training 1976–1977," *Ann Intern Med* 91 (1979):287–94 and Strickland, *Politics, Science, and Dread Disease*, 253.

126. Robert K. Merton, "The Matthew Effect in Science: The Reward and Communication Systems are Considered," *Science* 159 (1968):56–63.

127. Mel Bartley, "Coronary Heart Disease and the Public Health 1850–1983," *Sociol Health Illness* 7 (1985):289–313 and Howell, "Soldier's Heart."

128. Eric Hobsbawm, "Introduction: Inventing Traditions," in *The Invention of Tradition*, Eric Hobsbawm and Terence Ranger, eds. (Cambridge: Cambridge University Press, 1983), 1–14.

PART III

HISTORICAL PROBLEMS IN DIAGNOSIS AND THERAPY

9

Classifications in Medicine

STEPHEN J. KUNITZ

O body swayed to music, O brightening glance,
How can we know the dancer from the dance?

William Butler Yeats, "Among Schoolchildren"

In 1925 Alfred North Whitehead observed that "classification is a halfway house between the immediate concreteness of the individual thing and the complete abstraction of mathematical notions. . . . Classification is necessary. But unless you can progress from classification to mathematics, your reasoning will not take you very far."[1] In this chapter I suggest that disease classifications have functioned in just this way for physicians concerned with preserving their role as science-based diagnosticians against the encroachments first of laboratory scientists and then of family physicians. Indeed, the terms physician and diagnostician have often been used synonymously, and it is thus small wonder that classifications of disease should be so central to their concerns.

Classifications have served two functions: as guides to rational practice and as professional ideologies. By ideology I mean "a particular definition of reality . . . attached to a concrete power interest. . . . The distinctiveness of ideology is . . . that the *same* overall universe is interpreted in different ways, depending upon concrete vested interests within the society in question."[2]

As healers of all sorts are concerned with diagnosis, classifications of diseases and other misfortunes have been part of their armamentarium in all societies. The principles on which they are based have varied widely, however, both among and within societies. In our own culture, such systems have been based on notions of natural history, description of symptoms, and pathological anatomy. By the end of the nineteenth century, as the germ theory gained widespread acceptance, the principle of classification by etiology became common. So important did it become, indeed, that George Bernard Shaw satirized it in his Introduction to *The Doctor's Dilemma* as well as in the following passage.

> B.B. Overwork! There's no such thing. I do the work of ten men. Am I giddy? No. NO. If you're not well, you have a disease. It may be a slight one; but it's a disease. And what is a disease? The lodgment in the system of a pathogenic germ, and the multiplication of that germ. What is the remedy? A very simple one. Find the germ and kill it.[3]

It was against this sort of reification that the British physician F. G. Crookshank inveighed in a supplement to *The Meaning of Meaning* (by psychologist C. K. Ogden and literary critic I. A. Richards) when he observed:

> In modern Medicine this tyranny of names is no less pernicious than in the modern form of scholastic realism. Diagnosis, which, as Mr. Bernard Shaw has somewhere declared, should mean the finding out of all there is wrong with a particular patient and why, too often means in practice the formal and unctuous pronunciation of a Name that is deemed appropriate and absolves from the necessity of further investigation. And, in the long run, an accurate appreciation of a patient's "present state" is often treated as ignorant *because* it is incompatible with the sincere use of one of the few verbal symbols available to us as Proper Names for Special Diseases.[4]

Crookshank's point was that the application of a diagnostic label to a patient's problems was an example of the modern form of word magic, mistaking the word for the thing to which it referred. A diagnostic label was not simply a shorthand description of a process whose meaning was understood by all who heard it. In a complex, literate society learning is done largely in private and from books rather than publicly and by exemplification, and therefore multiple meanings attach to words.[5] Meanings are not shared and the illusion of understanding is created while the reality of the patient's experience becomes increasingly opaque.

Crookshank's was an extreme nominalist position. "It is a vulgar medical error," he wrote, "to speak, write, and ultimately to think, as if these *diseases* we name, these *general references* we *symbolize,* were single things with external existences."

> Teachers of Medicine . . . seem to share the implied belief that all known, or knowable, clinical phenomena are resumable, and to be resumed, under a certain number of categories or general references, as so many 'diseases'; the true number of these categories, references, or 'diseases' being predetermined by the constitution of the universe at any given moment.
>
> In fact, for these gentlemen, 'diseases' are Platonic realities: universals *ante rem*. This unavowed belief, which might be condoned were it frankly admitted, is an inheritance from Galen, and carries with it the corollary that our notions concerning this, that, or the other 'disease' are either absolutely right or absolutely wrong, and are not merely matters of mental convenience. In this way, the diseases supposed to be extant at any one moment are capable—so it is thought—of such categorical exhaustion as the indigenous fauna of the British Isles and the population of London. That our grouping of like cases as cases of the same disease is purely a matter of justification and convenience, liable at any moment to supersession or adjustment, is nowhere admitted; and the hope is held out that one day we shall know all the diseases that there 'are,' and all about them that is to be known.[6]

According to Crookshank, bacteriology encouraged the mistaken notion that diseases were discrete entities, that the same diagnosis in two different cases implied the same process, and that the application of a name—or diagnosis—was the same thing as understanding all there was wrong with a patient and why. His position was, I believe, an example of the ambivalence, if not hostility, with which many physicians confronted the bacteriologic revolution in the early decades of the century.

Russel Maulitz has described some of the ways in which bacteriology influenced clinical medicine. It was, he has suggested, "a vehicle for the infusion of the ideology of science into medicine."[7] But the effects were paradoxical, for although physicians stood to gain from the enhanced status of scientific medicine, many of them felt threatened, both by the emergence of bacteriologists as arbiters of diagnosis and management from their vantage point in the laboratory and by what they perceived as the growing irrelevance of clinical and interpersonal skills to diagnosis and the care of patients.

In an address in 1909, Humphrey Rolleston, later to become Regius Professor of Medicine at Cambridge, observed that classifications of disease had become harder to achieve than in the past as a result of the great advance of knowledge. "We realize that any scheme of classification adopted for convenience and practical purposes may almost any day be disturbed by a new discovery." He believed that not enough was yet known to classify diseases etiologically and that it was wise to use a mixed classification: etiological and regional. Peritonitis, for example, is a "group-disease," "a characteristic collection of symptoms which may be due to any one of a group of allied organisms."[8] Indeed, "Of the two essentials that go to make up our conception of a disease, (i.) the clinical aspect and (ii.) the etiological factor, the first is still more prominent in our minds."[9] He pointed out, however, that "the physician's field of activity" was becoming "narrowed" and that "his function as a diagnostician" was increasingly restricted by the importance of bacteriological tests and skiagraphy [Roentgenography], for the accuracy and value of which he must depend on experts."[10] He then went on to say: "The pure physician [i.e., internist], should he still survive, will be in a parlous plight between the surgeon and the deep sea of bacteriology."[11] Clearly, the rapid advances in bacteriology were perceived as a threat to the existence of the "pure physician" for whom diagnostic acumen was the essence of the professional persona. His recommendation was that in self-defense physicians develop surgical skills and specialize in some region or system of the body, much as obstetrician-gynecologists were already doing.[12]

It is an entertaining irony that even as bacteriology was exerting such a deeply disturbing effect on many physicians, the infectious diseases were becoming less and less significant as a leading cause of mortality. However, the principle of etiological classification, once established, had a lasting effect. In a presidential address to the American Society for Clinical Investigation in 1931, Francis Blake observed that under the influence of rapid advances in bacteriology in the late nineteenth century, the search for specific causes of diseases had become dominant. But, he continued, a real understanding of the etiology of disease requires "an understanding of all the conditions or circumstances under which it develops. Here we are concerned with pathogenesis, not etiology in the conventional usage of the word; the study of the interplay of specific agents, environmental factors, and human susceptibilities."[13] Clinical investigation, then, had to be construed broadly, for disease patterns were changing and those that had become important by the early years of the twentieth century were complex in origin. To investigate them, one had to be a clinician, not simply a laboratory worker, although the clinician might need to resort to the laboratory from time to time. "But when he does so let him remember that he has temporarily abdicated his position as a clinical investigator."[14]

There was conflict, however, about whether what came to be known as clinical investigation was most appropriately done at the bedside or the bench. The line was drawn clearly by Samuel Meltzer in a presidential address to the first meeting of the Association for the Advancement of Clinical Research in 1909 when he said,

> To my mind it is a fact that the leading clinicians of this generation do not compare favorably with their predecessors in this country, not to speak of a comparison with the leaders of clinical medicine in other countries. One of the reasons for the retardation in progress is the loss to clinical medicine of the brainy men who now devote their energies to the pure sciences of medicine.[15]

A decade later Knud Faber pointed out that there was "a signal difference between the physiological and the clinical study of functional disturbances," by which he meant disturbances that leave no anatomical trace.

> The main object of the clinical study is first to find what has caused the disturbance in the normal life of the organism, and then to understand how the cause has given rise to that series of law-directed phenomena designated by the name of disease. While the physiologist works back to normal function from the observed disorder, the clinician is primarily in quest of the cause of the disorder; the functional disturbance is chiefly of interest to him as a means to this end.[16]

He went on to say that functional diagnosis, though originally not concerned with classification, had "shared the fate of all other clinical methods; they all lead ultimately to new classifications, to the dissociation of non-homogeneous processes, and the consolidation of homogeneous ones." There were several reasons why the study of functional disturbance had led to greater progress in nosography than had been made when pathological anatomy was the only guide. First, "objective and measurable criteria have been provided which supplement and extend the information obtained through study of the subjective symptoms alone." Second, "the investigation of function has greatly contributed to the development of methods for locating the seat of disease." And finally, "through functional diagnosis, affections, functional disturbances, in organs or cells which never become the seat of anatomically demonstrable changes, can be demonstrated."[17]

Thus clinical research would both take its inspiration from and lead back to the bedside, for it was from the understanding of causes of functional disorders—which is to say, those in which no structural change is demonstrable[18]—that new and useful classifications for the clinician would emerge. This new etiological principle of classification was a legacy of bacteriology. It was important because proper classification allowed the physician to act by giving him a category which included not only cause but natural history and, therefore, prognosis. Faber was, however, too sophisticated to allow himself to fall into the realist trap satirized by Shaw and excoriated by Crookshank. He commented that

> All concepts of disease, like all other concepts denoting species, are human abstractions, not objective entities. Philosophically speaking, everything is fluent; but to the physician who is to live and act in the world, it is necessary to have definite categories of disease to serve as guides and tools.[19]

For Faber, then, classifications of disease were not classifications of real entities. The measure of their truth was the pragmatic one of the degree to which they improved the precision of prognosis and therapy, or prediction and control. They could always be changed when new information permitted "better" ways of classifying. Such pragmatic measures of truth seem particularly appropriate for practicing rather than learned professions, for the former act in and on the world whereas the latter are more likely to regard the world contemplatively.[20] Faber wrote,

> Every time any important advance is made in this field it is considered in the clinic to be a great feat, and the description of a new disease is of extremely great importance in practical medicine. To the physiologist and the worker in the laboratory, morbid categories are subordinate concepts, but to the physician, to the clinician, the reverse is the case; he cannot live, cannot speak, cannot act without them.[21]

For Faber nosographical entities made clinical work possible. Indeed, while drawing on the insights of the laboratory, it was the elucidation of specific diseases that justified the clinician's role, for it provided the means of classifying patients in ways that made rational action possible. Classification thus distinguished clinicians from laboratory workers and served as a rationale for their unique contribution.

It is significant, however, that Faber regarded etiology as an important classificatory principle, one that was necessary as a guide for appropriate action. As we shall see, more recently etiology has receded as a significant classificatory principle for some clinicians. Perhaps this is because in Faber's time etiology was still such a new principle that to be scientific one had to make it a central part of one's classification. Now that diagnostic tests and procedures are so much more advanced and have become so central to diagnostic work-ups, clinical information is less relevant to making an etiological diagnosis, and the clinician's task has been devalued. Reasserting the importance of the clinician means re-establishing the importance of clinical data.

Throughout the 1920s and 1930s, as concern with the laboratory study of functional disorders continued to expand with the newly developing schools of medicine, occasional voices of protest were raised both within the establishment and without, objecting that the individual patient was being lost from view. For example, in his 1927 address titled "The care of the patient," Francis Weld Peabody said, "The most common criticism made at present by older practitioners is that young graduates have been taught a great deal about mechanisms of disease, but very little about the practice of medicine—or, to put it more bluntly, they are too 'scientific' and do not know how to take care of patients."[22] He asked rhetorically, "In an era of internal medicine . . . which takes pride in the fact that it concerns itself with the functional capacity of organs rather than with mere structural changes and which has developed so many 'functional tests' of kidneys, heart, and liver, is it not rather narrow minded to limit one's interest to those disturbances of function which are based on anatomic abnormalities?"[23] He estimated that, excluding patients with acute infections, half the remaining patients seen by physicians "complained of symptoms for which an adequate organic cause could not be discovered. . . . Here . . . is a great group of patients in which it is not the disease but the man or the woman who needs to be treated."[24]

A decade later G. Canby Robinson's book *The Patient as a Person* appeared, which was a large study of the responses of patients to diseases.[25] He agreed with Peabody, as well as with Walter Cannon,[26] that emotions could cause functional disorders which could in turn cause anatomically observable diseases. In this context he made the by now familiar distinction between illness and disease. "Illness is subjective and consists of disturbances of health recognized and described or indicated by the affected individual, while disease is objective and is recognized by the observation of doctors."[27] He went on to say that "disease is only one element of illness, and is not the only cause of disturbances of the activities and functions of the body,"[28] by which he seems to have meant that mental processes—that is, illness—could cause physical disorders. He also argued, as did many of his contemporaries, that physicians had to be cognizant of functional disorders or else risk losing patients to unscientific healers such as Christian Scientists who would help them with their distress. He quoted the pragmatist philosopher John Dewey approvingly:

> Just in the degree in which a physician is an artist in his work he uses his science, no matter how extensive and accurate, to furnish him with tools of inquiry into the individual case, and with methods of forecasting a method of dealing with it. Just in the degree in which, no matter how great his learning, he subordinates the individual case to some classification of disease and some generic rule of treatment, he sinks to the level of the routine mechanic.[29]

Which is to suggest that classifications, while perhaps serving a useful purpose, could if mechanically applied obscure the individual patient's experience of disease. The distinction between illness and disease was thus an attempt to deal with both the uniqueness of the individual's experience (illness) and the more nearly universal functional derangement (disease). Significantly, however, when Robinson discussed the individual problems of the patients in his study, he classified them by disease, suggesting that the problems faced by people with a particular disease had much in common, no matter how much their individual circumstances might differ. More importantly, the patient's personal and social circumstances were not assimilated to the classification of diseases but remained unique and individual, the subject of the art of medicine.

These two examples could be multiplied several fold and are meant simply to suggest that some physicians believed that, to paraphrase Whitehead, medicine was being drawn to the pole of mathematical abstraction and away from the uniqueness of the individual patient. Robinson's efforts to create a taxonomy of patients was an attempt—finally unsuccessful—to resolve the tension. Indeed, within a decade laboratory research was to begin an unprecedented expansion, for after World War II the federal government became increasingly involved in fostering research through the development of the National Institutes of Health (NIH). Support was so generous, indeed, that Paul Beeson has observed elsewhere in this volume that he occasionally wondered what else he should be asking for.

The growth of NIH in the 1950s and 1960s produced more clinical investigators and more medical literature than had ever existed before, and led to considerable advances in knowledge of the etiology and therapy of a wide assortment of disorders.[30] Although opinions differed, clinical investigation was understood by many to mean that the relevant problems were related to diseases in human beings, and warnings against the separation of bedside and bench were made.[31] There was, however, evidence that an increasing number of investigators during the 1950s and 1960s were not dealing with either diseases or humans but rather with "nonhuman, nondisease" topics.[32]

In what was perhaps the most extensive discussion of clinical research, Alvan Feinstein argued that academic physicians had been attracted by NIH funding patterns to laboratory work, where they competed at a disadvantage with Ph.D. scientists, and had forsaken the bedside, where their expertise lay and where their contribution could be greatest.[33] Those contributions were not so much in explaining the etiology of diseases as in predicting their outcome and prescribing appropriate therapy.[34] The growing sophistication of laboratory research into etiology meant that physicians could not hope to do it as well as Ph.D.s and still retain their clinical competence. The physician's unique contribution would not be in studying etiology and pathogenesis but in studying the course of disease in human beings in order to improve prognostic and therapeutic capacities.

But for prognosis and therapy to be accurate, clinical observations had to be organized in ways that had not been given adequate attention, largely because clinicians had been diverted to laboratory work. Drawing on Boolean algebra and set theory, Feinstein suggested a "new taxonomic system for classifying the different clinical subgroups that constitute the diverse spectrum of a human disease. Without those classifications, clinicians had often analyzed each disease as though it were a single homogeneous fruit salad, rather than a mixture of heterogeneous fruits."[35] All other classifications had been designed for mutually exclusive categories[36] and had not considered the "overlappingness"[37] of things, something made possible by these new concepts and the use of computers. Clinical data are used to classify and stage patients' problems—for example, with regard to severity—in order to predict outcome and guide therapy. Set theory makes it possible for the investigator to do clinical staging and, once enough data are available, to assign outcome probabilities to each stage. Indeed, it is the clinician's job to collect such data and assign probabilities.

> If properly used, the computer will improve the practice of medicine by restoring attention to the *patient* in clinical science. The previous technology of the past century has pushed the patient out of the doctor's mind—replacing clinical evidence with the "scientific" data of disease or of human parts or fragments; replacing human symptoms and signs with the data of variables that had to be isolated and "controlled" be-

> cause no mathematical or technologic models existed to deal with multiple, overlapping, simultaneously independent, discrete categories of information. The computer can help expand the human horizon of clinical medicine by enabling scientific attention to be given to the clinical and personal descriptions of sick people, instead of restricting "science" to the dehumanized dimensions of laboratory data.[38]

It is not my intention to explicate Feinstein's work in any detail. The point is, simply, that by drawing on new technology and the new mathematics to classify clinical observations, he provided scientific legitimacy for clinical research aimed at removing the distinction between illness and disease[39] and by so doing improving prognostic and therapeutic ability. His use of the notion of illness was, however, different from the use to which Robinson had put it. Robinson meant that anxiety, family circumstances, and social situation all influenced the onset, course, and management of disease. Feinstein meant that subjective reports of the patient's state might be calibrated, at least roughly, and used in assessing prognosis.

Events were soon to make his proposals attractive to an increasing number of academic physicians, becoming part of the intellectual equipment of the new field of general internal medicine. The passage of Medicare and Medicaid in the mid-1960s, the escalation of the costs of care, and subsequent efforts at cost containment since the 1970s have had profound consequences and have ramified throughout academic medicine. Since the early 1970s NIH obligated funds have increased only slightly in constant dollars.[40] Fewer physicians are seeking academic careers as clinical investigators and more NIH grants are going to Ph.D.s. The clinical investigator is said to be an endangered species[41] and his habitat is said to be threatened as well.[42] As costs have risen, NIH support has become relatively less significant as a share of the budget of most academic medical centers, whereas clinical income has increased in both absolute and relative terms.[43] The result is a two-or three-track promotion system, with investigators and clinicians formally separated, and with more and more stringent requirements placed on entry into the research track.

Under such conditions, and as cost containment within hospitals has become more and more important, clinical epidemiology has become a way in which to do scientific research that is fundable because it may help to rationalize therapy and make it less expensive. Indeed, effectiveness of containing the costs of care is one of the rationales given for supporting programs in general internal medicine.

Related to changes in funding of research is the very profound impact of molecular biology on biomedical research. Gordon Gill has written in elegiac terms of the disappearance of the physician-scientist, who is no longer able to do basic research and remain a clinician both because the support of research and training have changed and because developments have moved too rapidly for clinicians to keep up with them.

> No one wishes to mourn the past. The new division of labor will likely bring about real benefits for the sick and afflicted more rapidly than ever before possible. It is worth marking, though, an era, a spirit, a time when those in academic medicine rightly or wrongly believed themselves in touch, in the mainstream of originality and creativity, when they were excited about what they were doing and religiously devoted to investigation; a time when this excitement was communicated to medical students, to the talented younger people; a time when one looked to colleagues for the next advance, the next theory, the next hypothesis, the next breakthrough. The advances in sciences will still be taught, but now those in academic medicine will look to their colleagues, not for exciting scientific ideas, but instead for ideas about delivery of health care, new diagnostic tests, new drugs for clinical use, faculty salary plans, hospitals, and medicare. As the private practice of medicine becomes more restrictive, academic medicine may again look more attractive to residents, but they will enter as academic physicians, not as physician-scientists.[44]

Thus, with the explanatory sciences moving rapidly in directions which clinicians find increasing difficult to follow, much less lead, the institutionalization of general internal medicine provides grounds for considering oneself a scientist even as one remains a clinician. Some, like Gill, view the change with regret; others have seized on it as an opportunity. Indeed, "clinimetrics" is proposed as yet another basic science of clinical medicine, one concerned with the methods by which reproducible observations may be made to enhance the physician's prognostic and therapeutic capabilities, rather than with explanation of etiology and pathogenesis.[45]

Finally, the growth of family medicine, originally stimulated by the cultural revolution of the 1960s and by state and federal concern with the distribution of primary care physicians, has resulted in defensive moves by internal medicine.[46] The professional ideology of the new specialty was holistic care of the individual patient. In this it was similar to, and influenced by, developments in British General Practice, of which David Armstrong has written, "GPs who attempted to measure morbidity in their practices, increasingly found themselves accepting the seeking of medical advice or 'spells of sickness' as the criteria of morbidity. In effect, patient-based criteria began to replace nosological referrents in the identification of illness."[47]

In response, it was acknowledged by a variety of academic internists that subspecialization has perhaps gone too far, that the generalist function must be reclaimed,[48] and that the Oslerian tradition is dead.[49] Edmund Pellegrino has made a case for the "generalist function" in primary, secondary, and tertiary care, which he believes differs from the primary care role of family physicians.

> What, then, is the generalist function? Specifically, it subsumes the whole train of processes—intellectual and practical—whereby the uncategorized patient is evaluated, his needs identified and placed in order of priority, and a plan and a set of decisions mapped out optimally to meet those needs. The subject is either the patient who has not yet been categorized as belonging to some specialty; or the patient who has been categorized, but develops new signs or symptoms; or finally, the patient who has problems simultaneously in more than one organ system or specialty. The intellectual function of the generalist is to categorize, continually to revalidate the categorization, and to relate categories to each other.[50]

At the primary care level the family physician may do many of these same things, as well as others for which the internist is not equipped. At secondary and tertiary levels of care, however, the general internist has a unique role to play: "The demands on the generalists in tertiary care are particularly rigorous and particularly necessary. Categorization of needs is more difficult and coordination of specialties and disciplines more complicated."[51]

Thus the general internist's job is one of classifying patients and their diseases. At the primary care level it may overlap with the responsibilities of the family physician. At secondary and tertiary care levels it is clearly different, and "sections of general medicine in departments of medicine or internal medicine . . . must not be eroded . . . by ill-advised attempts to teach family medicine or by being limited to primary care per se."[52]

To potential critics who argue that this new specialty with these new classificatory concerns is in danger of "further dehumaniz[ing] clinical medicine," Alvan Feinstein has replied that in fact concern with classifying symptoms and signs—which is to say, illness and disease—will have the effect of refocussing the attention of students, house officers, and physicians on patients and their subjective reports of the illness experience. Hence, he claims, it should help rehumanize rather than further dehumanize medicine.[53] Others have made similar claims, adding that the general internist is ideally suited to be the patient's advocate within the bewildering maze that medical care has become.[54]

Thus in response to changes in support for research, the rapid growth of laboratory science, increasing efforts at cost containment, and threats from other primary care specialties, general internal medicine has made an effort to reclaim its heritage as the premier clinical specialty for which diagnosis and prognosis are the hallmarks. Classification is therefore central to the concern of this specialty, for it is, to paraphrase Whitehead once more, a halfway house between the uniqueness of the individual patient and the abstractions of laboratory science.

The example of general internal medicine suggests that a new specialty may not arise only in response to the creation of new knowledge or new technology. It may arise in response to a perception that a new social or institutional problem has developed which must be solved. In this case knowledge is created after the fact by a group seeking to use it to gain legitimacy as a specialty. The development of new ways of classifying patients and diseases for managerial purposes is an example of what I mean. A similar example comes from an allied field, hospital management. I refer to the development of Diagnosis Related Groups (DRGs) and their use as a device by which costs, and physicians, may be controlled. I quote from one of the developers of this new classification system:

> Concern over the rising costs of medical care has resulted in increased pressure on hospitals to control patient care costs through the adoption of more efficient management techniques, such as those commonly employed by manufacturing firms. The successful transfer of these methods to the hospital sector requires a structure for examining utilization of services and for establishing standards and criteria for identifying areas which require improvement. The first step in providing this structure is to determine what the hospital is producing.[55]

DRGs constitute a classification of hospital products, "the goods and services (a hospital) provides its patients."[56] They are based on a limited set of variables: diagnosis, age, surgical procedures, and so on. Once the relevant data are entered into a computer, a ready-made program places the patient in the proper diagnosis-related group. Those patients whose costs and/or lengths of stay are beyond the norms established for the particular category may then be readily identified, along with the physician responsible for their care.[57] Education and even discipline of deviant practitioners thus becomes a real possibility, made easier by the fact that the growing number of physicians dependent on hospitals makes them increasingly vulnerable to the bargaining power of administrators and hospital chains.[58]

The analogy of the hospital as a manufacturing firm is instructive, for it calls to mind the useful point made by a number of (usually Marxist) observers of the health care system, that physicians, the archetypal free professionals, are not simply becoming bureaucratized by perhaps even proletarianized. Proletarianization, after all, refers to the loss of autonomy by craftsmen and the ability of their employers to exercise discipline when they do not conform to the rules of the factory. Although it is true that physicians produce much of the information on which DRGs are based, its codification and accessibility mean that no longer are they in control of the use to which it is put—far from it. There is considerable variability in the way different physicians treat the same conditions.[59] The ready availability of computer-generated profiles of treatment means that greater uniformity can be imposed on the system and that it does not require a physician to do it.[60]

The point is, simply, that we see in this brief example first, one of the ways new professions emerge and ascend to power and second, the part the power to define and classify relevant phenomena plays in the process. It was not that the growth of knowledge or technology made the ascent of hospital management inevitable. True, DRGs would be difficult to produce without computers, but computers alone were not sufficient. What was necessary was the development of the perception that medical care was costing the government too much money and the power acquired by government to manage the problem. This may seem so obvious as to be trivial, but I think not. We usually assume that it is the growth of knowledge and the development of technology that causes new specialties and new occupations to develop. That is only one way. Another way has to do with the creation of knowledge by groups concerned with the management of what is perceived to be a problem. In this case, as I have already suggested, knowledge is developed after the fact in order to acquire professional status and power.[61] If control over the definition and classification of a problem is one criterion by which professional status may be gauged, then Diagnosis Related Groups may be viewed as the means by which an increasingly powerful health care profession has advanced its claims.

Conclusion

The points I have wanted to make are the following. First, the division of labor is associated with the proliferation of technical vocabularies and classifications for pragmatic purposes, with the nominalism that characterizes most classifications, and with the fact that classifications may be used as professional ideologies to advance the claims and defend the interests of particular groups.

Second, there may well be a technological imperative that inevitably results in the division of labor, but there is also what might be called the professional imperative: the drive by groups of individuals to solve social or other kinds of problems by organizing into occupations that attempt to gain a mandate and license from society to be in charge of particular problems, which is to say, to become professions.[62] In this case the knowledge base often develops after the profession or specialty has been created. My impression is that this occurs primarily in the service professions, but I offer that as only a tentative suggestion. I do think it accurately describes the development of both general internal medicine and hospital management, among others.[63] In each case, the knowledge base that has been created includes a taxonomy of the problems of special concern to the group. In each case, too, the classification system has acquired ideological coloration as well as pragmatic value because it is used as a means of justifying the activities of the profession or specialty in addition to guiding its practice.

My final point has to do with the question raised by the quotation from Yeats which I have used as an epigraph: "O body swayed to music, O brightening glance, / How can we know the dancer from the dance?"—or the diseased person from the disease process? Classifications have been the way physicians and other healers have abstracted common qualities from otherwise unique sick individuals, no doubt doing violence to the special features of each person's experience.[64] It is evidently a necessary activity, however, not only for physicians but for patients as well. Applying a name to a previously disorganized complex of signs and symptoms may be word magic, as Crookshank insisted, but it creates order where before there was chaos. Sometimes it imposes a spurious order; at other times, presumably, it reflects, however imperfectly, an underlying order. Whatever the case, affixing a name universalizes the patient's condition. It is no longer unique and thus no longer uniquely terrifying. Naming and classifying imply dominion over that which is classified. The power may be illusory, but it is comforting nonetheless, for as T. S. Eliot has written,[65] "Human kind cannot bear very much reality."

I am grateful to Theodore M. Brown, Bradford H. Gray, Russell C. Maulitz, and Matthew C. Riddle for much useful advice, not all of which I have taken.

NOTES

1. A. N. Whitehead, *Science and the Modern World* (New York: The Free Press, 1967), 28.

2. P. L. Berger and T. Luckmann, *The Social Construction of Reality* (Garden City, NY: Doubleday Anchor Books, 1967), 123–24, italics in original.

3. George Bernard Shaw, *The Doctor's Dilemma* (Baltimore: Penguin Books, 1965), 107–8, written in 1913. See also J. Ettling, *The Germ of Laziness* (Cambridge: Harvard University Press, 1981) and K. C. Carter, "The Germ Theory, Beriberi, and the Deficiency Theory of Disease," *Med Hist* 21 (1977):119–36 and "Germ Theory, Hysteria, and Freud's Early Work in Psychopathology," *Med Hist* 24 (1980):259–74.

4. F. G. Crookshank, "The Importance of a Theory of Signs and a Critique of Language in the Study of Medicine," in *The Meaning of Meaning*, C. K. Ogden and I. A. Richards, eds. (New York: Harcourt, Brace and Company, 1930), 343 Suppl. II. Emphasis in original. See also F. G. Crookshank, introductory essay on the relation of history and philosophy to medicine, in *An Introduction to the History of Medicine*, C. G. Cumston, ed. (New York: Alfred A. Knopf, 1926).

5. Indeed, one function of clerkships and residency training is to reduce this sort of ambiguity by teaching through exemplification.

6. Crookshank, "Theory of Signs," 342.

7. R. C. Maultiz, "'Physician versus Bacteriologist': The Ideology of Science in Clinical Medicine," in *The Therapeutic Revolution*, M. J. Vogel and C. E. Rosenberg, eds. (Philadelphia: University of Pennsylvania Press, 1979), 92.

8. H. D. Rolleston, "The Classification and Nomenclature of Disease, with Remarks on Diseases Due to Treatment," *Lancet* May 22 (1909:1437).

9. Rolleston, "Classification and Nomenclature of Disease," 1437.

10. Rolleston, "Classification and Nomenclature of Disease," 1439.

11. Rolleston, "Classification and Nomenclature," 1438–39.

12. Something very like what Rolleston advocated seems to be emerging in the form of procedure-based subspecialties in internal medicine, such as pulmonary disease and gastroenterology, which "experienced a great fillip when the flexible endoscope came into use." See P. B. Beeson, "The Natural History of Medical Subspecialties," *Ann Intern Med* 93 (1980):624–26.

13. F. G. Blake, "Clinical Investigation," *Science* 74 (1931): 27–29.

14. Blake, "Clinical Investigation," 28.

15. S. J. Meltzer, "The Science of Clinical Medicine," *JAMA* 53 (1909):511.

16. K. Faber, *Nosography: The Evolution of Clinical Medicine in Modern Times* (New York: Paul B. Hoeber, 1930), 163–64.

17. Faber, *Nosography*, 165–67.

18. F. K. Taylor, *The Concepts of Illness, Disease, and Morbus* (Cambridge: Cambridge University Press, 1979).

19. Faber, *Nosography*, 207–8.

20. C. I. Lewis, "A Pragmatic Conception of the *a priori*." *J Philos* 20 (1923): 169–77, especially 174.

21. Faber, *Nosography*, 211.

22. F. W. Peabody, "The Care of the Patient," *JAMA* 88 (1927):877.

23. Peabody, "Care of the Patient," 880.

24. Peabody, "Care of the Patient," 879–80.

25. G. C. Robinson, *The Patient as a Person* (New York: The Commonwealth Fund, 1939).

26. W. B. Cannon, "The Role of Emotion in Disease," *Ann Intern Med* 9 (1936):1453–65. I am grateful to Theodore M. Brown for calling this reference to my attention and for suggesting to me the significance of psychosomatic medicine for internal medicine and physiologic research in the 1920s and 1930s. His own work on this topic is currently in preparation.

27. Robinson, *Patient*, 4.

28. Robinson, *Patient*, 4.

29. Robinson, *Patient*, 6.

30. P. B. Beeson, "How to Foster the Gain of Knowledge About Disease." *Perspect Biol* 23 (1980) (Suppl.):9–24.

31. D. W. Seldin, "Some Reflections on the Role of Basic Research and Service in Clinical Departments," *JCI* 45 (1966):976–79 and P. B. Beeson, "The Academic Doctor," *Trans Assoc Am Physicians* 80 (1967):1–7.

32. A. R. Feinstein, N. Koss, and J. H. M. Austin, "The Changing Emphasis in Clinical Research, I. Topics Under Investigation," *Ann Intern Med* 66 (1967): 396–419.

33. A. R. Feinstein, *Clinical Judgment* (Baltimore: Williams & Wilkins, 1967), 35.

34. Feinstein, *Clinical Judgment*, 25.

35. Feinstein, *Clinical Judgment*, 11.

36. Feinstein, *Clinical Judgment*, 10. See also L. D. Stoddard, "Toward a New Human Pathology: I. Biopathological Populations, or Sets: A Substitute for the Old Pathology's Diseases," *Hum Pathol* 11 (1980):228–39.

37. A. O. Lovejoy, *The Great Chain of Being* (Cambridge: Harvard University Press, 1936), 57.

38. Feinstein, *Clinical Judgment*, 370–71. Emphasis in original. See also M. A. Woodbury, J. Clive, and A. Garson, "Mathematical Typology: A Grade of Membership Technique for Obtaining Disease Definition," *Comput Biomed Res* 11 (1978):277–98 and J. Clive, M. A. Woodbury, and I. C. Siegler, "Fuzzy and Crisp Set-theoretic-based Classification of Health and Disease," *J Med Syst* 7 (1983): 317–32.

39. Feinstein, *Clinical Judgment*, 24–25.

40. D. S. Fredrickson, "Biomedical Research in the 1980s," *N Engl J Med* 304 (1981):509–17.

41. J. B. Wyngaarden, "The Clinical Investigator as an Endangered Species," *N Engl J Med* 301 (1979):1254–59.

42. R. S. Ross, "Boundaries of the General Clinical Research Center in an Academic Medical Center," *Clin Res* 33 (1985):105–10; D. E. Rogers, *American Medicine, Challenge for the 1980s* (Cambridge: Ballinger Publishing, 1978), part II; D. E. Rogers and R. J. Blendon, "The Academic Medical Center: A Stressed American Institution," *N Engl J Med* 298 (1978):940–50; and W. B. Schwartz, J. P. Newhouse, and A. P. Williams, "Is the Teaching Hospital an Endangered Species?" *N Engl J Med* 313 (1985): 157–62.

43. R. H. Ebert and S. S. Brown, "Academic Health Centers," *N Engl J Med* 308 (1983):1200–8.

44. G. Gill, "The End of the Physician-Scientist?" 368.

45. A. R. Feinstein, "An Additional Basic Science for Clinical Medicine," *Ann*

Intern 99 (1983):393–97, 544–50, 705–12, 843–48. D. L. Sackett, R. B. Haynes, and P. Tugwell, *Clinical Epidemiology: A Basic Science for Clinical Medicine* (Boston: Little, Brown, 1985).

46. R. G. Petersdorf, "Internal Medicine and Family Practice; Controversies, Conflict and Compromise," *N Engl J. Med* 293 (1975):326–32.

47. D. Armstrong, *The Political Anatomy of the Body* (Cambridge: Cambridge University Press, 1983), 79.

48. D. E. Rogers, "On Technologic Restraint," *Arch Intern Med* 135 (1975): 1393–97.

49. W. Regelson, "The Weakening of the Oslerian Tradition: The Changing Emphasis in Departments of Medicine," *JAMA* 239 (1978):317–19.

50. E. D. Pellegrino, "Internal Medicine and the Functions of the Generalist: Some Notes on a New Synergy," *Clin Res* 24 (1976):253.

51. Pellegrino, "Internal Medicine and the Generalist," 256.

52. Pellegrino, "Internal Medicine and the Generalist," 256.

53. Feinstein, "An Additional Basic Science," 848.

54. J. M. Eisenberg, "The Sculpture of a New Academic Discipline: Four Faces of Academic General Internal Medicine," *Am J Med* 78 (1985):283–92.

55. R. B. Fetter, "Diagnosis Related Groups: The Product of the Hospital," *Clin Res* 32 (1984):336–40.

56. Fetter, "Diagnosis Related Groups," 336.

57. L. F. McMahon, Jr., "Diagnosis-Related Group Prospective Payment: Effect on Medical Quality Assurance," *Eval Health Prof* 7 (1984):25–41.

58. G. S. Omenn and D. A. Conrad, "Implications of DRGs for Clinicians," *N Engl J Med* 311 (1984):1314–17.

59. J. E. Wennberg, K. McPherson, and P. Caper, "Will Payment Based on Diagnosis-Related Groups Control Hospital Costs?" *N Engl J Med* 311 (1984): 295–300.

60. B. E. Spivey, "The Relation Between Hospital Management and Medical Staff Under a Prospective-payment System," *N Engl J Med* 310 (1984):984–86.

61. I have dealt with this issue at greater length in the following article: "The Historical Roots and Ideological Functions of Disease Concepts in Three Primary Care Specialties," *Bull Hist Med* 57 (1983):412–32.

62. E. Friedson, *Profession of Medicine* (New York: Dodd Mead, 1970).

63. For example, family medicine, psychiatry, nursing, and social work.

64. R. Baron, "An Introduction to Medical Phenomenology," *Ann Intern Med* 103 (1985):606–11.

65. T. S. Eliot, "Murder in the Cathedral," in *The Complete Poems and Plays, 1909–1950* (New York: Harcourt, Brace and Company, 1952).

10

Notes from the Underground: The Social Organization of Therapeutic Research

HARRY M. MARKS

In the latter half of the twentieth century, physicians benefit from a miraculous array of drugs and devices capable of altering the course of disease at the cellular, even the molecular, level. Accompanying these developments have been a series of innovations in the evaluation of new therapies, culminating in the randomized controlled trial (RCT). The contemporary clinical trial, incorporating randomized assignment of patients and "blinded" assessment of outcomes, represents an unparalleled technique for measuring the value of novel treatments: "No other method for studying the merits of clinical treatment regimens can approach the precision of estimating effects and the strength of inference permitted by sound RCTs."[1]

Historical accounts of the clinical trial have followed the lead of statisticians in presenting a tale of forgotten ancestors and notable conceptual breakthroughs.[2] The insights and methodological innovations of these intellectual pioneers form an essential part of the story. When they take center stage, however, a peculiar narrative results in which history is blindly driven forward by scientific progress.[3] Yet it is difficult to read repeatedly about James Lind's prophylactic trial for scurvy in the eighteenth-century British navy or Pierre Louis' experiments with blood-letting in nineteenth-century Paris without beginning to wonder, What took everybody else so long to catch on?[4]

In this chapter I argue that clinical researchers conceived of controlled clinical studies before they had the means to carry them out. The obstacles they faced were as much social and organizational as conceptual. Researchers desiring to conduct a well-planned therapeutic experiment not only had to develop the necessary financial and institutional resources to initiate such studies, but they had to adopt social norms and organizational controls which would ensure that a plan of study, once agreed on, would be carried out according to that agreement. The modern RCT, with its management in the hands of a coordinating bureau of statisticians, ultimately offered the most secure guarantee of such cooperative behavior.

In 1975 Harry Dowling drew attention to a series of now forgotten efforts at clinical research, commencing with the Cooperative Clinical Group's investigation of syphilis treatments (1928–1935) and culminating in the studies of tuberculosis treatment and prevention by the Veterans Administration (VA) and the Public Health Service (PHS) after World War II.[5] In a subsequent era of randomized, double-blinded trials, these investigations represented mistakes of the past which statisticians were eager to forget. What makes them historically interesting is the possibility that their defects had little to do with any intellectual failings on the investigators' part, and very much to do with the social conditions under which therapeutic research was then conducted.[6]

The history of these studies is nonetheless not without intellectual interest. What made them stand out in the eyes of contemporaries was, in part, that they were collaborative enterprises. Earlier generations of researchers held no particular ideological brief for the virtues of cooperation. Rather, cooperative studies were a unique device for overcoming the limited vision and opportunities of individuals. Their special appeal was in promising to combine several investigative virtues in one: gathering large numbers of patients to offset the effects of spontaneous recoveries; bringing the combined judgments of experienced investigators to bear on a problem to offset the effects of individual bias; and, so far as was possible, specifying in advance the means and techniques for selecting patients, delivering treatment, and evaluating results. Where we rely on method and procedure to secure the intellectual integrity of therapeutic research, our predecessors relied on organization and experience.

In the following account, experimental controls, in anything like the modern sense, make their appearance rather late. This is not because therapeutic researchers failed to understand the role of chance in creating the illusion of effective treatment—quite the opposite. The ideas that patients undergo spontaneous recoveries, that physicians often credit these recoveries, mistakenly, to treatment, and that large numbers of patients must be studied to offset these effects occur in tandem in critical discussions of therapeutic research. But in the protostatistical intellectual universe that these scientists inhabited, chance was an enemy of knowledge rather than an ally, working its most powerful effects when the researcher was ignorant of "true" causes.[7] In the evolution of therapeutic experimentation, the deterministic world of the laboratory served as a model which clinical research could only approximate:

> Clinical observations can be made . . . just as accurate as laboratory observations; but in the human subject, observation cannot be as readily controlled, the conditions cannot be easily kept uniform or varied—in one word, the problems cannot be analyzed, as they can be in the animal.[8]

Unable to stabilize the conditions of clinical research, investigators sought to master an irreducible uncertainty by accumulating experience. Experience brought detailed knowledge of the vagaries of specific disease and the opportunity to make continued observations on large numbers of patients. This made therapeutic evaluation a task for the specialist. The inexperienced, those with too diverse a clinical practice, and those without access to laboratory and hospital facilities were unsuited for the task.[9] By convening groups of experts, cooperative studies further enhanced specialists' ability to assess the value of new therapies and establish their most appropriate uses.

The following section takes up the story of the Cooperative Clinical Group, which pioneered in the development of multi-institutional therapeutic investigations. Their efforts foundered on a series of deficiencies, not the least of which was a lack of institutional and financial resources for conducting therapeutic research. Cooperative investigations during and after World War II did not, by and large, suffer from a comparable lack of money or qualified personnel. Those directing research into the value of penicillin and streptomycin still found it difficult to restrain physicians unwilling to relinquish control of patient management to an investigative protocol. The scope of these difficulties, and organizers' efforts to overcome them, are described in later sections of this chapter.

The Cooperative Clinical Group

In March 1928 John H. Stokes, Professor of Dermatology and Syphilology at the University of Pennsylvania and scientific advisor for the newly organized Committee on Research in Syphilis, invited a small group of colleagues to join him in a multiclinic "attack" on the problems of treating syphilis.[10] The opportunity Stokes envisioned promised little money but offered "perhaps a little glory and certainly a wonderful chance to do something in research in syphilis in this country."[11] If the experts could agree on uniform standards for selecting, classifying, treating, and evaluating patients, then the effects of various treatments might be reliably compared.[12]

Stokes' associates were among the country's leading clinical specialists in syphilis: Udo Wile, Professor of Dermatology and Syphilology at the University of Michigan; Joseph Earle Moore, Professor at Johns Hopkins who, like Stokes, was at work on one of the first textbooks to summarize the "modern" treatment of syphilis; Paul O'Leary, who had taken over from Stokes as Head of the Dermatology Section at the Mayo Clinic in 1924; Harold Cole, a respected dermatologist at Western Reserve, and a close associate of the therapeutic reformer, Torald Sollman; and Thomas Parran, Jr., New York State's Commissioner of Health.[13] By coordinating their efforts, the Cooperative Group could provide an authoritative basis for judging the merits of both current and future syphilis treatments: "We want very much to get the cooperation of certain recognized syphilis clinics which can come up to the standard required for this type of investigative work."[14]

The physician treating syphilis in the late 1920s faced an embarrassment of riches: a diversity of drugs and an even greater diversity of opinions about how to use them. To Paul Ehrlich's salvarsan (arsphenamine), introduced in 1910, pharmaceutical research had added neoarsphenamine and a variety of other arsenical compounds designed to potentiate the more toxic effects of Ehrlich's drug.[15] Easier to prepare and safer to administer, the newer arsenicals were especially favored by practitioners who did not specialize in treating syphilis. But their value was doubted in turn by some who had mastered the art of using the more potent drug.[16] Along with development of the arsenicals came improvements in more traditional treatments. Heavy metals, such as mercury, with limited powers to attack the infecting spirochetes, were nonetheless believed to promote local and general resistance to the disease, complementing the arsenicals' specific spirocheticidal effect.[17]

Even for those physicians content to work with arsphenamine, the difficulties of keeping patients in treatment once they were asymptomatic led some physicians to favor short, intensive bouts of therapy. Others held just as strongly to the need for continued long-term treatment with breaks at planned intervals.[18] Depending on a patient's symptomatology, serologic findings, and initial reactions to treatment, each physician might favor up to half a dozen treatment regimens.

The variety of remedies and treatment schedules compounded the already technically complex problem of evaluating syphilis treatments. Patients whose symptoms had cleared in the early stages of treatment were understandably reluctant to return for continued therapy and observation. Only a few clinics specializing in syphilis managed to accumulate a sufficient number of observations over a long enough period of time to distinguish the effects of treatment from those of spontaneous recovery. In the opinion of specialists, the average practitioner lacked both the resources and training to judge the value of treatments: "It does not suffice for a physician to say, 'In my experience neoarsphenamine is better than arsphenamine.' How does he know? Has he followed patients treated with one drug or the other for 5, 10, 15 years?"[19] Practitioners, it was argued, should take their lead from the experts. But apart from a general consensus about their special competence, even the experts did not agree about the merits of specific treatments.[20]

The members of the Cooperative Clinical Group, by reviewing the records of their own experiences, meant to provide a more authoritative basis for recommending one syphilis treatment over another. Once successful in their initial endeavors, they hoped to become a national resource for the evaluation of new syphilis remedies as they were developed. Studies conducted by experienced specialists would, they anticipated, be of much greater value than the haphazard evaluations sponsored by the manufacturers of new remedies.[21] The first stage of their investigation, however, would be a retrospective inquiry of treatment results at their respective clinics. The analysis of past experience would guide both future research and current clinical practice.

Questions Without Answers The simplicity of their objectives belied the complexity of the task. Awaiting the Cooperative Group were numerous unresolved questions: Which stages of syphilis and what combinations of treatment should be studied first? Which patients should be included and which kept out? Who should perform the assessments of outcomes? What constituted a treatment success and what a failure? What kinds of ancillary data, clinical and laboratory, were needed to make sense of the results? Deciding such questions is a necessary stage in any therapeutic investigation, but the characteristic that made the Cooperative Study unusual was the requirement that the investigators agree on the answers.

From the beginning the Cooperative Group was plagued with the problem they had set out to resolve: the lack of uniformity among physicians in approaches to treating syphilis. "Astonishing variations between the course pursued by different patients in the same clinic as well as between the practice of individual clinics frequently disclosed themselves."[22] Unlike the majority of physicians, the specialists in the Cooperative Group favored arsphenamine, the original and more difficult to handle arsenical. But a reliance on arsphenamine was all they had in common: how frequently they used it, the preferred dosages, and the choice of cotreatment (mercury or bismuth) varied from clinic to clinic and patient to patient.[23] Irregularities of patient attendance and the vagaries of clinic record-keeping compounded the problem of intentional variations in therapeutic practice.

Analysis of treatment outcomes proved no less problematic than the classification of regimens. Differences among the clinics in referral sources and record-keeping made it extremely difficult to document the extent of prior treatment that patients had received. Some clinics relied on the patients' reports of their prior history, while others were reluctant to do so.[24] Without consistent data about treatment history, it was difficult to say anything reliable about treatment failures. Patients who had relapsed after an initial round of treatment might easily be confused with patients who had been successfully treated and then reinfected.[25] About all that could be concluded is "that no clinical case thus far reported, including our own material satisfied all the criteria that have been proposed by students of the subject as tests for a valid reinfection."[26]

Conclusions about the rates of treatment success were similarly at risk; without consistent data on treatment history, it might be difficult to distinguish between patients in the first stage of syphilis who had been successfully treated and patients in the early stage of secondary syphilis. Both groups might appear disease-free on serological data, but one would be cured and the other would be simply at an advanced stage of the disease in which serological testing was often negative.[27]

If the difficulties of classifying patients by stage of disease, regimen, and treatment outcome were merely technical, they might have been readily resolved. Yet each time a question seemed to be settled, it arose again.[28] Differences of opinion about how to classify patients, treatments, and outcomes were at the heart of existing therapeutic controversies: "It seems as if the question of interpretation is an individual matter for every case and accordingly the abstracting of each case would have to be conducted by the head of the department personally and then would reflect to a considerable extent his particular slant on the treatment of syphilis."[29]

The difference between an inadequate mode of treatment and the failure of an adequate treatment to cure a particular patient also depended on how different regimens were classified. Were patients who received five doses of arsphenamine in a short amount of time to be considered in the same group with patients who received more of the drug over a much longer period? It all "depends on whether from a medical angle five doses of arsphenamine in one to three months is as efficacious as fifteen doses spread through a period of six to twelve months. Doctor Stokes feels that it is, while Doctor Moore feels that it is not."[30]

The Division of Labor The organization of the work hampered efforts to arrive at a permanent consensus. Individual members took principal responsibility for specific articles: in conjunction with statistical and clerical staff provided by the Public Health Service, records were abstracted and coded according to a prearranged scheme. Questions arising from ambiguities in the data were resolved by consultation with one or, at most, two of the principals. Only when draft papers were circulated did others in the group examine in detail the improvised revisions in methods or definitions; accommodating their criticisms meant not merely redrafting the paper, but redoing the analysis.[31] Successful completion of a paper required getting "the whole thing shipped off before anyone has a chance to find some other point on which a difference may be raised."[32]

Among more pressing obligations, the project's senior investigators were unable to find time for the cooperative study. Over time, the lure of other research "work of a more spontaneous nature" grew stronger, and more of the daily work in coding and analyzing the data fell to the statistical clerks provided by the Public Health Service.[33] In the opinion of the senior physicians, these clerks lacked the clinical experience to make judgments about classifying patients and interpreting treatment outcomes. In the absence of "adequate medical counsel and constant supervision," the statistical workers were "forced by circumstances to call in what help [was available] on the spot."[34] Such delegation

> introduces into the whole study a problematical inaccuracy which, to the minds of many of the readers of the papers, may invalidate the whole material. From the records which I have reviewed with Miss Usilton . . . I know that some of them are inaccurately classified. How many are in this category and to what extent the final classification would be changed if the material were reviewed by a physician, I am unable to say.[35]

One alternative to depending on the statistical staff was to delegate the classification and coding of patient records to the more junior physicians in the clinics. Early in the study, this option was foreclosed.[36] In preparing the group's initial paper, John Stokes relied heavily on two associates he wished to reward by granting them senior authorship: "We pull together as a team, we put our shoulders to the wheel and see the drudgery through and I cannot understand why I or Wile or anyone else is entitled to absorb the glory of authorship, leaving young, enthusiastic and wholehearted co-operators with nothing but a few shekels for their side of the account."[37] Stokes saw little point in "men of established reputation" holding "tight to what little property in ideas" they had managed to accumulate.[38] His collaborators did not entirely agree: "The directors of the various schools who have collected their records over a long period of years, are entitled to more consideration than is the feeling of some assistant or graduate student who has spent a few weeks helping to compile the statistics."[39]

The basic issue, Stokes' colleagues argued, was not one of rights to intellectual property but of keeping "track of the purpose" for which the money was raised—to demonstrate that a group of physicians could see a collaborative investigation through to the end. Authorship of papers derived from jointly produced materials belonged to the Cooperative Group: "This, of course, means that the deductions made from a survey of this material are to be the combined impressions of the group and not of any single individual."[40]

Getting Out the Word Ensuring that cooperative publication reflected the group's "combined impressions" required substantial adjustments to the customary norms of writing scientific papers. The critical review of the literature, accompanied by authoritative pronouncements based on the author's experience would not work. Such summaries were "controversial," "speculative," and inevitably "a one-man" affair, entering "the uncharted field of other people's uncontrolled and uncontrollable observation." It would be better, Stokes advised, to stick to the facts revealed in the group's own records.[41]

But getting to the "facts" was not an easy matter. Stokes and Moore, the two members who had worked most with the data, were especially cognizant that behind each "fact" lay a series of decisions, often controversial and sometimes inconsistent, concerning the classification and interpretation of the data. Where they differed was on how to handle the problem. Moore held out for a uniform methodology across all their publications, an approach which Stokes deemed quixotic in the face of the group's experiences to date.[42] The best that might be done, Stokes argued, was to give prominence in their reports to the way in which the data were obtained, grouped, and interpreted.[43] In his view, only a methodical self-consciousness about its limitations distinguished the "scientific" work of the Cooperative Group from that of others:

> a scientific as distinguished from a popular standard in work of this sort demands the publication of method with fact in the first instance, even though subsequent summaries and re-statements allow the methodological part to sink into the background. We are not in this work, as I conceive it, attempting a series of syphilogical [*sic*] barber shop harmonies to be sung around a lamp-post for the edification of a public that knows no better. We are aiming at the highest standard of scientific, statistical effectiveness in critical problems, and every statement we make deserves an exhibition of the method by which it was derived.[44]

For his part, Moore worried that an overemphasis on method and the publication of numerous tables would prevent any nonexpert reader from obtaining the desired clinical information.[45]

At the Public Health Service's request, the group's initial studies were published in *Venereal Disease Information*, the house organ of the Service's Venereal Disease Division.[46] Two years after publication, Thomas Parran expressed concern that

> the detailed reports have made very little impression upon the medical profession. . . . I think a large part of the practical value of our studies will be lost unless a concerted effort is planned and put into practice for persistent propagandizing of the medical profession with the facts elicited by the studies.[47]

Publishing their findings in an obscure journal, further concealed by the detailed presentation of the methodology, did not help. But for all their careful work, the Cooperative Group did not have much to show: "We found ourselves in the unique situation of measuring one type of treatment, namely that administrated in high type clinics, while in this country at least, a large part of the syphilis treatment is in the hands of private practitioners using quite another type of treatment."[48]

The study clinics principally used arsphenamine, a drug "too complex for the practicing physician" to handle. Meanwhile, they had produced little or no data on the merits of the most commonly used treatments—neoarsphenamine, silver arsphenamine, or bismarsen—much less how these compared with arsphenamine.[49] Arsphenamine *was*, in the opinion of specialists, the treatment of choice, and establishing more precisely its therapeutic value remained a desirable objective from the Cooperative Group's point of view.[50] But they had also planned to examine the relative merits of simpler, if less effective, treatments which "would enable us to outline for the vast army of physicians who treat the majority of patients with early syphilis, if not the ideal treatment scheme, at least the best treatment scheme which they are capable of carrying through."[51] Their plans for a more comprehensive, prospective, therapeutic research foundered repeatedly on an inability to find a stable source of funding.

A Small Question of Money In financial as well as intellectual terms, therapeutic evaluation in this period resided in a no man's land between laboratory research and public health projects aimed at demonstrating the benefits of community programs in the detection or prevention of disease. The interest of foundations was either in subsidizing new advances in medical knowledge or in convincing communities to devote their energies and resources to proven interventions.[52] The Cooperative Group's emphasis on the more rigorous evaluation of existing and novel treatments for syphilis fell somewhere between the two.[53]

Heads of clinics looked to the cooperative study as a means to fill the existing gaps in research support, which fell mostly in the area of clinical investigation.[54] Stokes and Moore, especially, were not merely looking for someone to subsidize the evaluation of specific antisyphilitic remedies but to underwrite their general program of clinical research.[55] A lack of funding nearly derailed the Cooperative Group at the start, when sponsors of the Committee on Research in syphilis developed second thoughts about putting their money into clinical, rather than laboratory research.[56] Only a generous donation from H. H. Timken of "Timken Roller Bearing" fame enabled the retrospective studies of arsphenamine to begin.[57]

If finding interested money was difficult, getting money from sources that were interested *and* respectable was even more problematic. Whenever the group's finances seemed shaky, Stokes and Moore suggested an approach to "responsible" drug firms.[58] At present, Moore argued, a manufacturer with a promising new drug had

> two alternatives. He can either ship small quantities of the drug to several hundred Dr. Whose-and-whats in small towns throughout the country, subsequently foisting the drug upon the medical public on the grounds of such reports as, 'I have treated three patients with your drug and think that it is better than arsphenamine'; or he may make a se-

> rious effort to interest one of the six or eight larger syphilis clinics in the country in carrying out a detailed and respectable trial. All of these clinics find themselves in the same difficulties that we are, namely, that such trials are time-consuming, expensive and not at present adequately financed.[59]

If the Cooperative Group would make their clinics available for therapeutic research, then manufacturers might do well by doing good, that is, by meeting the gaps in the clinics' funding and obtaining authoritative evaluations of new products in the bargain. Parran, who did not operate a clinic of his own, was not convinced. Like other potential sources, drug firms lacked the appearance of disinterestedness: "I have always thought that manufacturers of pharmaceuticals are the least desirable of all possible sources of funds for syphilis research."[60]

As Stokes and Moore recognized, individual firms might easily be tempted to exploit sponsored research in subsequent promotions.[61] One possible solution was to establish a consortium of firms and clinics interested in "securing research advantages which both of them desire and which can be very much more easily obtained through cooperation than otherwise." The firms of Merck, Searle, Parke-Davis, and the Dermatological Research Laboratories, Stokes suggested, might be interested in such an arrangement.[62] Others in the group were agreeable, so long as it was possible to "avoid the stamp of any one organization pushing our project."[63]

In selecting prospective donors, the appearance of impartiality was crucial. The Dermatological Research Laboratories, which figured prominently in Stokes' proposals, were closely associated with their own version of arsphenamine.[64] Harold Cole, acting on Torald Sollman's advice, suggested the Chemical Foundation "which is backed not only by the manufacturers of arsphenamine, but of various types of chemicals" and has "plenty of money, oodles of it." The Chemical Foundation, a consortium established to handle foreign chemical patents during World War I, served as general spokesman for the industry's public relations but had limited success in subsidizing medical research.[65] Moore countered with a proposal to channel corporate funds through a committee of physicians composed of "persons who would not be so situated as to profit individually from any grants."[66]

Drug manufacturers *might* be interested in the proposed arrangements for future research.[67] But after four years of working with the Cooperative Group, Thomas Parran was beginning to weary of the gap between promise and performance. The participating clinics had a talent for using up the funds at their disposal without necessarily producing the work.[68] By the spring of 1932, Parran was inclined to let the individual clinics seek funding on their own:

> If I had the control over the expenditures for syphilis research I would not be inclined to recommend considerable grants over a long period to these clinics for clinical researches projected into the future. I was not very convinced by the projects submitted in advance of the last meeting or discussed there. They appeared to be trying hard to think up things which needed to be done.[69]

Despite his reservations, Parran was obligated and interested in seeing the work of the Cooperative Group completed. Having the Group around was useful, both to the Public Health Service and the Milbank Fund: "If we try, however, to require these clinics to produce results in cooperative researches planned for the future, I feel sure we shall fail."[70]

Legacies With the publication of studies on syphilis in pregnancy and cardiovascular syphilis, the active phase of the Cooperative Group began to wind down.[71] Their reports did not take the medical world by storm. Outside of a few specialized areas, their therapeutic pronouncements contained few surprises. By and large, their recommendations echoed the previous convictions of the collective authors: treat syphilis frequently and, when possible, with arsphenamine.[72] The uniqueness of their enterprise was nonetheless duly noted, and over the years their results became a benchmark against which other studies could compare themselves.[73] Clinicians who relied on the Cooperative Group as an authoritative source were sometimes "surprised," on closer examination, "to see what a relatively small number of cases the [critical conclusions about] neoarsphenamine are based on."[74]

The Cooperative Group's historical importance rests not so much on what they accomplished as on what they tried to do and the reasons for their failure. The greater availability of public funding during and after World War II removed at least one of the obstacles to conducting prospective, multicenter studies. But as the experiences of subsequent collaborations suggest, the absence of money was not, in the final analysis, the principal barrier to successful cooperative investigations in medicine. Rather it was the difficulty of getting research physicians who were drawn to cooperative research to surrender their intellectual autonomy in carrying out their commitments. As chiefs of prestigious clinics, the members were good at giving orders, and as former interns they were good at taking orders, but neither experience equipped them to share authority. They excelled at originating novel ideas and at criticizing other people's work, but not at jointly resolving differences of opinion.

In organizing their work, the Cooperative Group lacked examples to follow, and they lacked what development economists call an "infrastructure": a network of resources, personnel, and opportunities on which to draw and the ability to use them productively. The ideological barriers that prevented the principal investigators from leaving the statisticians in charge of the data analysis were every bit as real as the material lack of time available to the principals for doing the research on their own. Moreover, these barriers made difficult intellectual questions about measuring the outcomes of treatment or the severity of disease practically impossible to solve.

The Fortunes of War

During World War II the cause of cooperative clinical investigation received a substantial boost when decisions about medical research were centralized in the Committee on Medical Research (CMR) of the Office of Scientific Research and Development (OSRD). CMR in turn relied heavily on the distinguished committees of the National Research Council's (NRC) Division of Medical Sciences in selecting deserving problems and investigators.[75] Military exigencies dovetailed neatly with the medical elite's prewar convictions regarding cooperative research: putting a group of specialists to work on well-defined problems was deemed both efficient and scientific. Cooperative studies, by virtue of their ability to accumulate large numbers of patients treated by a common regimen, were thought to yield the most reliable answers in the shortest time.

Among CMR's numerous tasks was the evaluation of the therapeutic potential of penicillin. Rationing the drug's limited supply to a handful of "experienced investigators" who agreed to work under "[CMR's] direction and supervision," the research program focused first on the most serious infections and those for which other drugs performed poorly.[76] For the military, syphilis was as serious a medical problem as any, and existing therapies were quite inadequate. The time-consuming arsenical treatments endorsed by experts strained operating units and medical facilities alike. Initially, military research focused on accelerated arsenical treatments deemed too experimental for civilian use.[77] But in the summer of 1943 John F. Mahoney, a Public Health Service researcher, demonstrated that contrary to earlier reports penicillin had a pronounced spirocheticidal effect in experimental infections.[78]

Mahoney's subsequent report that the initial syphilitic lesions in four sailors had promptly disappeared on treatment with penicillin heightened military interest in the drug.[79] By the fall of 1943, increased production made possible plans for a study of penicillin in syphilis treatment under the direction of Joseph Earle Moore, Chairman of the NRC's Subcommittee on Venereal Disease and an alumnus of the Cooperative Clinical Group.[80] At the Army's request, the NRC would determine the optimal use of penicillin and evaluate its efficacy under more carefully controlled circumstances.[81]

Researchers participating in the NRC study agreed in advance to "cooperate in a planned investigation, [with] each clinic utilizing a treatment scheme indicated to it by the steering panel." A cooperative study, operating according to a fixed plan, would accumulate results much more quickly than a series of less focused individual inquiries. Standardized data collection and laboratory procedures were decided at the outset.[82] Final decisions about the conduct of the research were in the hands of the CMR, whose virtual monopoly over the civilian distribution of penicillin greatly enhanced its authority.[83]

The participating clinics represented a handful of elite investigators, selected for their expertise either in syphilis or in the study of anti-infectious agents.[84] Unlike the Cooperative Clinical Group, they did not lack funds or manpower in pursuing their researches. But more favorable circumstances found researchers no less reluctant to surrender their intellectual autonomy, even in the pursuit of agreed on goals. The study began by examining the value of penicillin in a range of doses up to 1.2 million units. Mahoney had demonstrated that 1.2 million units would work, but no one knew if lesser amounts would do as well. Participating clinicians, wishing to cure as many patients as possible, resented the protocol's requirement to employ the lower dosages.[85] Even after dosages below 1.2 million units were abandoned, investigators objected to "merely acting as technicians, each dealing with a small phase of a large experiment."[86]

Researchers' requests to use a portion of their penicillin allocations for autonomous investigations were repeatedly rejected by senior CMR officials.[87] Not surprisingly, individual physicians followed promising leads anyway, with the result that their pursuit of scientific curiosity led to the neglect of patient follow-up in the cooperative study.[88] Nearly half the cases accumulated during the war had to be discarded due to incomplete information or failure to follow the protocol.[89] Loss of patients to follow-up made interpretation of the remaining data difficult.[90] Although the study was intended to compare standardized treatments across clinics, individual clinics were rarely assigned more than two or three of the numerous regimens being tested. Variations in race, gender, and stage of disease among the clinics further complicated efforts at interpretation by confounding treatment with clinic effects.[91]

Despite their problems, cooperative studies had an appeal which the outbreak of peace did little to reduce. As military pressures abated, the NRC's attention turned to evaluating treatment schedules and modes of administration that might prove useful in postwar civilian practice.[92] But with penicillin supplies increasing, getting investigators to follow the research protocols became even more difficult, NRC exhortations notwithstanding:

> Since money is provided for a particular purpose, it should so be employed. The individual clinics should resist pressure to abandon a given treatment method 'because we have already so treated 100 patients with it,' and to adopt a new one, perhaps because of the latest publication of a new penicillin fraction, of methods of administration or of absorption delaying.[93]

In 1947, projected cutbacks in funding led to a phasing out of the cooperative study in favor of individual investigations, both laboratory and clinical.[94] Well after the war, the Central Statistical Unit continued to churn out publications on the study's behalf.[95] But despite the impressive numbers enrolled in the study, the cooperative investigators were forced to draw heavily on speculation and ad hoc interpretations of the data in defending specific findings against the conclusions of other researchers.[96] For the study's statisticians, the most important result had been learned much earlier:

> It is less important to get very large numbers of patients on a particular schedule and then not pay much attention to following them, than it is to get a smaller number who are followed through. There is a balance between the two problems of getting large numbers and devoting enough energy to following them up, so that conclusions are not based primarily on pure assumptions.[97]

The need for more planning and better follow-through was an experiential lesson, not easily taught in the textbooks. For it to fully take hold, many more studies would have to share the frustrations of the penicillin investigators. Meanwhile, despite its difficulties, the systematic approach pioneered in the NRC's studies of penicillin served as a testimony to the virtues of cooperative research:

> The first step in the evaluation of a chemotherapeutic agent is the discovery that X drug is "good" in the treatment of Y disease. In the past, once that step has been made, there has been a great tendency for the responsible leaders of the medical profession to lose interest in the subsequent all important but infinitely less dramatic subsequent steps. These include attempts to decide: *how* "good" is X drug? in what forms is it of little value? does one administer it by the pound or by the ton? daily, weekly or for 18 month periods?; under what circumstances is the treatment definitely worse than the disease. . . .
>
> Mahoney made the X-Y step for penicillin in syphilis less than four years ago and by means of the cooperative approach a vast amount of information on the subsequent steps has already been accumulated.[98]

A Tale of Two Studies

The introduction of streptomycin toward the close of the war provided a ready-made opportunity to continue the tradition of cooperative investigation. Like penicillin, streptomycin was initially in short supply, and its distribution was restricted. To CMR officials in charge of rationing supplies of the drug, using the available streptomycin to determine its most beneficial uses seemed the appropriate response. In the spring of 1946, they began planning an organized program of research to investigate the drug's potential in treating tuberculosis.[99] Preliminary research identified tuberculosis as one of the conditions for which streptomycin showed therapeutic promise. For advanced stages of the disease such as military tuberculosis, the drug demonstrated dramatic and unquestioned effects. For the initial stages, its advantages over conventional therapies were far from clear-cut. Additional research was needed to specify the precise benefits (and hazards) of treating tuberculosis with streptomycin.[100]

As originally planned, the proposed study was intended as a joint venture between the Veteran's Administration (VA), the Army, the Navy, and the Public Health Service (PHS). Modeled on the wartime penicillin investigations, the research strategy placed a premium on efficiency; by accumulating more patients and handling them in a uniform manner, a cooperative study could produce quicker and more reliable answers than any independent, albeit coordinated, series of researches.[101] Lack of funding prevented the PHS from immediately joining a major research initiative.[102] But with

9,000 tuberculosis patients in its hospitals, and more on the way, the VA could not afford to wait: in June of 1946, the first of its studies began.[103]

Research in the Bureaucracy The VA may have seemed like the ideal organization to conduct a controlled investigation of streptomycin treatment—a centralized bureaucracy, newly invigorated by an infusion of medical and scientific talent.[104] The reality was somewhat different. The VA medical system operated more like a confederacy of independent fiefs than like a model Weberian bureaucracy. Political end runs by local VA officials were an ever-present danger, making office staff in Washington acutely self-conscious of the VA's public image. The very idea that they were conducting experiments had to be approached gingerly: "We don't like to use the word 'experiments' in the Veterans Administration; 'investigation' or 'observations,' I believe is the approved term for such a study in the VA hospitals."[105]

The VA's delicacy in these matters presented problems for what was initially planned as a controlled experiment.

> It was the original decision of the Committee to have the units select suitable cases and divide them at random into two groups, the one to be treated with streptomycin, the other to provide controls. It seemed a feasible procedure at the time. The very scanty supplies of streptomycin and the real ignorance of its effectiveness made it reasonable to leave half the patients without treatment or rather, to treat them by other methods than streptomycin.[106]

Within several months it became apparent that there was a shortage of eligible patients in the designated study hospitals, too few to sacrifice half their number for a control group.[107] Yet the VA's reluctance to employ an (untreated) control group was due as much to political considerations as to more technical concerns.[108]

What began as a pragmatic decision, motivated by a desire to get answers about streptomycin as quickly as possible, soon became a matter of policy:

> In general, and in particular with a disease as various and unpredictable as pulmonary tuberculosis, there can be no doubt as to the theoretical desirability of untreated controls, selected by alternation or randomization. In the laboratory, this is axiomatic. In the clinic, however, such a series seems justifiable to us on only one of two grounds: (1) a genuine ignorance or doubt that the drug in question has any therapeutic value; or (2) a shortage of supply which, by making it *impossible* to treat all cases, makes it fair to treat alternate cases. Although one or both of

> these conditions may have existed at the commencement of our study, they were very transient and, for reasons which can be visualized, we did not adopt the method.[109]

The VA officials in charge of the study were well aware of the intellectual difficulties of interpreting treatment results without an untreated control group for comparison. But without some externally imposed constraint, neither the VA investigators nor their patients were willing to abandon existing treatments in the interests of better science. Despite the arguments of some consultants that a control group was necessary, the study proceeded without such a safeguard.[110] In the absence of an untreated control group, VA investigators were forced to rely on ad hoc comparisons of study patients with the results of conventional therapy obtained in the recent past on comparable patients.[111] The difficulties of interpreting such comparisons soon became evident.[112] Despite these shortcomings, the VA study remained the largest, if not the only, program investigating streptomycin: "Absolutely the whole profession is going to have to depend on the Veterans Administration to tell us what we are going to be able to learn about streptomycin. There is no other organization which is likely to be able to learn about streptomycin on such a wide scale."[113]

The value of the VA study to the community of tuberculosis researchers depended on the VA's ability to treat large numbers of patients according to a standardized protocol. So long as little streptomycin was available, it proved possible to restrict its use to the elite group of VA hospitals "most competent" to assess the drug. But as supplies improved, regulating the use of streptomycin in the larger VA system became increasingly difficult. This, in turn, threatened investigators' ability to enroll sufficient patients. With the drug generally available, they feared, patients might be more reluctant to enlist in the study.[114]

Restricting the use of streptomycin within the VA system did not present the only problem, however. Getting participating researchers to follow the protocols proved equally difficult. Like the penicillin investigators, they wanted to pursue their own ideas about the drug.[115] With more VA hospitals joining the study, ability to ensure compliance with the protocol diminished.[116] As reports from other, smaller, studies became available, the impetus to explore new directions suggested by these findings grew.[117] The participation of university-based VA affiliates posed a particular problem: "Streptomycin is a new toy with a lot of our attending men and in one of our hospitals I think our Dean's Committee has been wanting to use it.

We are not particularly sure about the type of cases in which they are using it."[118]

Politics in the Service of Science While the VA study was getting underway, the Public Health Service was planning its own investigation of streptomycin.[119] Mindful of the penicillin experiences, they emphasized the need to decide on a research plan and stick to it:

> Innumerable physicians throughout the country will be treating small series of patients with this or that regimen and will be publishing their results. This will constitute a pressure in the form of competition which is most difficult to resist. We must be prepared, however, to accept the risk that some one of these unsponsored programs may discover something which we have not yet had an opportunity to study. We can do this only if we are secure in our minds that what we are studying, limited in scope as it will be, should provide us with some tangible answers at the end of a net period of time.[120]

The planners called for a strictly defined protocol, to be policed by a central statistical unit which might also assist in designing the study. Participating physicians would be required to continue treating patients on a given regimen until authorized by a steering committee to discontinue treatment.[121] Individual tuberculosis researchers, however, wanted the PHS to sponsor a free-ranging program of investigation, not purely confined to evaluating streptomycin treatment in humans.[122] The announcement of cutbacks in Congressional appropriations for studying tuberculosis forced a change in

> philosophy from free research to a target [*sic*] study directed at the specific question of the merit of streptomycin in tuberculosis therapy. . . . The essence of this portion of the program, as distinguished from the various proposals of the Study Section, is that a group of special experts in the field of clinical tuberculosis, in different institutions, in different parts of the country, agree to cooperate in a large scale, rigidly controlled project, which is operated in such a way as to insure the collection of uniform observations that may be combined or pooled to furnish statistically significant evidence in the treatment of certain well defined types of pulmonary tuberculosis.[123]

The Bureau of the Budget (BoB) approved funding for the PHS study on condition that the research would "be carefully coordinated with similar work by other government agencies . . . and be closely controlled in extent and direction by the Study Section, the [National Health Advisory] Council and appropriate specialists in the Public Health Service." BoB's principal concern was that appropriations for medical treatment not be slipped in under the guise of research.[124] But BoB's insistence on a carefully planned study provided PHS officials with an opportunity to engage the contentious issue of experimental controls. They insisted that the PHS study, unlike the VA investigation, contain a preselected control group of patients who did not receive streptomycin: "The cases chosen by the Panel shall, by proper random device, to avoid all possibility of bias, be divided by the Central Unit into cases for treatment and cases for control."[125]

A Clash of Cultures In principal, the arguments for a control group were well understood. The course of tuberculosis was highly erratic. In the absence of an untreated control group, crediting improvements to streptomycin, or any novel treatment, was problematic.[126] In practice, however, the PHS anticipated difficulties from physicians asked to withhold streptomycin from one group of patients while treating another with the drug:

> It seems very likely that the men responsible for various phases of this project may encounter criticism from people who are already convinced of the value of streptomycin, or who for some other reason do not consider necessary a program providing for withholding the drug from one group of patients. Since we have agreed to go ahead with such a program, it is important to protect the individual investigators from possible serious consequences of this criticism.[127]

Advocates of a control group wanted backing from the authorities on the study's Steering Committee, in the form of a statement justifying the withholding of streptomycin. As in the VA's case, the limited amounts of streptomycin available, coupled with uncertainty about the drug's precise value, could serve as an initial justification. Skeptics were not sure that any such statement would serve its purpose, which was to stiffen the backbone of investigators faced with a patient whose condition was deteriorating.[128] The proposed compromise was "that physicians do not communicate to patients the fact that they are being considered for inclusion in this series. Hence patients who are in the control group are not to realize that they have been denied streptomycin."[129]

The majority of investigators participating in the PHS study proved willing to go along with the idea of a control group.[130] What remained unresolved was the handling of control patients whose disease worsened substantially during the study. Should they receive the drug, and under what circumstances? PHS representatives proposed that investigators submit such cases to an Appeals Board which would decide if an exemption was warranted. Provided the exemption criteria were sufficiently narrow, and specified in advance, only a few patients would be lost and the research design need not be compromised.[131] This proposal only altered the terms of the debate. According to one dissenting study section member, it all boiled down to a question of clinical integrity:

> As a matter of fact I do not believe it is possible to give a definition [of life-threatening conditions] which would cover all the possibilities. Fundamentally, it rests on the judgement of the physician who is treating the case and who knows the patient best. He is in a far better position than anyone else to make the decision. If he is capable of undertaking a clinical investigation of therapy, he is certainly capable of assuming the responsibility for such judgement.[132]

To advocates of experimental controls, this approach, if allowed free rein, "would completely invalidate the control study" and "jeopardize the entire program of the Study Section."[133]

The PHS officials in charge of the study exercised an unusual degree of influence over the conduct of the research. But centralized control of treatment assignment could not forestall the investigators' desire to raise questions that were not contemplated in the original research plans. Nearly eighteen months into the study, the Evaluation Policy Committee proposed that "an adequate evaluation [of outcome] must take into account everything that can be known about a patient," including data that only the treating physician could provide.[134] The VA study had begun to demonstrate problems with the traditional reliance on roentgenographical measures of outcome.[135] Holding an improvised case conference on each patient, clinicians argued, would "lend greater accuracy to interpretations of questionable features and in the long run give greater significance to the interpretation of results."[136]

As with the syphilis studies of a generation earlier, reaching agreement on a measure of outcome was hampered by a lack of understanding of the factors which made the disease progress. Lacking more knowledge about the disease, only time would provide a "true" measure of outcome: "In the final analysis, survival without detectable reactivation of the disease under essentially 'normal' socio-economic conditions is the criterion for success of therapy."[137] Meanwhile, short-run answers were needed about the value of streptomycin and other drugs in treating tuberculosis. The clinician's inclination was to bring into the account those signs which, while difficult to standardize, were used to interpret the course of individual patients, "for no sets of figures can completely represent clinical experience."[138]

To the statisticians in charge of the PHS study, such data was at best of secondary importance and at worst inherently unreliable. There were enough difficulties producing trustworthy scores for data they had agreed to collect, without trying to introduce clinical material that was neither standardized nor uniformly available: "It would be a tragic mistake to distort the original pattern of the study now to try to make it yield information it was not designed to produce, because in so doing, the kind of answers it can give will lose their validity."[139] Their inclination was to distrust measures that could not be reliably reproduced: in this, as in other respects, the future belonged to the statisticians.[140]

The Appearance of Truth

> *Q*: Are we in favor of this, trying to do better on the follow up?
> *A*: Who isn't against sin?[141]

In keeping curious and independent researchers in line, the directors of the VA and PHS studies faced difficulties reminiscent of earlier collaborative investigations. Even under the most favorable circumstances—and for getting scientists to cooperate, national emergencies *were* the most favorable circumstances—obtaining the sustained cooperation of clinical investigators had been difficult to engineer. But those directing the streptomycin studies also faced changing beliefs about the purpose and character of cooperative investigations, changes which they themselves had helped to bring about. The continuing operation of the PHS and VA groups over the next two decades, evaluating newer drugs and regimens in the treatment of tuberculosis, testifies to their ability to provide new solutions to old problems.

The original impetus for these projects arose from the need to find fast and reliable answers to questions about the use of streptomycin. Cooperative studies were, by nature, more efficient; they were also believed to be more credible. For an earlier generation of clinical researchers, the participation of specialists in joint projects was in itself a partial guarantee of a study's scientific merit. Along with other therapeutic trials in the postwar era, the VA investigations of streptomycin demonstrated that specialists, no less than anyone else, were capable of self-deception, selecting the most or least promising cases for treatment, depending on their particular prejudices.[142]

Both the VA and PHS testified favorably on behalf of streptomycin, but it was the PHS studies, properly randomized, that received credit for demonstrating the new drug's benefits in treating tuberculosis. The methodological innovations adopted by the PHS researchers—randomization and standardized measures of outcome—gave their reports greater credibility. The VA investigators were no less confident of their conclusions, but they were unable to convince others; without sufficient methodological safeguards, their findings were suspect. For the VA researchers to be as influential as they wished, they would have to adopt the use of randomized controls in future trials.[143] The virtue of randomization, properly executed, was to free the investigator from the charge of bias as well as the act: "The random method removes all responsibility from the observer."[144]

The PHS's studies of streptomycin served as an example of scientific progress in therapeutics, long after the results they reported ceased to be of clinical interest and the technical procedures they employed to assign patients were obsolete. Along with centrally controlled randomization, the use of objectively measured indicators of response to treatment and blinded assessments of therapeutic outcomes represented the future of clinical experimentation. The rationale offered for all these innovations was that they would limit the exercise of subjective judgment; rather than pitting the clinical acumen of one physician against another, studies conducted according to the canons of experimental methodology would provide an objective measure of therapeutic progress. The unmentioned aspect was that these procedures also reduced the clinician's ability to deviate spontaneously from an agreed on plan of research, whatever the reason.

The adoption of controlled experimentation in medicine has generally been interpreted as a triumph for the intellectual power and cogency of statistical concepts and theory. Yet physicians' appreciation for the concepts of statistics generally followed, rather than preceded, the adoption of procedures advocated by methodological reformers. Statisticians' arguments about the need for centrally controlled randomization, the simplification of experimental objectives, and a greater reliance on impersonal measures of clinical improvement drew their force from the experiences of the past twenty years, in which well-intentioned researchers had repeatedly undermined the designs of cooperative experiments. To contemporaries, the improvements in experimental method offered by statisticians represented an elegant technical fix for a host of previously insoluble organizational and social problems. By taking a multitude of decisions out of the hands of participating investigators, these innovations removed a series of opportunities for clinicians to frustrate the plans of cooperative experiments and their own best intentions.

As the outcome of subsequent decades demonstrated, centralizing the management of therapeutic studies did not eliminate the physician's conflict between loyalty to the needs of patients and to the objectives of research. Someone would still be required to enforce the details of the experimental protocol. But putting the central statistical office in charge of this task relieved participating clinicians of the duties of policing themselves. If statisticians had not already gained respect among medicine's scientific elite, through their participation and criticism of cooperative studies, then they would not have been placed in such positions of authority.[145] But once in office, they served to draw the fire that had formerly been directed at the investigating physician. Thirty years later, cracks would appear in the edifice erected by the statisticians, as a younger generation of clinical investigators grew restive under their hegemony.[146] But for the moment, the new science brought a welcome social peace to the community of therapeutic researchers.

I, if not my work, have benefited from the advice and criticisms offered by readers of previous drafts: John Bailar III, Peter Buck, William Coleman, Diana Long, Russell Maulitz, Frederick Mosteller, Charles Rosenberg, and John Swann. Portions of this work were completed with the support of a grant from the Health Services Improvement Foundation, Inc., New York, and grant No. HS-05151-01 from the National Center for Health Services Research.

NOTES

1. John C. Bailar III, "Introduction," in *Clinical Trials: Issues and Approaches*, Stuart Shapiro and Thomas Louis, eds. (New York: Marcel Dekker, 1983), 1. Other useful discussions of the RCT include Jerome Cornfield, "Recent Methodological Contributions to Clinical Trials," 104(1976):408–21; Sonja M. McKinley, "Experimentation in Human Populations," *Milbank Mem Fund Q Health and Society* 59(1981):308–23; and Paul Meier, "Statistics and Medical Experimentation," *Biometrics* 31(1975):511–29.

2. J. P. Bull, "The Historical Development of Clinical Therapeutic Trials," *J Chron Dis* 10(1959):218–46 and Abraham M. Lilienfeld, "Ceteris Paribus: The Evolution of the Clinical Trial," *Bull Hist Med* 56(1982):1–18.

3. Intellectual history, no less than social history, is poorly served by the obsessive "precursoritis" that besets this literature. Contrast Lilienfeld's essay with the more resolutely historicist approach of Edwin G. Boring, in his general history of experimental controls, "The Nature and History of Experimental Control," *Am J Psychol* 67(1954):573–89.

4. The recent attempts of historians such as John Warner and William Coleman to evaluate the specific intellectual and social circumstances that affected the reception of quantitative, experimental evaluations in nineteenth-century medicine have yet to show signs of reaching the hagiographical literature. See William Coleman, "Experimental Physiology and Statistical Inference: The Therapeutic Trial in Nineteenth Century Germany," in *The Probabilistic Revolution,* Lorraine Daston, Michael Heidelberger, Lorenz Kruger, eds. (Cambridge: MIT Press, 1986); John Harley Warner, "The Selective Transport of Medical Knowledge: Antebellum American Physicians and Parisian Medical Therapeutics," *Bull Hist Med* 59(1985): 213–31; and idem, "Therapeutic Explanation and the Edinburgh Blood-Letting Controversy: Two Perspectives on the Medical Meaning of Science in the Mid-Nineteenth Century," *Med Hist* 24(1980):241–58.

5. Harry Dowling, "The Emergence of the Cooperative Clinical Trial," *Trans Stud Coll Physicians Phila* 43(1975):20–29. I am grateful to Allan M. Brandt for calling my attention to this essay and, more generally, for insisting on the importance of the Cooperative Clinical Group to the history of the randomized controlled trial. Although there are numerous differences on matters of fact as well as interpretation between Dowling's account and mine, his article introduced me to the wartime studies on penicillin and the postwar studies on streptomycin that are discussed in the latter half of this chapter. I am especially indebted to Dowling's work for identifying the published transactions of the VA's streptomycin researchers, which form the principal primary source for my analysis of their study.

6. The other respect in which these studies are important is as historical influences in their own right: Dowling's essay traces the manner in which one or two individuals from each study play important roles in subsequent landmark investigations. Although the networks of influence were larger and more complex than Dowling indicates, it would be a mistake to entirely neglect the role of individual influences.

7. A distinction should be made between a handful of writers who by the mid-1930s accepted the probabilistic character of these recoveries and those who, while continuing to disparage the value of a purely statistical knowledge, insisted on the necessity of larger series of patients and the use of a control series. The recommendations of both groups were similar but the understanding was not. Compare the arguments of W. D. Sutliffe, an advocate (and practitioner) of controls, with those of F. T. Jung and Donald Mainland, the latter two working in the tradition of Pearson and R. A. Fisher. W. D. Sutliffe, "Adequate Tests of Curative Therapy in Man," *Ann Intern Med* 10(1936):89–96; Frederick T. Jung, "Centripetal Drift: A Fallacy in the Evaluation of Therapeutic Results," *Science* 87(1938):461–62; and Donald Mainland, "Problems of Chance in Clinical Work," *Br Med J* ii(Aug. 1, 1936):221–24.

8. Torald Sollman, "Experimental Therapeutics," *JAMA* 58(1912):243.

9. See especially Torald Sollman, "The Evaluation of Therapeutic Remedies in the Hospital," *JAMA* 94(1930):1279–81 and Harry Gold, "Recent Advances in Drug Therapy," *Int. Clin* (Dec. 1930):96–97.

10. As chair of the Scientific Committee of the Committe on Research in Syphilis (CRS), Stokes expected to command ample funding: the Committee held the pledge of half a million dollars from Averill Harriman. Shortly thereafter, Thomas Parran, Jr., took over from Stokes as chair of the Scientific Committee of CRS and, subsequently, as director of the Cooperative Group study. Parran to Hugh S. Cumming, 3 January 1931, Box 325, Record Group (RG) 90, Public Health

Service, Venereal Disease Division 1918–1936: National Archives (hereafter cited as "NA"); Edward L. Keyes to Parran, 27 December 1928 (F 235) and Parran to Paul O'Leary, 12 March 1929 (F 221): Thomas Parran, Jr. Papers, University of Pittsburgh (hereafter cited as "Parran Papers").

11. Stokes to O'Leary, 26 March 1928 (F 235): Parran Papers.

12. Committee on Research in Syphilis, Scientific Committee. *Draft Agenda for Session on Clinical Problems. April 30, 1928* (F 220): Parran Papers. On the need to study large numbers of patients and the advantages of expert determination of patient outcome, see Taliaferro Clark, Thomas Parran, Jr., Harold N. Cole, et al., "Cooperative Clinical Studies in the Treatment of Syphilis. I. Introduction," *Ven Dis Info* 13(1932):135–37.

13. For the initial reactions to Stokes' invitation see Wile to Parran, 20 March 1928 (F 237) and O'Leary to Stokes, 30 March 1928 (F 235): Parran Papers.

14. Stokes to O'Leary, 26 March 1928 (F 235). On the scope of the initial program, see also *Report of the Conference of Clinicians. 5–6 January 1929* (F 226) and Parran to O'Leary, 7 May 1929 (F 235): Parran Papers.

15. On the initial evaluation of salvarsan, see Patricia Spain Ward, "The American Reception of Salvarsan," *J Hist Med* (January 1981):44–62 and Charles F. Craig and Henry J. Nichols, *Studies of Syphilis,* War Department, Office of the Surgeon General, Bulletin No. 3 (Washington: Government Printing Office, 1913).

16. From the outset, specialists advocated that physicians receive hands-on training in administering salvarsan. Henry Eksber, "The New Treatment of Syphilis (Ehrlich-Hata): Observations and Results," *JAMA* 55(1910):2053. On the difficulties of using the drug, see Oliver S. Ormsby, "Salvarsan and Neosalvarsan in Syphilis," *JAMA* 68(1917):949–50. On the pros and cons of endorsing the use of neoarsphenamine, see "Abstract of Discussion," *Trans Sec Pharmacol Ther AMA* (1920):217–28. Although various improvements in the manufacture and technique of administering arsphenamine occurred following its introduction, it remained a trickier drug to administer. See Joseph Earle Moore, Harold N. Cole, J. F. Schamberg, et al., "The Management of Syphilis in General Practice," *Ven Dis Info* 10(1929): 66–73. On the production of arsphenamine in the U.S., see Jonathan Michael Liebenau, *Medical Science and Medical Industry, 1898–1929: A Study of Pharmaceutical Manufacturing in Philadelphia* (Ph.D. dissertation, University of Pennsylvania, 1981), 313–51, and on the relative use of sulpharsphenamine and neoarsphenamine to arsphenamine, see George H. Bigelow and N. A. Nelson, "The Distribution of Arsenicals by the Massachusetts Department of Public Health," *N Engl J Med* 201(1929):761–63.

17. Interest in new mercury compounds was stimulated by Ehrlich's own work prior to the development of salvarsan. Jay Frank Schamberg, John A. Kolmer, and George A. Raiziss, "The Chemotherapy of Mercurial Compounds," *Am J Syphilis* 1(1917):1–6. On combination treatments, see John H. Stokes, "The Application and Limitations of Arsphenamine in Therapeutics," *Trans Sec Ther Pharmacol AMA* (1920):194–97. The introduction of bismuth, less toxic than mercury, in 1922 further assisted the resurgence of interest in combined treatments. See Carroll S. Wright, "The Effect of Bismuth Alone and in Combination with the Arsenobenzenes on the Wasserman Reaction," *Am J Med Sci* 173(1927):232. While few experts recommended treatment with mercury alone, it was still preferred by some physicians as an initial treatment. Jay F. Schamberg and Carroll S. Wright, *Treatment of Syphilis* (New York: D. Appleton and Company, 1932), 3.

18. The requirement of rest intervals in therapy was premised not only on the

belief that the body needed time to recover from the toxic build-up of arsenicals but that breaks provided an opportunity for natural resistance to develop. Some specialists advocated alternating heavy metals and arsenicals to avoid toxic reactions but saw no justification for a break in treatment.

19. Joseph Earle Moore, "Clinical Investigation in Syphilis," *Ven Dis Info* 9(1928):529 and Louis Chargin and Abraham Stone, "The Therapy of Syphilis," *NY State J Med* 26(1926):551. The problem was not unique to syphilis: see Sollman, "Evaluation of Therapeutic Remedies," 1279–81.

20. Compare the conclusions of Louis Chargin, favoring the use of intensive therapy with rest periods, with Joseph Moore's advocacy of continuous alternating treatment. Louis Chargin, "Early Syphilis: Results," *Arch Dermatol Syphilis* 19(1929):750–63 and Joseph Earle Moore and Albert Keidel, "The Treatment of Early Syphilis. I. A Plan of Therapy for Routine Use," *Bull J Hopkins Hosp* 39(1926):6–8.

21. *Report of the Conference of Clinicians. January 5–6, 1929,* (F 226) and Parran to O'Leary, 7 May 1929 (F 235): Parran Papers.

22. John H. Stokes, Harold N. Cole, Joseph Earle Moore, et al., "Cooperative Clinical Studies in the Treatment of Syphilis: Early Syphilis," *Ven Dis Info* 13(1932):208.

23. Stokes et al., "Cooperative Studies in Treatment of Syphilis."

24. See Stokes to Parran, 16 August 1929 (F 236) and Lida Usilton to Parran, 15 March 1930 (F 231): Parran Papers. On the grounds for distrusting patients' reports, see John H. Stokes, *Modern Clinical Syphilology* (Philadelphia: W. B. Saunders, 1927), 30–31, 39.

25. See Wile to Stokes, 14 March and 27 March 1930, with Stokes' reply 24 March (F 231) and Stokes to Parran, 23 May 1930 (F 230). The problem of distinguishing relapses from reinfections continued to recur in discussions of later papers. See Moore to Stokes, 23 March and 1 April 1932 (F 224): Parran Papers. On the difficulties of determining from clinical data whether treated syphilitics had been reinfected, see Alan M. Chesney, *Immunity in Syphilis* (Baltimore: Williams & Wilkins, 1927), 36–37.

26. Stokes to Parran, 23 May 1930 (F 230): Parran Papers.

27. Moore to Stokes, 23 March 1932 (RG 90): Public Health Service, Venereal Disease Division, 1918–1936. Committee on Research in Syphilis, Box 326: NA. Stokes to Cole, 8 March 1932 and to Moore, 7 March 1932 (F 228): Parran Papers.

28. Lida J. Usilton, Memorandum for Doctor Joseph Earle Moore, 15 January 1935 (F 223): Parran Papers.

29. Stokes to Parran, 16 August 1929 (F 236): Parran Papers.

30. The alternative under consideration, to give prominence to the number of treatments without regard to the duration of treatment, proved equally problematic. The difficulty was in determining where the cutoff between "little" and "much" treatment lay. Usilton to Taliaferro Clark, 9 April 1932 (RG 90): Public Health Service, Venereal Disease Division, 1918–1936. Committee on Research in Syphilis, Box 326: NA. The final solution was to analyze treatments both on a frequency basis, taking account of the duration of treatment, and by the total number of treatments received. This "solution" made the resulting paper close to unintelligible for anyone unable to devote the time to follow the logic and detailed calculations presented for each option.

31. For an explicit discussion of the problem, see Moore to Stokes, 1 April 1932 and to Parran, 2 April 1932 (F 224) and Stokes to Moore, 4 April 1932 (F 228). See

also Stokes to Parran, 23 May 1930 (F 230). Experience was no teacher in this regard; the same problem recurred in developing the group's later papers on cardiovascular syphilis. Cole to John McMullen [Assistant Surgeon General], 20 April 1935 (F 223). All references to Parran Papers.

32. Stokes to Parran, 2 June 1930 (F 230): Parran Papers.

33. Wile to Parran, 9 March 1932 (F 231) and Moore to Parran, 21 January 1932 (F 228): Parran Papers.

34. Stokes to Parran, 12 April 1930 (F 230): Parran Papers.

35. Moore to Stokes, 6 April 1932 (RG 90): Public Health Service, Venereal Disease Division, 1918–1936. Committee on Research in Syphilis, Box 326: NA. See also Moore to Stokes, 25 July 1934 (F 222): Parran Papers. The physicians were handicapped by a corresponding lack of familiarity with the intellectual complexities of handling statistical data. The ideal solution, to identify someone competent to handle both aspects, never materialized, although at various times they considered recruiting the advice of a more senior statistical consultant or trying to enlist one of their own members to greater involvement. See Moore to Stokes, 30 March 1932 and Stokes' reply, 4 April 1932 (F 224) and Stokes to Parran, 12 April 1932 (F 230): Parran Papers. None of these efforts came to much.

36. Junior clinical staff *do* appear to have done some of the initial record abstracting before sending data to Washington, but they were not available for the subsequent work of classifying and interpreting the records.

37. Stokes to Parran, 9 October 1929; for an earlier proposal along similar lines, see Stokes to Parran, 9 January 1929. Both letters (F 230): Parran Papers.

38. Stokes to Parran, 9 October 1929 (F 230): Parran Papers.

39. O'Leary to Parran, 15 October 1929 (F 236): Parran Papers.

40. O'Leary to Parran, 15 October 1929 (F 236): Parran Papers. Udo Wile had raised the initial objections to Stokes' proposal. Parran, who served as arbitrator for the group on this and numerous other occasions, shared Stokes' reservations about the general practice of exploiting the labors of "young men." He accepted O'Leary's contention, however, that this was a "pioneer venture to demonstrate a new method of approach to the problem of syphilis through concerted action": such a special case required that "sacrifices in individual identity" be made. Parran to Stokes, 14 October 1929 (F 230): Parran Papers.

41. Stokes to Moore, 29 February 1932 (F 228): Parran Papers.

42. Moore to Stokes, 30 March 1932 and Stokes' reply, 4 April 1932 (F 228): Parran Papers. Stokes' objections were not purely practical: he held onto the idea that for the group to dictate method would sacrifice too much "individual autonomy" and that all the group could require was that the members restrain themselves in drawing conclusions from the data.

43. Stokes to Moore, 4 April 1932 (F 228): Parran Papers.

44. Stokes to Taliaferro Clark, 29 March 1932 (F 224): Parran Papers.

45. Moore to Stokes, 23 March, 25 March, and 30 March 1932 (F 224): Parran Papers.

46. Moore was especially reluctant to "smothering" his paper in *Venereal Disease Information*. Taliaferro Clark to Parran, 29 October 1931 (F 221); Stokes strongly objected when the Public Health Service indicated it would be unable to provide substantial numbers of reprints at a subsidized price, which "seems to me to be one unintentional method of blanketing the work so far as its popularization and dissemination among the medical profession is concerned." See Stokes to Clark, 21 June 1932 (F 230): Parran Papers.

47. Parran to John McMullen, 9 May 1934 (F 222). Ironically, one of Joseph Earle Moore's initial objections to Public Health Service sponsorship was that its "prestige . . . in this country was so great" that if it endorsed "incomplete or erroneous conclusions it might take years to remove the impression created on the medical profession." Moore to Stokes, 16 November 1928 (F 228): Parran Papers.

48. *Minutes of the Fourth Meeting of the Cooperative Clinical Group, May 6, 1931* (F 220): Parran Papers.

49. Moore to Parran, 20 December 1930 (F 228): Parran Papers.

50. From the Public Health Service's perspective, even the reserved endorsement of arsphenamine presented problems: "All health officers know that few physicians in private practice will go to the trouble of making up old arsphenamine even though they are qualified to do so. If we are to succeed in our campaign to encourage physicians to administer intravenous treatment for syphilis, I believe it is necessary that we recommend neo-arsphenamine because of its simplicity of administration until some drug of much greater efficacy is discovered." R. A. Vonderlehr to Moore, 29 February 1936 (F 223): Parran Papers.

51. Moore to Parran, 21 January 1932 (F 228): Parran Papers.

52. For examples of each approach, see Robert E. Kohler, "A Policy for the Advancement of Science: The Rockefeller Foundation, 1924–1929" *Minerva* 16(1978):480–515 and Peter Buck, "Why Not the Best? Some Reasons and Examples From Child Health and Rural Hospitals," *J Soc Hist* 18(1985):413–29. By the late 1920s, the laboratory side of the therapeutic research had begun to cultivate a variety of funding sources, largely commercial in origin. See John Patrick Swann, *The Emergence of Cooperative Research Between American Universities and the Pharmaceutical Industry, 1920–1940* (Ph.D. dissertation, University of Wisconsin, 1985). I am indebted to Swann for making a copy of his thesis available to me.

53. Even the Milbank Memorial Fund, which Parran convinced to pick up the financial holes left by the decline in Timkin's finances and interest, thought the most interesting aspect of the Cooperative study would be to have the findings "tried out in a community such as Cattaragus County, New York, to test its real effectiveness particularly with reference to diagnosis of early syphilis and the treatment of it." *A Report of the Fourth Meeting of the Cooperating Clinical Group . . . March 18, 1932* (F 226). Parran had obtained funding from the Milbank in part by emphasizing the public health importance of evaluating syphilis treatments. See Parran to John A. Kingsbury, 12 January 1931 (F 222): Parran Papers.

54. Harold Cole, for example, sought to stretch the Cooperative Group funds by using them to keep "at least one doctor through the coming year" rather than purchasing an automobile and hiring an additional nurse as budgeted. See Cole to Parran, 24 November 1930 (F 228). On lack of support for clinical investigation, see Cole to Parran, 29 January and 18 February 1929 (F 227); O'Leary to Edward L. Keyes, 16 April 1929 (F 235); and Stokes to Moore, 8 February 1929 (F 228): Parran Papers. The lack of stable funding was a generic problem in medical research prior to 1930, with short-term grants predominating. See Richard H. Shryock, *American Medical Research* (New York: Commonwealth Fund, 1947), 107.

55. Moore to Parran, 7 October 1931 (F 222): Parran Papers. See Parran to Cole, 25 January 1929 and Cole's reply, 29 January (F 227): Parran Papers; Parran to Hugh S. Cumming, 31 January 1931 and Parran to O'Leary, 8 January 1931 (RG 90): Public Health Service, Venereal Disease Division, 1918–1936, Box 325: NA.

56. O'Leary to Parran, 27 March 1929 and 27 February, 8 March, and 26 April 1929 (F 221): Parran Papers.

57. *Report of the Conference of Clinicians. January 5–6, 1929* (F 226); Moore to Parran, 21 January 1932 (RG 90): Public Health Service, Venereal Disease Division, 1918–1936, Box 324: NA.

58. Moore to Parran, 3 January 1932 (F 228): Parran Papers.

59. Parran to Moore, 13 October 1931 (F 222): Parran Papers. Harold Cole was similarly suspicious of subsidies from commercial firms. In this he was probably following the lead of his mentor, Torald Sollman, who as the leading figure of AMA's Council on Pharmacy and Chemistry had ample reason to suspect the motives of individual firms. See Cole's objections to accepting a subvention from Abbot Laboratories to publishing the Cooperative Group's studies under their auspices: Cole to O'Leary, 16 February 1935, and to John McMullen [Assistant Surgeon General] (RG 90): Public Health Service, Venereal Disease Division, 1918–1936, Box 325: NA.

60. An alternative funding source, the Public Health Institute in Chicago, was also rejected because it was "at war with the medical profession" over the issue of providing dispensary care to syphilis patients, among others. The prospect that the Institute's bad odor might rub off on the Cooperative Group was too great to risk taking "money from them, much as we would like to have it." See Sollman to Cole, 26 November 1930 and Cole to Parran, 28 November 1930 (F 227): Parran Papers.

61. See the extensive correspondence between Stokes and Parran in the fall of 1929 regarding the misrepresentation of some of Harold Cole's work by Loeser Laboratory, manufacturer of a bismuth solution for treating syphilis (F 221): Parran Papers. Both Moore and Stokes were willing to work in support of the FDA's regulation of drug claims; at the same time, both had research clinics to support and did not think it amiss to seek funding from reputable firms. On cooperation with the FDA, see Parran to Moore, 22 September 1930 (F 228) and *Report of the Conference of Clinicians. January 5–6, 1929* (F 226): Parran Papers.

62. Stokes to Parran, 18 December 1930 (F 236): Parran Papers.

63. Parran was agreeable to trying Stokes' proposal, but wanted to defer action until other options were exhausted. See Parran to Stokes 31 December 1930 (F 230). Cole was also sympathetic, especially if the alternative was the Public Health Institute. Cole to Parran, 21 January and 24 February 1931 (F 227): Parran Papers.

64. On DRL's relations with the profession, see Liebenau, *Medical Science and Medical Industry*, 313–51.

65. Cole to Parran, 7 March 1931 (F 233): Parran Papers. On the Chemical Foundation's interests in medical research, see John Parascandola, "Charles Holmes Herty and the Effort to Establish an Institute for Drug Research in Post World War I America," in *Chemistry and Modern Society*, John Parascandola and James C. Whorton, eds. (Washington: American Chemical Society, 1983), 94–96.

66. Moore to Parran, 7 October 1931 (F 222). Moore proposed having Wade Brown from the Rockefeller Institute and Paul O'Leary on the committee, as both came from well-endowed institutions and were therefore not likely to personally benefit "from any grants which the committee might make." Moore to Parran, 3 January 1932 (F 228). Both Moore and Stokes had recently obtained grants from individual firms without strings attached. Moore to Parran, 3 January 1932 (F 228); Stokes to Parran, 8 March 1932 (F 230); and *An Agreement Between Abbott Laboratories, Inc. and the Department of Dermatology and Syphilology of the University of Pennsylvania*, (n.d.) (F 230). All references to Parran Papers.

67. Merck officials, for example, expressed some interest, provided the arrangement was sufficiently long term and that "it might rebound to their ultimate

commercial benefit." Moore to Parran, 19 January 1933 and R. E. Gruber (of Merck) to Moore, 7 March 1933 (F 228). A successful arrangement, however, depended on Parran's backing and possibly that of the National Research Council. See Moore to Parran, 13 March 1933 (F 228). All references to Parran Papers.

68. Parran to Taliaferro Clark, 24 March 1932 (F 224): Parran Papers.

69. Parran to Taliaferro Clark, 15 April 1932 (F 221): Parran Papers.

70. Parran to Taliaferro Clark, 15 April 1932 (F 221): Parran Papers.

71. Harold N. Cole with Lida J. Usilton, Joseph Earle Moore, et al., "Syphilis in Pregnancy," *Ven Dis Info* 17(1936):39–46 and idem, *Cardiovascular Syphilis," Ven Dis Info* 17(1936):91–118. As late as 1939, however, the group was still formally in existence, but the founding members were hoping to pass on their responsibilities to a younger generation of syphilologists. The difficulties of doing so while continuing to benefit from the reputations and experience of the senior members raised again the old question of collective versus individual responsibility for cooperative projects. See especially R. A. Vonderlehr to Moore, 22 August 1939 and Moore's reply, 28 August (RG 90): Public Health Service, General Classified Files, 1936–1944, Box 53: NA.

72. "The Treatment of Early Syphilis," *Ven Dis Info* 15(1934):313–16 and Austin W. Cheever, "Progress in the Diagnosis and Treatment of Syphilis, 1934," *N Engl J Med* 212(1935):882.

73. Louis Chargin, William Leifer, and Theodore Rosenthal, "Marpharsen in the Treatment of Early Syphilis: Comparison of Results in One Hundred and Eighty-Eight Cases with Those of the Cooperative Clinical Group," *Arch Dermatol Syphilol* 40(1939):208–17.

74. [Cornell] Conferences on Therapy, "Evaluation of Drugs Used in the Treatment of Syphilis," *JAMA* 112(1939):2417. As late as 1937, even PHS officials were sceptical about the strength of the evidence on which claims for the superiority of arsphenamine rested. R. A. Vonderlehr to Joseph Earle Moore, 21 August 1937 (RG 90): Public Health Service, General Classified Files, 1936–1944, Box 53: NA.

75. As a nongovernment body, the NRC could not officially allocate government funds, but the overlap in membership between its committees and CMR eroded much of the distinction between them. From its first meeting, the CMR decided to rely heavily on the NRC's committees: the Chairman of the NRC'S Division of Medical Sciences, Lewis Weed, was appointed Vice-Chairman of the CMR, and the head of each of the NRC's major medical subject committees was appointed a CMR consultant. Although the two organizations differed at times, much of CMR's routine business was channeled through the NRC's committees. See A. N. Richards, "Foreword," in *Advances in Military Medicine,* E. C. Andrus et al., eds. (Boston: Little, Brown, 1948), vol. I, xliii–xliv and Irvin G. Stewart, *Organizing Scientific Research for War: The Administrative History of OSRD* (Boston: Little, Brown, 1948), 45–46, 98–101.

76. See Chester S. Keefer, "Penicillin: A Wartime Achievement" in *Advances in Military Medicine,* Andrus et al., eds., vol. II, 719 and Chester S. Keefer, Francis G. Blake, E. K. Marshall, Jr., et. al., "Penicillin in the Treatment of Infections: A Report of 500 Cases," *JAMA* 122(1943):1217–24.

77. Paul Padget, "Diagnosis and Treatment of the Venereal Diseases," in U.S. Army Medical Service, *Internal Medicine in World War II,* vol. II: *Infectious Disease* (Washington: Office of the Surgeon General, 1963), 419–23.

78. After demonstrating its effects in rabbit syphilis, Mahoney obtained au-

thorization to try the drug in humans. [Chester Keefer], *Memorandum on Use of Penicillin in Syphilis* [late October 1943]. NRC Program Files: DIV NRC: Medical Sciences: Committee on Medicine, Subcommittee on Venereal Diseases: Correspondence, Archives, National Academy of Sciences (hereafter "NAS"). Approval for Mahoney's human trial was granted over the objections of J. E. Moore, who thought that additional animal investigations would be more productive and reliable. Moore to E. C. Andrus (of CMR), 13 July 1943 (RG 227): OSRD/CMR, F Penicillin VD, Box 67: NA.

79. Padget, "Diagnosis and Treatment of the Venereal Diseases," U.S. Army Medical Service, *Internal Medicine in World War II*, vol. II: 419–23; William S. Middleton, "European Theater of Operations," U.S. Army Medical Service, *Internal Medicine in World War II*, vol. I: *Activities of Medical Consultants* (Washington: Office of the Surgeon General, 1961), 291–99. Both accounts make it clear that extensive informal contacts between NRC committee members and military consultants served to keep the latter abreast of new developments, despite wartime restrictions on reporting penicillin research.

80. Pilot studies on humans were being explored as early as August, but detailed planning of a cooperative investigation did not begin until October. [Chester Keefer], *Memorandum on Use of Penicillin in Syphilis*. Moore's committee was under the jurisdiction of the NRC Committee on Chemotherapeutic Agents, chaired by Chester S. Keefer. As Special Advisor and Consultant to CMR and, after 1944, their Chief Medical Administrative Officer, Keefer provided the necessary links to OSRD.

81. Although the Army did not wait for the results of NRC investigations to initiate use of penicillin in treating syphilis, they did initiate the series of NRC studies to investigate optimal use of the drug. See NRC-USPHS *Meeting of Pencillin Investigators: 7 and 8 February 1946*, 1–2. On the limitations of the Army's own studies, see Donald M. Pillsbury, "Penicillin Therapy of Early Syphilis in 14,000 Patients: Follow-Up Examination of 792 Patients Six or More Months After Treatment," *Am J Syphilol Dermatol* 30(1946): 134–35.

82. OSRD/CMR, *Agenda for Penicillin Conference Nov 9, 1944* (RG 227): OSRD/CMR, Box 67: NA; *Minutes of a Conference on Penicillin in the Treatment of Syphilis in Human Beings: October 29, 1943*, NAS. NRC Program Files: DIV NRC: Medical Sciences, Committee on Medicine, Subcommittee on Venereal Diseases: Minutes, 1940–1943.

83. Through April 1944, Keefer and CMR were exclusively in charge of allocating civilian supplies of penicillin, which essentially was distributed for the research program and on an emergency basis only. U.S. Senate, Committee on Education and Labor, *Wartime Health and Education: Part 7. Hearings on Medical Research*, 2205–7. 78th Congress, 2nd Session; J. Solon Mordell, Conference on Requirements and Distribution, 3 December 1943 (RG 179): Box 75. Chemicals: Drugs: Penicillin. Keefer continued as advisor to the War Production Board on policy for penicillin distribution at least through April 1945. War Production Board, *Report of the Operations, from April 1944 to April 1945 . . . Office of Civilian Penicillin Distribution* (RG 179): Box 379, 052.528. All references NA.

84. Ultimate decisions concerning the study, while strongly influenced by the specialists on the Subcommittee for Venereal Diseases, were controlled by CMR's Keefer who added the clinics of Francis Blake and W. Barry Wood to the study. *Twenty-First Meeting, Subcommittee on Venereal Diseases: 11 November 1943*, NAS, NRC Program Files: DIV NRC: Medical Sciences: Committee on Medicine,

Subcommittee on Venereal Diseases: Minutes: 1940–1943. Blake's and Wood's expertise, like that of Keefer's, was in the more general domain of chemotherapy and infectious disease. An undercurrent of tension between general infectious disease and venereal disease specialists runs through the wartime and postwar discussions. These differences in perspective deserve more careful examination than I have been able to provide.

85. The use of lower dosages was also influenced by the initial shortages of penicillin. See NRC, CMR, *Minutes on a Conference on Penicillin in the Treatment of Syphilis in Human Beings, 29 October 1943*. NAS, NRC Program Files: DIV NRC: Medical Sciences: Committee on Medicine, Subcommittee on Venereal Disease: Minutes: 1940–1943; and OSRD/CMR, *Agenda for Penicillin Conference November 9, 1944* (RG 227): OSRD/CMR, Box 67, NA.

86. J. E. Moore, Memorandum, 9 May 1945 (RG 227): OSRD/CMR Correspondence, Box 67, F Penicillin VD, NA.

87. The NRC Subcommittee on Venereal Diseases passed these requests on to the NRC Committee on Chemotherapeutics chaired by Chester Keefer. Keefer's committee insisted that any proposed studies would have to come up through NRC and CMR for a full review. J. E. Moore to members, Penicillin Panel, Subcommittee on VD, 24 January 1945 (RG 227): OSRD/CMR Correspondence, Box 56 and J. E. Moore, Memorandum, 9 May 1945 (RG 227): OSRD/CMR Correspondence, Box 67, F Penicillin VD (both references are to NA).

88. See the remarks of Joseph Earle Moore, U.S. PHS, FDA, and NRC, *Penicillin Conference 26–27 March 1946* [mimeo text] (Washington: n.p., n.d.), 159.

89. For specific examples of shortcomings in the data, see Otis L. Anderson to Medical Officers in Charge, 24 June 1944 (RG 90): PHS, General Classified Files, 1936–1944, Box 56, NA. As late as 1945, Moore reported that the initial 6,000–8,000 cases would need to be reabstracted and reanalyzed. J. E. Moore to A. N. Richards, 2 May 1945 (RG 227): OSRD/CMR, Box 67, F Penicillin VD, NA. Only 6,000 of 11,000 cases proved useful in the end. See Margaret Merrell in "General Discussion," NRC, U.S. PHS, *Meeting of Penicillin Investigators: 7 and 8 February 1946*, 147.

90. Overall loss to follow-up averaged 9.5% but was as high as 43.5% in one clinic. See J. E. Moore, "Preliminary Statement," U.S. PHS *Conference of Investigators of Penicillin Therapy* (7–8 February 1946), 4.

91. Assignments were based on estimates of the numbers of patients available in individual clinics and, presumably, on the willingness of investigators to try specific regimens, although this is not explicitly stated in the records. Variability in follow-up rates only increased the "noise" in the data present from the initial experimental design. Other problems evocative of the Cooperating Clinic Study were the inclusion in the study of patients who had been treated prior to entry, and differences of opinion regarding the distinction between relapse and reinfection. See Paul D. Rosahn, "The Treatment of Early Syphilis with Penicillin Alone and Combined with Mapharsen and with Bismuth: Results of a Nation-Wide Study." In U.S. PHS *Conference of Investigators of Penicillin Therapy* (7–8 February 1946) and the comments of Joseph Earle Moore and Margaret Merrell in the discussion at this conference: NRC, U.S. PHS, *Meeting of Penicillin Investigators: 7 and 8 February 1946* (n.p.), 146–47.

92. In January of 1946, OSRD/CMR turned responsibilities for the study over to the Public Health Service, which simply added two or three members to the existing NRC subcommittee overseeing the study, christened it an advisory study

section to the National Institutes of Health, and continued operating as before. For a list of committee members, see J. E. Moore, "Preliminary Statement," U.S. PHS, *Conference of Investigators of Penicillin Therapy* (7–8 Feburary 1946), 1.

93. J. E. Moore, "Preliminary Statement," U.S. PHS, *Conference of Investigators of Penicillin Therapy* (7–8 February 1946), 4.

94. There is some evidence that Surgeon General Parran was more concerned with protecting funding for the federal program of venereal disease case finding than with the research program. U.S. Congress, House of Representatives, Committee on Appropriations, *Hearings: Department of Labor-Federal Security Appropriation Bill for 1948: February–March 1948*. Part 2, 282–85, 80th Congress, 1st Session. The study responded to cutbacks by eliminating clinics with poor track records in following protocols and finding patients; support for the Central Statistical Unit was maintained to allow for continuing analysis. [Anonymous], "Financial Support for Medical Research in the Venereal Diseases," *Am J Syphil Gonorr Ven Dis* 31(1947):664–68.

95. Margaret Merrell, "Estimates of Relapse and Reinfection Rates in Early Syphilis Treated with Penicillin," *Am J Syphil Gonorr Ven Dis* 35(1951):532–43.

96. Frank W. Reynolds, "Penicillin in Early Syphilis: An Analysis of the Discrepancies Between the Results of Arnold et al. and Those of the Central Statistical Unit," in U.S. PHS, *Recent Advances in the Study of Venereal Diseases: A Symposium: April 8–9 1948* (Washington: Venereal Disease Education Institute, 1948), 113–21. In comparing the cooperative study with the superior results obtained by John Mahoney and his colleagues, Reynolds notes that Mahoney's superior "cure" rates may have been due to the cooperative study's greater diligence in following patients, which lowered their overall success rate.

97. Margaret Merrell in "General Discussion," NRC, U.S. PHS, *Meeting of Penicillin Investigators: 7 and 8 February 1946* (n.p.), 147–48. Interestingly, the postwar cutbacks in funding for the study apparently concentrated the mind: "The fact that only two issues instead of a battery were under investigation meant that the material was not fractionated so many ways. There were about 3,000 cases, of which over two thirds were concentrated at three large clinics which distributed their cases almost equally over the 4 schedules. Thus the cases under these 4 treatments were almost identical in their distribution as to color, sex and admission diagnosis." Margaret Merrell, "Report from Central Statistical Unit on Comparative Failure Rates for Early Syphilis Treated with Penicillin," *A Symposium on Current Progress in the Study of Venereal Diseases: April 7–8 1949* (Washington: Public Health Service, 1949), 40.

98. [Walsh McDermott] to Doctors Palmer, Bogen, Barnwell, Hinshaw, Willis, and Long (27 March 1947), *Suggestion for the Report from the Panel on Dose Regimens to the Tuberculosis Study Section*, Esmond Long Papers, National Library of Medicine, Box 15 (hereafter cited as Long Papers).

99. Although as of January 1946, CMR no longer controlled research funds, it continued to be in charge of allocating scarce drugs. The publicity given streptomycin prior to establishing production facilities on an industrial scale led producers to request that distribution of the drug be regulated. Apart from a few researchers supplied directly from drug firms, civilian allocations of streptomycin through October 1946 were to be made by Chester Keefer. See *Initial Report on Operations: July 1, 1945 to March 31, 1946*, Drug Section, Chemicals Division, Civilian Production Administration (CPA) (RG 179): Box 73; Streptomycin Industry Advisory Committee, CPA, *Meeting: January 15, 1946* (RG 179): 533.8405; CPA, Memo,

13 February 1946 (RG 179): 533.845; and Ernest M. Allen to R. E. Dyer, 20 February 1946 (RG 443): NIH, Office of the Director, Box 142 (all references are to NA). Keefer continued to wear two hats and as an NRC official was involved in planning the cooperative study. See Chester Keefer to Esmond Long, 9 March 1946, Box 15, Long Papers.

100. H. Corwin Hinshaw, et al., "Report of the Committee on Therapy" [American Trudeau Society, 11–12 January 1946], *Am Rev Tubercul* 54(1946):442; H. Corwin Hinshaw and William H. Feldman, "Streptomycin in Treatment of Clinical and Experimental Tuberculosis," *Ann NY Acad Sci* 48(1946):177–82; and H. McLeod Riggins and H. Corwin Hinshaw, "American Trudeau Society: The Streptomycin-Tuberculosis Research Project," *Am Rev Tubercul* 56(1947):168–73.

101. *Projected Plan for a Joint Study of TB: April 25, 1946,* Box 15, Long Papers. Of the key figures involved in planning the study, Arthur Walker had just come from writing a history of the penicillin investigations for OSRD. Esmond Long had spent the war as a consultant on tuberculosis to the U.S. Army; he joined the planning at the request of Lewis Weed, head of the NRC's Division of Medical Sciences. John Barnwell had newly joined the VA as head of its Tuberculosis Division. William B. Tucker, "Evolution of the Cooperative Studies in the Chemotherapy of Tuberculosis of the Veterans Administration and Armed Forces of the U.S.A.," *Adv Tubercul Res* 10(1960):3–4; Veterans Administration, *Minutes of the Third Streptomycin Conference: May 1, 2 and 3, 1947* (St. Louis: Veterans Administration, 1949), 7.

102. In June 1946, the Public Health Service refrained from adding streptomycin to its research program due to "conditions prevailing in Congress at that time." Discussions of a study within the PHS and by the Bureau of the Budget continued, however. National Health Advisory Council, *Minutes: December 6–7, 1946,* Vol. 1: 51 (RG 443): Box 2, NA. Meanwhile, PHS members continued to participate in an advisory capacity with the VA study, along with various NRC members. See William B. Tucker, "Evaluation of Streptomycin Regimens in the Treatment of Tuberculosis: An Account of the Study of the Veteran's Administration, Army and Navy, July 1946 to April 1949," *Am Rev Tubercul* 60(1949):716.

103. Tucker, "Evolution of the Cooperative Studies," 6. While the Army and the Navy continued to participate in the VA study, the latter organization was in a position to provide most of the patients.

104. Paul R. Hawley, "Medical Problems of the Veterans Administration," *JAMA* 129(1945):521–22 and Paul Hawley, "New Opportunities for Physicians in the Veterans Administration," *JAMA* 130(1946):403–5.

105. [John Barnwell] in Veterans Administration, *Minutes of the First Streptomycin Conference: December 12, 13, and 14, 1946* (Chicago: Veterans Administration, 1949), 29. See also U.S. Army–U.S. Navy–Veterans Administration–U.S. Public Health Service–National Research Council–National Tuberculosis Association, *Streptomycin Conference: May 10, 1946,* Box 15, Long Papers.

106. Streptomycin Committee, "The Effect of Streptomycin upon Pulmonary Tuberculosis in Man—Preliminary Report of a Cooperative Study of 223 Cases by the Army, Navy and Veterans Administration," *VA Tech Bull* TB 10-37 (24 September 1947), 4.

107. Streptomycin Committee, "Effect of Streptomycin upon Pulmonary Tuberculosis," 4.

108. The VA's subsequent decision not to participate in the Public Health Service study of streptomycin was based in part on the conviction that the use of con-

trol groups would produce "undesirable repercussions" from "certain groups in this country." Veterans Administration, *Minutes of the Fourth Streptomycin Conference: October 9, 10, 11, and 12, 1947* (St. Louis: Veterans Administration, 1947), 61. The issue was so sensitive that John Barnwell, head of the VA Tuberculosis Division, withdrew from the review panel handling appeals from physicians in the PHS study who wished to provide streptomycin to control group patients. Despite the fact that it was not Barnwell's study, he wished to avoid "situations" which "would be embarrassing to him" as "an employee of a tuberculosis service of the federal government." Tuberculosis Study Section, *Report of Informal Meeting: June 17, 1948*, Box 16, Long Papers.

109. Arthur M. Walker and John Barnwell, "Clinical Evaluation of Chemotherapeutic Drugs in Tuberculosis," *Ann NY Acad Sci* 52(1949):746.

110. If the VA officials in charge of planning the study had not recognized the scientific importance of controls, then the insistence of Carroll Palmer, PHS representative to the planning group, on the need for controls would have made the point clear. At the same time, the difficulties of conducting controlled studies in the VA overrode these considerations. Veterans Administration, *First Streptomycin Conference*, 5–6, 42–43; for Palmer's views, see especially Veterans Administration, *Third Streptomycin Conference*, 155–56. As new regimens came under consideration, the issue of controls recurred, with the same themes being sounded. See the discussion on a control group for thoracoplasty: Veterans Administration, *Third Streptomycin Conference*, 33–34. For an additional discussion of the issue of controls in the VA study, see idem, 34–35.

111. Veterans Administration, *First Streptomycin Conference*, 5.

112. In an effort to prevent knowledge of treatment from influencing assessments of outcome, "blind" evaluations of X ray results were obtained from observers who did not know whether they were scoring cases that had received streptomycin. Statisticians reviewing these results reported that interobserver agreement about the degree of improvement was no better than might have been expected by chance. See Veterans Administration, *Third Streptomycin Conference*, 147–65, especially 150–52, and Streptomycin Committee, "The Effect of Streptomycin," 6. The study was further compromised by the decision, in October 1947, to no longer require individual investigators to collect a two-month baseline period of observations on patients before beginning treatment. Veterans Administration, *Fourth Streptomycin Conference*, 67.

113. The importance of the VA program only increased as other projects encountered funding difficulties. [H. Corwin Hinshaw] in Veterans Administration, *Minutes of the Second Streptomycin Conference: January 23 and 24, 1947* (Chicago: Veterans Administration, 1949), 87, 50–51; see also [Esmond Long], Veterans Administration, *Minutes of the Fifth Streptomycin Conference: April 15, 16, 17, and 18, 1948* (Chicago: Veterans Administration, 1948), 149. Apart from having greater numbers of patients available, the VA could also expect a greater proportion of their patients to return for follow-up, as such examinations were a condition of receiving disability checks. Walker and Barnwell, "Clinical Evaluation of Chemotherapeutic Drugs," 742–43.

114. Veterans Administration, *Second Streptomycin Conference*, 5–6, 69, 84–85. Discussions of the implications of increasing streptomycin supply began almost as soon as the study started. See A. M. Walker to John B. Barnwell, Esmond Long, and George Owen, 17 June 1946. In November 1946, less than six months into the

study, the VA decided to make streptomycin generally available for all non-TB uses, while keeping the Streptomycin Committee in charge of allocations for TB cases. Paul Hawley to Long, 25 November 1946 (both references from Box 15, Long Papers).

115. Investigators were granted permission to use the drug on ineligible patients at their discretion, so long as they did not include those patients in their reports on the study. Streptomycin Committee to Study Units, 20 December 1946, Box 15, Long Papers.

116. In general, there were two distinct kinds of protocol violation: one involved continuing the study at sites without the correct laboratory facilities to monitor the drug, the other involved selecting patients who did not fit the protocol's rules of eligibility, or varying the treatment regimen in some fashion. It was the latter type of deviation that caused difficulties in interpreting results. Veterans Administration, *Third Streptomycin Conference*, 63, 67, 69, 152–53, 157.

117. See the discussion in Veterans Administration, *Fifth Streptomycin Conference*, 147–50.

118. [H. L. Mantz], Veterans Administration, *Third Streptomycin Conference*, 66 and discussion, 57–58.

119. The overlap in membership between the VA's Streptomycin Committee, the Tuberculosis Study Section of NIH, and the Committee on Research of the American Trudeau Society makes it difficult to determine at times *which* study is being discussed, especially in the spring and summer of 1946 when the VA study was just getting underway. The NRC's continuing involvement only complicates the problem. The key players with multiple hats were John Barnwell, who served as head of the VA's TB Division and on the NIH's TB Study Section; Esmond Long, a key figure in the American Trudeau Society, who served as the NRC's representative to the VA study and later helped design the PHS investigation; and Carroll E. Palmer, who headed the PHS TB Division and consulted frequently to the VA study. Other ubiquitous players included H. Corwin Hinshaw, J. Burns Amberson, Chester Keefer, and Walsh McDermott.

120. [Walsh McDermott] to Doctors Palmer, Bogen, Barnwell, Hinshaw, Willis, and Long, *Suggestions for the Report from the Panel on Dose Regimens to the Tuberculosis Study Section* 27 March 1947, Box 15, Long Papers.

121. [Walsh McDermott], *Dose Regimens.*

122. The initial request to Congress was for an appropriation of $3 million, of which $1.25 million was intended for research on streptomycin independent of the cooperative project. See testimony of R. E. Dyer, U.S. Congress, House of Representatives, Committee on Appropriations, *Hearings: Department of Labor–Federal Security Appropriation Bill for 1948: February–March 1946*, Part II, 491. 80th Congress, 1st Session. I have been unable to trace the records of the TB Study Section's deliberations; however, it appears as if a Steering Committee consisting of Esmond Long, Walsh McDermott, H. Corwin Hinshaw, Carroll Palmer, H. McLeod Riggins, and H. Stuart Willis found itself in the position of having to trim the study plans without help from the Study Section. See Willis to Long, 16 May 1947 and Long's reply, 19 May. Box 15, Long Papers.

123. National Health Advisory Council, *Minutes: June 6–7, 1947*, vol. 1, 168 (RG 443): NIH Office of the Director, Minutes, National Advisory Health Council, 1945–1960, Box 2, NA.

124. National Health Advisory Council, *Minutes: June 6–7, 1947*, vol. 1, 167–68 (RG 443): NIH Office of the Director, Minutes, National Advisory Health

Council, 1945–1960, Box 2, NA; the concern of the Bureau of the Budget that the project be conducted "wholly on an investigative basis" was also made clear to the officials managing the VA study, who warned researchers that funding would be cut off "if it [streptomycin] gets too widely disbursed." [John Barnwell], Veterans Administration, *Third Streptomycin Conference*, 51.

125. *Minutes: Meeting of the Tuberculosis Study Section Steering Committee and Special Consultants* 24–25 May 1947, Box 16, Long Papers. The PHS' Carroll E. Palmer, along with statisticians from the VA and NRC, were highly critical of the VA's decision to proceed without controls, and generally pessimistic about the "fruitfulness" of the VA study "as presently conceived." It was Palmer who finally managed to convince Esmond Long of the need for controls in the PHS research "in spite of the difficulties." Subcommittee on Tuberculosis, *Minutes: May 2, 1947* and Gilbert Beebe, *Memo for Lewis Weed on Organization of Research in Use of Streptomycin in TB, June 11, 1947*, NRC: Division of Medical Sciences: Committee on Medicine: Subcommittee on TB, NAS.

126. Esmond R. Long and Shirley H. Ferebee, "A Controlled Investigation of Streptomycin Treatment in Tuberculosis," *Public Health Rep* 65(1950):1421–22.

127. Carroll E. Palmer to Long, 21 October 1947, Box 15, Long Papers.

128. Palmer to Long, 21 October 1947; H. C. Hinshaw to Palmer, 29 October 1947; Walsh McDermott to Palmer, 3 November 1947, Box 15, Long Papers. Hinshaw's and McDermott's letters make it clear that both were uncomfortable with signing a statement denying that streptomycin had *any* value, but whereas Hinshaw proposed a modified statement justifying a control group, McDermott thought that the best approach was saying nothing at all on the subject.

129. H. C. Hinshaw to Palmer, *Proposed Statement of Investigations . . .* , 29 October 1947. Box 15, Long Papers.

130. It appears, however, that both control patients and those receiving streptomycin were permitted to have other traditional treatments such as "collapse therapy"; when the control group is referred to as "untreated" it is the use of streptomycin which is meant. In the event, 79.2 percent of the streptomycin patients and only 73 percent of the controls received *no* surgical intervention. Long and Ferebee, "A Controlled Investigation," 1424.

131. TB Study Section, Steering Committee, *Minutes: November 22, 1947*, 6 Long Papers, Box 16; Shirley H. Ferebee to Long, 2 December 1947, Box 15, Long Papers.

132. J. Burns Amberson to Long, 18 December 1947, Box 15, Long Papers. The continued obstructions placed by Amberson in the face of maintaining effective controls are all the more striking as in 1931 he had conducted what appears to be the first U.S. clinical study employing an untreated control group where the assignment of treatment/no treatment was left to chance. J. Burns Amberson, B. T. McMahon, and Max Pinner, "A Clinical Trial of Sanocrysin in Pulmonary Tuberculosis," *Am Rev Tubercul* 24(1931):401–35.

133. H. McLeod Riggins to Long, 14 November 1947; Riggins to H. Stuart Willis, 10 November 1947, Box 15, Long Papers. The subsequent decision to create an Appeals Board did not, however, permanently resolve the underlying issue: questions about the scope and operating procedures of the appeals process continued to recur. See Tuberculosis Study Section, *Report of Informal Meeting: June 17, 1948*, Box 16, Long Papers. The discussion implies that some physicians were referring cases which could not possibly meet the appeals criteria, perhaps in the hopes of having the Appeals Board take responsibility for withholding the drug. This

document also raises questions about the investigators' understanding of the concept of blind allocation to treatment and controls.

134. Shirley H. Ferebee to J. Burns Amberson, 20 October 1948, Box 15, Long Papers.

135. William B. Tucker, "Evaluation of Streptomycin Regimens in the Treatment of Tuberculosis: An Account of the Study of the Veterans Administration, Army and Navy, July 1946 to April 1946," *Am Rev Tubercul* 60(1949):745–46; Lawrence B. Hobson and Walsh McDermott, "Criteria for the Clinical Evaluation of Antituberculosis Agents," *Ann NY Acad Sci* 52(1949):782–87. On Carroll Palmer's scepticism about the VA's outcome measures, see Gilbert Beebe, *Memo for Lewis Weed on Organization of Research in Use of Streptomycin in TB, June 11, 1947*, NRC: Division of Medical Sciences, Committee on Medicine, Subcommittee on TB, NAS.

136. Amberson to Long, 3 November 1948, Box 15, Long Papers.

137. Tucker, "Evaluation of Streptomycin Regimens," 745.

138. Tucker, "Evaluation of Streptomycin Regimens," 745.

139. Ferebee to Amberson, 20 October 1948, Box 15, Long Papers.

140. The soliloquy of Emil Bogen on the subject of clinician's reliability is quite interesting in this regard. To the statisticians' plaint that experienced clinicians cannot agree even in judging X rays, Bogen replied, in effect: They can if you throw out the bad films. Veterans Administration, *Minutes of the Eighth Streptomycin Conference: November 10, 11, 12, and 13, 1949* (Washington: Veterans Administration, 1949), 279.

141. *Transactions of the 14th Conference on Chemotherapy of Tuberculosis: February 7–10, 1955* (Washington and Atlanta: Veterans Administration, 1955), 372.

142. [Morris C. Thomas], Veterans Administration *Fifth Streptomycin Conference*, 15; William Stead, "A Suggested Change in the Method of Randomization of Patients in Therapeutic Trials," Veterans Administration, *Transactions of the 16th Conference on the Chemotherapy of Tuberculosis: February 1957* (Washington: Veterans Administration, 1957), 117–19. Manipulation of treatment assignment by physicians who "randomized" on the basis of patients' chart numbers was widely suspect in another VA study, a study of anticoagulants, conducted in the 1950s. See Louis Lasagna, "The Controlled Clinical Trial: Theory and Practice," *J Chron Dis* 1(1955):357–58.

143. The PHS shared credit for demonstrating the value of streptomycin with the British Medical Research Council, whose trials also used randomized controls. The VA decision to "finally" adopt randomization was influenced by disagreements between the three cooperative groups (VA, PHS, and MRC) concerning the relative value of isoniazid versus streptomycin plus para-amino salicylic acid (PAS). William B. Tucker, "A Controlled Study of the Variables in the Chemotherapy of Pulmonary Tuberculosis: An Account and Critique of the Investigation by the Cooperative Group of the Veterans Administration, Army and Navy, 1946–1953," Veterans Administration, *Transactions of the 12th Conference on the Chemotherapy of Tuberculosis: February 1953* (Washington: Veterans Administration, 1953), 31–32; Tucker, "Evolution of the Cooperative Studies," 28. It is difficult to reconcile Tucker's claim in 1960 that "repeated checks" found only "minor deviations" from randomization (30) with William Stead's observation as late as 1957 that statistically significant differences existed among the treatment arms in severity of disease. What is clear is that even "internal" critics of the VA study, such as Stead and

Tucker, continued to believe in the VA findings—the adoption of centralized randomization was to convince others. Stead, "Change in the Method of Randomization," 119.

144. A. Bradford Hill, "Assessment of Therapeutic Trials," *Trans Med Soc Lond* 68(1953):132. Hill continued to insist that one of the main points in using randomization was to convince others: A. B. Hill, "Aims and Ethics," in *Conference on Controlled Clinical Trials: Vienna, 1959* (Oxford: Blackwell Scientific Publishers, 1960), 5.

145. The repeated proposals to improve the statistical competence of research design and review at the NIH suggest that progress in this field was slow. See, National Advisory Health Council, *Minutes: February 20–21, 1953*, vol. 2, 4–5 and *Minutes: October 23–24, 1956* (RG 443): NIH Office of the Director. Meetings, National Advisory Health Council 1945–1960, Boxes 3 and 4, NA. Certainly, the news of their elevation might have come as a surprise to most statisticians working in medical fields prior to 1960. See Donald Mainland, "We Wish to Hire a Medical Statistician: Have You Any Advice to Offer?" *JAMA* 193(1965):289–93.

146. Alvan R. Feinstein, "An Additional Basic Science for Clinical Medicine: II. The Limitations of Randomized Trials," *Ann Intern Med* 99(1983):544–50; idem, "Clinical Biostatistics: VI. Statistical Malpractice—and the Responsibility of a Consultant," *Clin Pharmacol Ther* 11(1970):898–913.

PART IV

A CONCLUDING VIEW

11

The Curious Career of Internal Medicine: Functional Ambivalence, Social Success

ROSEMARY STEVENS

Internal medicine is an American specialty that has long drawn on British organizational models but was based originally on German ideas about medical knowledge and technique. It is not surprising that, from its formal beginnings in the 1880s, it has been marked by contradictions and ambivalence. As a would-be "general specialty," internal medicine has been in constant search of its own definition. As a would-be consulting field along British lines, internal medicine defined a role for which there was no obvious niche. In other respects, too, inconsistencies mark its organizations. Early leaders of internal medicine, including Francis Delafield and William Osler, took pride in standing apart from medical politics.[1] Nevertheless, the history of internal medicine as a specialty has been largely driven by external influences, including the politics of other specialty fields. Although leaders of internal medicine have sought flexibility, the field has become locked into a bureaucratic network of subspecialties, of which there are now eleven.[2] Meanwhile, internal medicine is distinguished as a basic field of primary care. For its ambivalence alone—in its attempts to encompass distinct, sometimes competing, notions about the nature of medicine—internal medicine offers a rich and challenging historical field.

Yet internal medicine has also become enormously successful as an organizational entity within American medicine. Indeed, a major task for the historian is to reconcile the ambiguities of internal medicine with its organizational success. Today approximately a fourth of all residents are in approved internal medicine programs; decisions about the focus of training and the number (and funding) of these residents send ripples across the whole of medicine. University departments of medicine have become powerful centers of prestige. The American Board of Internal Medicine (ABIM) granted almost 40 percent of all primary specialty certificates in the last decade,[3] and the American College of Physicians is one of the largest and most influential medical organizations in the country. Here, in short, is a field marked both by definitional ambivalence and by institutional importance within American medicine.

This chapter focuses on the organizational development of internal medicine within the context of its search for definition. By setting out the general organizational development of the field I hope to provoke interest in its institutional history among both historians and practitioners. A second aim is to sketch, tentatively, the relationships between organizational goals and the tensions inherent in internal medicine as a field. I will first discuss the history and then consider briefly some contemporary questions in historical perspective.

Early Definition

Internal medicine exists because it is organized. There might well have been a field of general medicine, with or without subspecialties, had internal medicine not developed with all its present ramifications. But it is the actions of individuals, grouped into specific organizations, that have shaped the contours and set up the dynamics of internal medicine as we now know it. Of particular importance in its history have been the founding of the Association of American Physicians (1885), the American College of Physicians (1915), and the American Board of Internal Medicine (1936). The comparatively late dates of all of these organizations should be stressed. There has been nothing in American medicine to compare with the dominant role of the British Royal Colleges, which provided both the authority and an umbrella framework for the development of the specialties in Britain. Indeed one useful organizing framework for the history of American medicine is to see the American medical profession as a profession that developed without the establishment of strong centralized guilds and has spent much of its history trying to invent them.

Thus, although internal medicine with its subspecialties has much in common *substantively* with the field of general medicine in Britain, American medicine developed *organizationally* its own idiosyncratic patterns and stresses. In Britain the consultant physician has a clear role as a hospital-based specialist who accepts patients on referral from family practitioners and returns them when an episode of treatment is completed. This system, marked by the institutional relationships of the major medical guilds in Britain, was formalized between 1880 and 1914 under the joint pressures of specialization and national health insurance.[4] In the United States, where no such formal division of roles developed, internists compete for patients directly with other practitioners. As a result, internal medicine—an American specialty—has long been beset by two historically rich issues toward which it has been ambivalent: the relationship between internal medicine and other specialties, and its role in primary care.

Proposals for a divided profession in the New World were doomed to failure. John Morgan's attempt in the eighteenth century to establish a national College of Physicians on the model of the Royal College of Physicians of London was vetoed by Thomas Penn. The College of Physicians of Philadelphia was finally established in 1787, but it was not to play a role in national licensing as the English College did.[5] Thus it had no power to regulate the profession by providing a cadre of high status physicians, marked by educational attainment and prestige, whose role was separate both from general practitioners and from surgeons. Nor, in a country that consisted of a federation of largely independent states, was the College a ready base for a national organization of an educated physician elite. There was, therefore, no tradition of a ranked profession or consultant practice within which internal medicine could later be developed as a formal, consulting elite. This lack of tradition may have been all to the good, but it provided no foundation for any future consulting field in general medicine.

Instead, the control and regulation of physicians through licensing devolved on the states, while the American medical profession remained, formally, egalitarian. Despite the establishment of the American Medical Association in 1847, it was not until the late nineteenth century that there were any effective demands for national medical organizations. These were spurred on by exuberant, unbridled specialization in practice; by huge variations in the standards of medical education; by the development of new scientific and craft elites, notably in laboratory medicine and surgery; by the rapid development of hospitals and surgical enthusiasm among ill-equipped practitioners; by the Johns Hopkins model of medical education as an exemplar of reform; and by the shared European educational experience of hundreds of American physicians. It was in this turbulent and rapidly changing environment, an organizational free-for-all of professional divisions and allegiances, that modern internal medicine was invented.

The seven physicians who came together in 1885 in Francis Delafield's office to form the nucleus of the new Association of American Physicians (AAP) were distinguished by their common experience and skill in pathology, by foreign postgraduate study, by their investigative interests as well as private practice, and by the fact that all taught and had part-time academic positions.[6] They represented the new generation of European-trained scholar-clinicians, linking the skills of clinical medicine with pathology. They were scientifically oriented generalists. They can also be seen as members of a new, well-educated professional elite, based in New York, Boston, and Philadelphia. Perhaps unconsciously echoing John Morgan's much earlier proposals, the AAP defined a separate caste of educated physicians. This caste was distinguished from the mass of practitioners by its superior professional preparation, research interests, and diagnostic skills. Drawing on the prestige system of the time—German education and technique—these physicians, like Morgan, sought to establish a new prestige system within medicine.

However, there were immediate structural problems in defining internal medicine as an elite form of generalism. Internal medicine as a special focus, rank, or field had to be invented in an organizational environment that was discouraging in at least two respects. First, it lacked the benefit of a long-established institutional base, such as a national College of Physicians, which could sustain and justify the emergence of the field. Second, internal medicine was in direct competition with other rapidly organizing specialties. Thus from the beginning, internal medicine could neither claim a monopoly as "consultant medicine" nor truly be "general medicine." By the late 1880s, pediatrics, dermatology, and neurology, each of which might legitimately be considered a subfield of general medicine, were already embarked on separate organizational careers, forming a model for the later development of other fields. Internal medicine had to carve out its own field under less than ideal organizational conditions.

Internal medicine has also to be seen in relation to—and in reaction to—professional developments in American surgery. In England the prestige of the "physician" long antedated that of the surgeon. In the United States the positions were reversed. The AAP developed in a period of exceptional surgical expansion, attuned to the American "can-do" ideology in the "fast" modern age of the 1880s and marked by the skills, success, flamboyance, and self-glorification of leading surgeons. Although research needs to be done on the specific role and dominance of surgery in American medicine from the 1880s to the present, especially as it affected perceptions and structures in the nonsurgical specialties, it is significant that surgery was successfully organized before internal medicine attempted to develop its own definition. If internal medicine was to succeed in America as a field based on the German scientific style of careful investigation, logic and exact methods, it had to develop its own articulated purpose and ideology, either by analogy to surgery or in open competition with it. The drama and seductive imagery of surgery, its base in the new hospitals, the boldness and arrogance of its technique, and its exploitation of the body for the patient's good caused it to have a special hold on the American imagination.

Three years before the AAP was founded, Samuel D. Gross, in his address of welcome as the first president of the American Surgical Association (1882), waxed lyrical about the progress of American surgery and its relevance to the American spirit and American life. The new association was to be an "altar" to surgical science, with science based squarely on experience: "Theory has given way to fact, and nothing that cannot withstand this test is worthy of acceptance."[7] It is reasonable to assume that practitioners of internal medicine went out of their way to define their field as a branch of medicine that also stressed facts (pathology) and skills (diagnostic acumen), in an effort to challenge American surgery head on. Otherwise, the new physicians might lay themselves open to criticism in the American professional environment as being academic, ineffective, and effete.[8] A reluctance to tangle with the power politics of surgery probably strengthened the AAP's resolve to be an apolitical organization. Meanwhile, the link between clinical medicine and laboratory investigation gave internal medicine a knowledge base competitive with surgical empiricism.

Under these conditions, external events triggered responses from the AAP from its beginning; it was impossible to be truly apolitical. Aside from a natural inclination to define the new field as having a mission and intellectual roots distinct from surgery, there was organizational potential for an elite organization of physicians that would match the national organization for surgeons. Thus the American Surgical Association invited the AAP to assist it in approaching other specialized societies to form a Congress of Physicians and Surgeons, whose first meeting was in 1888. The AAP could probably have developed such national leadership in other ways, too, taking on a role more like the present American College of Physicians. Instead, another set of external pressures confirmed its role as an intellectual focus for the linking of pathology and clinical medicine. By the mid-1890s there was a recognized shortage of well-trained pathologists and bacteriologists to teach in the rapidly reorganizing medical schools.

It was in this context that William Osler, in his presidential address to the AAP in 1895, called for the training of "able young men" in "internal medicine as a specialty."[9] These new specialists were to be seen as "special clinical physicians," whose work was based on pathology, and whose career was to pass through the laboratories to the wards, applying laboratory science directly to clinical medicine.

Quite apart from the cognitive implications of this definition, the acceptance of internal medicine as a specialty had two immediate structural advantages. First, it distinguished internal medicine from the domain of general practice, thereby giving it a unique professional turf. Osler made this point explicitly by remarking that special clinical physicians could not develop readily in the "routine of family practice." Second, it gave internal medicine, like surgery, a hospital base. Osler saw the opportunity for a career in internal medicine in "every city with a hospital of fifty beds." Thus the AAP could be seen as the apex of a field that was functionally distinguished from surgery, gynecology, and general practice, and substantively distinguished by its links with the biomedical sciences. A later AAP president confirmed these expectations in 1899, linking the clinician with the pathologist, bacteriologist, and chemist.[10]

By these moves internal medicine gained its tortuous definition, both as a specialty and as a field that was more general than other specialties, which were seen, in turn, as marred by narrow-minded routine and devotion to technique.[11] However, such a definition of internal medicine as a general specialty—that is, as a general consulting elite justified by special competence—could only thrive under two continuing conditions, one qualitative and one functional. First, the definition assumed that general practitioners had an inadequate medical education in the basic medical sciences or, at least, demonstrably inferior skills to internists; second, it assumed that there was room for the consulting practitioner, idealized in the example of William Osler and his work. History was soon to challenge both of these conditions.

The University Base

The reform of American medical schools, both before and after the Flexner report of 1910, provided internal medicine with a powerful institutional foundation. With the growing authority of university departments of medicine, the hospital became less important as a seat for professional definition.[12] Full-time academic medicine became well established by 1920.[13] As the departments in the leading schools linked laboratory medicine and clinical facilities around research interests, leadership in internal medicine moved from practice to the schools. In turn, the AAP became a center for full-time academicians. This early divergence of academic medicine and medical practice was to provide lasting questions for internal medicine that have never been fully addressed or resolved: How was internal medicine to develop as a major field? Or was it? Were the university departments primarily for research or to educate general medical practitioners, or both? Were they to assume two ranks of physician, the general practitioner and the internist? Was internal medicine primarily an investigative field? While the answers to these questions varied over the years, the identification of internal medicine with the university departments of medicine in these formative years gave internal medicine a peculiar and persistently academic tone.

Ironically, the establishment of the American College of Physicians in 1915 came in the midst of the rising power of the university departments. The irony lay in the fact that, to the professors, a College now had little relevance. The foundation of the College was also curiously repetitive. Once again the physicians followed the path of the surgeons; the American College of Surgeons had been established two years earlier in 1913. Here also was John Morgan's idea of a national elite college for physicians, this time reflected in the vision of Heinrich Stern, who saw an American college as parallel to the Royal College of Physicians of London. However, the British model had come far too late to provide a prestige system based on guilds. American medicine was being reformed along German lines, through a major refocusing in and on the schools.

Furthermore, the physicians' College could not compete with the driving success of the College of Surgeons. Stern's personality and influence made him an ineffective leader in comparison with the more charismatic Franklin Martin of the American College of Surgeons. The question was not, of course, merely one of character, but also of potential purpose and mission. The American College of Surgeons spoke for standards of surgery as a whole. There was a recognized need to limit surgical excess, that is, to upgrade the standards of surgery across the country, to reduce unnecessary procedures, and to restrict the performance of surgical operations wherever possible to the properly trained. These were democratic and public service goals. The American College of Surgeons' standards were to provide a discriminating mark by which the better trained could be identified from the mass, but the aim was to upgrade the entire practice of surgery. Practitioners of internal medicine, however, never saw themselves as a force for reform across the whole of medicine. In standing apart from (and above) general practice, they continued to adopt an elitist point of view. Thus there was no urgent reason in internal medicine, as in surgery, to establish professional standards from within. Surgical reform, although originating from the university departments of surgery, centered on community hospital practice, whereas the focus of internal medicine was the laboratory and clinics of the university.

Leaders in the emerging departments of medicine had little interest in Stern or his apparent status-seeking. To the stars in academic medicine, the new College appeared pretentious, irrelevant, unnecessary, and perhaps even faintly absurd. Academic medicine was sui generis, looking for intellectual and scientific measures as the gauge of medicine's success. Osler spoke proudly of the results of experimental and chemical research that were reported in the medical journals as evidence of the increasing stature and success of internal medicine; he praised the reorganization of practical subjects on university lines.[14] While the universities were expanding and developing a clinical research emphasis, the intellectual focus served well to define internal medicine as a serious, difficult, and aristocratic discipline.

Charles S. Martin, recollecting the early days of the American College of Physicians, reported that academic support was slow, development unsatisfactory, and "mediocrity seemed its only destiny."[15] By 1925 College membership was almost 1,000, but leaders of the profession and heads of university departments were conspicuous by their absence. There was an obvious tension, still largely unexamined, between two competing concepts of internal medicine: that of a consulting hierarchy whose stature was so far above the mass that its excellence needed no further organizational definition, and that of a specialty of internal medicine whose needs were not unlike those of surgeons, seeking recognition for their skills in the marketplace of medical care.

The American Society for Clinical Investigation, organized in 1908, provided another focus for the academic and scientific development of internal medicine as a specialty. The Society's membership linked clinical science and clinical medicine. Thus the Society's first president defined clinical medicine, after all the specialties had divided off, as the study of the natural history of diseases: their "physiology and their pharmacology."[16] These definitions suggest that the shift in leadership from the consultants to the professors was also a shift in focus from diagnosis to research. However, it is probably more accurate to say that the growing concentration of individuals and resources in medical schools and their associated hospitals and clinics in the early twentieth century changed the meanings of both diagnosis and research.

The leading physicians in academic medicine did not need professional organizations to define their field; they were already defined by virtue of their rank in university departments of medicine and their positions on national networks. The academics have indeed remained, in some ways, resistant to organizations by avoiding formal classification of internal medicine wherever it has been feasible to do so. However, external events were, once again, to intervene. The widespread organization of specialist organizations, including the specialty boards, in the 1920s and 1930s, forced internal medicine to define itself in order to defend a generalist position, through the competing activity—indeed the encroachment—of other specialist fields.

The Practice Specialty

In 1920 the American Medical Association (AMA) Council on Medical Education and Hospitals organized fifteen specialist committees, drawing the members from universities and major specialty associations.[17] These committees were to develop, first, curricula for undergraduate medical courses and, second, programs to mark specialist skills. Both tasks impinged on the actual and potential power of university departments of medicine. The committees also threatened internal medicine as a substantive field that was both wide-ranging and based on the clinical sciences. The establishment of separate committees for the basic medical sciences, including pathology and bacteriology, removed them from the imputed domain of internal medicine. The basic medical sciences were recognized, in effect, as the property of the whole of medicine, subjects on which every clinical specialty had a right to speak. At the same time, committees for pediatrics, dermatology, urology, and ophthalmology, as well as internal medicine, put the latter on the same organizational level—essentially denying internal medicine a special niche as a superior elite or even as an umbrella organization under which other medical fields might be sheltered.

These AMA committees were important because they formed the nucleus for the gradual development of specialty certifying boards, each with its own national specialist allegiances and each pressing to set up its own university programs and curricula and specially defined residency positions. True to its form as a university-based field, the 1920s committee on internal medicine favored recognition of specialists through a university degree, as well as by certification by a body similar to that of the American College of Surgeons. However, the American College of Physicians was not seen as a natural focus for this effort; instead, the committee suggested certification through the AMA's Council on Medical Education and Hospitals. There is clearly a good story in these debates.

The plight of general practice and its relations with specialties raised other problems of definition for internal medicine in the 1920s. General practice was becoming a field defined functionally by omission and educationally by inferiority. Without a separate committee of investigation in the AMA reports in the early 1920s, general practice could be defined as something left over after each special field had carved out its domain. How general practice was to be defined in terms of education was moot. University-based physicians tended to see general practice as a relatively comprehensive medical education before the selected few went on to specialize; in other words, they tended to see general practice as a preliminary, inferior brand of education, with specialists representing the intellectual elite. Yet, it was not clear whether this meant that specialists in internal medicine were to be regarded as super general practitioners, that is, as a small group of consultants in a two-tier system of general medicine.

Such questions appear to have been of little interest within university departments of medicine in the 1920s, which continued to focus on clinical medicine in an expanding context of clinical research. However, the fact that internists lacked a single, recognized organization to represent their interests left the field open for unilateral action by the Council on Medical Education and Hospitals of the AMA. In a world driven by the political rivalries of organization and specialization, it was no longer possible to maintain an aristocratic aloofness. The AMA Council began to investigate hospitals offering residencies in 1924 and published its first list of residencies in 1927. The Council was by then firmly of the view that it was not necessary for a hospital offering residency training to have a medical school affiliation, and certainly not necessary for the resident to work for a university degree. Thus, as residencies moved to independent hospitals, the links between internal medicine and universities were attenuated. University departments of medicine were not, in short, to have a monopoly on deciding who was to be trained as a specialist in their field. Moreover, compared with other specialties, there was an obvious and growing gap in authority over residency education in internal medicine.

Specialty certification arose initially out of the recognized need to define and regulate the practice of surgery. The strong early role played by the American College of Surgeons was soon echoed by the American Board of Ophthalmology (1917) and the American Board of Otolaryngology (1924). Most of the other specialty boards developed in the 1930s. The goals of the new boards were twofold: to provide a hallmark of quality in fields that were a prime target for practice by general practitioners (including appendectomies and tonsillectomies) and by other health professionals (including optometrists) and also to establish monopolies based on specialist techniques. In establishing certification requirements, leaders in the specialties sought to raise the prestige of their field above that of general practice and assure it a major place in university medical schools. Ironically, such moves were largely irrelevant to internal medicine. Its academic leaders were already prestigious within the schools. Furthermore, with their emphasis on research-based practice, academic physicians did not consider themselves to be competing in the same domain as general practitioners, whereas other specialties were. Indeed, specialists in internal medicine had little interest in curtailing the activities of general practitioners; it would make more sense to expand the role of general practitioners as providers of primary care who would refer difficult patients to internists for an expert opinion.

It is not surprising, then, that internal medicine was a late and reluctant entry to specialty certification. The American Board of Internal Medicine was the twelfth approved specialty board. The board fit into the strenthening and emerging agenda of the American College of Physicians, which was becoming for the first time a legitimate voice within internal medicine. Despite strong views that internal medicine was not a specialty, in the sense of a narrow technique or restricted area of practice, there were equally strong views that if the College did not participate with the AMA in founding a specialty board it might well be bypassed, either by the AMA or by public licensing agencies.[18] Such views were realistic. The Association of American Physicians, long proud of its isolation from medical politics, took no official action. However, the College was becoming a central force for internal medicine as both an academic and a practice discipline. Professors and the College were finally linked.

The American College of Physicians' leadership in specialty certification gave the College a majority vote in the new specialty board and ensured a university rather than a practice flavor. As far as possible, certification would reflect the prevailing values of academic internal medicine. For example, it was agreed that College fellowship should be contingent on certification from the Board, a measure achieved in 1940. This link ratified the idea of an elite community of physicians, identified by quality and organized in a college. The examination was also to be patterned after those of the British Royal Colleges. John Morgan's wish for a national elite was thus finally attained within a uniquely American setting.

Significantly, it was also agreed that eventually the new board would set up procedures for additional certification in medical subspecialties. Such moves undoubtedly prevented the fragmentation of separate boards in gastroenterology and tuberculosis, which existed in embryonic form in the late 1930s.[19] Subspecialty certification was put into effect in 1941 for allergy, cardiovascular disease, gastroenterology, and tuberculosis. Despite the wishes of early leaders of the Board to retain internal medicine as a flexible field, based on general principles, the development of the Board and its subspecialties inevitably implied that internal medicine could be defined by the acquisition of certain techniques and skills. The structural definition of internal medicine was hard to resist. The Board's existence also proclaimed that internal medicine was strategically different from general practice and that internal medicine was a field that had subspecialties, to which entry could only be made after a period in general internal medicine.[20] General internal medicine had been placed on a lesser rung of the ladder of academic prestige than the evolving subspecialties. New problems had been created. If internal medicine was a general specialty, why have subspecialties at all? If internal medicine was a consulting specialty, did this mean consulting primarily at the subspecialty level? The future role of general internal medicine became increasingly ambiguous.

What self-described specialists or diplomates in internal medicine were actually doing in the 1930s demands special investigation. There were few effective medical techniques available to general physicians in the 1930s beyond diagnostic acumen, good patient-physician communication, and supervision of nursing care. None of these applications should be downplayed. Nevertheless, the primary attributes of the good physician were knowledge, logic, common sense, and judgment—skills of personality, experience, and intellect.

The introduction of the sulfonamides in the late 1930s and the development of antibiotics and mood-altering drugs during and after World War II, respectively, changed the picture significantly by giving physicians, for the first time, a powerful technological armamentarium. At the same time, the drugs downplayed the role of general internal medicine by vastly increasing the capabilities of general practitioners and physicians in other specialties who were also providing primary care. These movements coincided with the early years of the American Board of Internal Medicine and confounded its effects.

It is easy to identify the establishment of the Board as the beginning of regimentation in medicine and as shifting internal medicine towards a focus on procedures and away from the art of doctoring, the best of science and the best of humanism. However, such criticisms need to be placed in their appropriate framework. It was not possible to sustain the Oslerian tradition of the consultant-generalist in the rush to specialist definition in the 1930s and 1940s and in the face of changes in medical technique.

Leaders of the Association of American Physicians continued to describe it as an elite club devoted to the cultivation of medical learning and to exactness and perfection in medicine through pure science.[21] However, clinical practice had become the "medicine of multiple maneuver," in which the patient was "clinicked," organ by organ, piece by piece.[22] The new generalist, it appeared, would have to be both a sorter of gratuitous information and a guide for the patient through a network of specialists. This was a role for the primary care physician.

At the same time, the specialty board gave the American College of Physicians a renewed sense of purpose and a central role in the organization of professional structures of internal medicine. The College became an active force in the field: it brought together the academic and practitioner interests and was strongly associated with the new specialty certifying machinery. Thus, although none of the ambivalences in internal medicine were resolved by World War II, the organizational structure was becoming streamlined. Internal medicine had become a medical specialty, involved in politics and turf battles across all of medicine. Internal medicine was now a practitioner's field.

Internal Medicine in the Past 40 Years

The great burst of specialization accompanying the war, the enormous increase in the number of residencies after the war, and the development of new techniques such as cardiac catheterization in the 1950s and flexible endoscopes in the 1960s and 1970s gave new meaning to the old debates. Was internal medicine general medicine, academic medicine, a holding company for the subspecialties, or merely one form of primary care? And could it continue as an uneasy blending of all of these missions?

By the late 1950s debates over the nature of internal medicine were in full flower. The number of residencies offered in internal medicine grew from approximately 700 in 1940 to over 3,700 in 1950 and on to 5,500 in 1960. The number of board-certified specialists in internal medicine increased from 2,158 in 1940 to 11,155 in 1961, representing 41 percent of all internists in the United States.[23] An increasing number of these internists were engaged in primary care. Irrespective of their training, their function was little different from that of the general practitioner.

At the same time, general practitioners were rising in organizational strength and pushing for separate specialty recognition, a new banner, and new forms of education. The foundation of the American Academy of General Practice in 1947, in combination with interlocking pressures for recognition of primary care as a distinctive field of practice, eventually led to the foundation of the American Board of Family Practice in 1969. Internal medicine was challenged to distinguish its role both from other specialties and from a new form of general medicine—family practice. Indeed, because family practice also included the care of children (the domain of the pediatrician) it was, in fact, more "general" in its applications than internal medicine, which had long ceded children to the pediatricians. Family practice also emphasized its "humanistic" focus, by stressing the importance of the physician-patient relationship and psychological skills.[24] Internal medicine's special claim to represent both the science and the art of medicine was thereby undercut and perhaps preempted.

If family practice was a specialty, there would be no physicians who were *not* specialists; the medical army would be all officers with no one in the ranks. Internal medicine was therefore faced with definitional problems in three interconnected spheres: its place as a consulting specialty (or elite), its future as a general specialty, and its evolving role in primary care. The least ambiguous category was the traditional yearning for a consulting elite. In the future, it seemed, the only true consultants would be the subspecialists.

Attempts to define internal medicine during the 1950s and 1960s reveal the strains and stresses on internal medicine as its leaders and organizations struggled to define and defend a special mission. There were claims that the field was at the crossroads of survival, even that it was a dying specialty, and suggestions that the specialty be refocused, for example, by renaming the board the American Board of Diagnostic Medicine. Concern about the future of the internist in primary care was joined by dismay at the discovery that the general, unspecialized internist was no longer in power—and was generally on the wane—in university departments of medicine.[25] The internist with subspecialty training was taking over the hallowed ground in the medical schools, which had been the center for internal medicine's image since at least the 1920s. Calls for a new role for the mass of internists, including the lingering and nostalgic claim to reinvent internal medicine above family practice as a consulting specialty, were sharpened by the implied insult of third party insurance schemes, which assumed internists and general practitioners provided equal services in primary care. The American Society of Internal Medicine was formed specifically to represent practitioner interests.

As James Warren observed in the mid-1960s, internal medicine was now divided into two major and different kinds of internists: the generalists in primary care, who no longer acted as consultants, and an increasing number of subspecialists, such as cardiologists and hematologists, who were consultants but not generalists.[26] There was real concern that the division of internal medicine into subspecialties would destroy the integrity of internal medicine as a field. I agree with Alvin Tarlov, who has labeled the period 1955 to 1975 as one of a major shift toward the subspecialties, that the shift was a response in large part to the great enlargement and growing prestige of subspecialty sections in medical schools, stimulated by the growth of research sponsored by the National Institutes of Health (NIH) and by the appointment of formally trained subspecialists as department chairmen.[27] Because internal medicine had a strong research focus since its inception, it was not surprising that as research interests changed so would leadership in the field. For whatever reason, young internists were rushing away from general internal medicine. In the first half of the 1970s, 80 percent of residents in internal medicine selected additional subspecialty training.[28]

The preceding chapters have illuminated the historical development of selected subspecialties and the general rise of the medical subspecialties from World War II to the present, including their roles, their techniques, their institutions, their relative prestige, and their organizational jostlings within internal medicine. Two important confounding factors prevent any simple interpretation of the changing balance of generalists and subspecialists. These are, respectively, the influence of incentives within the health care system and the dynamics of specialty certification.

The number and distribution of residency positions, which are the base for specialist education, are determined in large part by the service demands of hospitals, the medical power structures of hospital medical staffs, and the availability of funds through third party reimbursement. These choices are tempered by the residency review committees, including the residency review committee in internal medicine, which must approve individual programs. However, because virtually all physicians after World War II went on from their medical education to graduate education in hospitals, the hospitals, collectively, have had a strong role in determining the structure of specialty education. Since hospitals provided 75 percent of the revenue of residency training in internal medicine at the height of subspecialization in the mid-1970s, their influence has been critical. Third party reimbursement enabled high cost, high technology services in hospitals, including the blossoming of cardiology around specialized cardiac intensive care and widespread cardiac catheterization.

The American Board of Internal Medicine appears to have swung from one position to another, responding to strategic interest and environmental pressures, rather than to any consistent philosophical position. In 1967, the board modified its requirements, as did the American Board of Pediatrics, to certify family physicians. However, this failed to stem the establishment of a separate board of family practice. Instead, the ABIM developed a complex set of pathways to specialist certification, adding six more subspecialties in the 1970s, each with its own subspecialty board. Thus the Board itself was becoming increasingly bureaucratic, rigidly structured, and divided by strong vested interests. In these respects the board reflected the status of internal medicine as a whole.

In turn, a new generalist movement was launched in the 1970s to reinvent general medicine as a legitimate academic field within university departments of medicine, through the establishment of general internal medicine units. Before 1970 there were only five organized general internal medicine units in the primary teaching hospitals; by the end of the 1970s most such hospitals had general internal medicine units.[29] Apart from the obvious goal of sustaining general internal medicine in an increasingly specialized professional environment, these new units were supported for a variety of reasons: to provide faculty for general training of internal medicine residents and training in primary care, to manage and staff general medical clinics, and to respond to concerns among leading internists that general medicine could be redefined as a legitimate intellectual field. Behind these issues were other questions of balance and relative power within internal medicine.

General internal medicine is still defining its focus and field and attempting to develop a clear-cut power structure as a primary care specialty. John Eisenberg, a leading advocate for general internal medicine, has called primary care the "flagship for general internal medicine."[30] Yet the diversity of potential roles in primary care—and the often trivial nature of the complaints presented by patients—make it difficult to establish a monopoly of practice, a set of unique skills, or a turf that would place general internal medicine as a specialty comparable with the subspecialties, which are defined by referrals, specialized equipment, and technique. Eisenberg has argued for a new kind of practitioner who can address the social as well as the biological missions of internal medicine and who is comfortable with scholarship in the social sciences and humanities as well as in the medical sciences; this physician would also be a clinical investigator and have a role in "secondary" or consulting care. Such ideas suggest a new role for a humane, well-educated diagnostician—William Osler reinvented. However, the picture becomes confused when it is also suggested that the general internist may have a specific area of expertise and when general internal medicine units are challenged to define their specific areas of research interest.

General internists in the academic units have stopped short of claiming that theirs is a medicine based on skills in the social sciences. Meanwhile the field lacks the clarity and sense of intellectual colleagueship that distinguished the founders of internal medicine or, for that matter, that distinguish current medical subspecialties. It is significant that a recent survey of chairmen of departments of medicine overwhelmingly stressed research capability and potential as a primary factor affecting the academic viability of general internal medicine in the future.[31] How faculty in the general units define research, how far chairmen of departments of medicine encourage research over the demands for teaching and service in primary care, and how far research by generalists can be presented as a unified body of work of unquestioned intellectual and scientific excellence, form major problems in academic internal medicine for the 1980s and 1990s.

For internal medicine as a whole, questions of generalism and specialism have formed continuous themes over the past forty years, taking on new meanings as the context of medicine has changed. The image of the general physician as consultant—that is, as a highly trained physician able to generalize across the broad scope of internal medicine, who is recognized as a consultant by other physicians—has largely disappeared, although it reappears from time to time as an ideal to be reinvented. The situation is complicated because there are outstanding individual physicians in academic settings, great general diagnosticians like Jack Myers, who continue to play a consulting role for their peers, in careers forged through special talents and individual experience. Attempting to legislate a general consultant role through the professional structures of medicine (i.e., board certification) would be a losing proposition in the 1980s. Indeed the general internist is now in an organizational relationship, vis-à-vis the subspecialties, similar to that of the family physicians to the early internists. The consultant role has largely moved to the subspecialties, confirming general internal medicine as concerned mainly with primary care.

Redefining Generalism

The relationship between general internal medicine and the subspecialties has dominated the development of the field in the past forty years, while the major external defining forces have been fiscal incentives within the health care system. Now, arguably, the relative influence of the board is on the wane. However, the meaning of "generalism" continues to be vexing. Indeed, new questions of generalism and specialism have arisen out of recent changes within the practice fields.

The early leaders of internal medicine assumed that the specialist was, inevitably, narrowly focused. Now the superspecialist, like the generalist, is frequently required to generalize across the whole of medicine and to take into account a complex array of facts and risks in caring for an individual patient. It is not clear how far the image of the subspecialist should now be equated with the supertechnician. For example, managing a difficult carcinoma requires physician skills of knowledge, science, judgment, humanism, empathy, and communication—the same skills as those emphasized by the great practitioners of the late nineteenth century. Thus, in some ways, the subspecialists, as well as the general internists, can be seen as the inheritors of the Oslerian tradition. How far the subspecialists will be defined as generalists, in this context, is an interesting question that will be addressed in the next twenty years.

The appearance of new general fields, cutting across the established specialties, muddies the issues even further. Because the lines of the specialty examining boards were largely laid down before World War II, it is not surprising that new fields of "general medicine" arose outside the organizational boundaries of internal medicine or have competing sponsorship by other specialties. For example, allergy, immunology and nuclear medicine have attained independent board status. Emergency medicine is virtually autonomous as a conjoint board. Toxicologists, with an as yet unapproved board, are waiting in the wings. What to do about other cross-cutting fields, including critical care, clinical pharmacology, and nutrition, is a major contemporary issue. Each of these fields eats into the territory of internal medicine as it is organizationally defined by its specialty board structures. As defined by these structures, internal medicine and general medicine have significantly diverged.

There are now twenty-three approved medical specialty boards; internal medicine is only one of these. Most boards have subspecialties. As a result, the present array of specialist qualifications is fraught with competing and overlapping jurisdictions. For example, both internal medicine and family practice are seeking what they call "added qualifications" in geriatric medicine, and critical care has been approved by the American Board of Medical Specialties—the "holding company" for all the boards—as appropriate for a special certificate by five boards, including internal medicine, anesthesiology, neurological surgery, pediatrics, and surgery. As a result of these changes, the definition of a specialty as a single disciplinary unit, identified through board status, is seriously threatened.

For the past forty years, whatever the crises and turmoil in the field, internal medicine has been structurally defined by its residencies and certifying machinery. Today all of the definitional questions are once more open. More important, the frame of reference demands reexamination. In the past forty years, the term internal medicine has been considered synonymous with the professional structures of specialization. However, in the future it is quite possible that new organizations will arise that will not accept this narrow definition or that will invent a new field of "general medicine."

Conclusions in Late Twentieth-Century Perspective

One solution to the present divisions within internal medicine would be to dissolve it altogether, that is, to dissolve internal medicine as an organized specialty. General internal medicine might, logically, merge with family practice. Each of the subspecialties could decide whether to develop independently or continue under the present board. University departments of medicine would continue to act as an umbrella for the pursuit of investigation, teaching, and clinical practice across a wide array of disciplines. Within their boundaries might emerge a new, broad definition of "general medicine."

Such observations, however rational, ignore the other side of the coin of the specialty's history: its organizational success within the profession of medicine, buttressed by continuing self-questioning of its aims. The historical record suggests at least four reasons for preserving internal medicine as a mix of a general and subspecialist fields, with all its internal inconsistencies.

First, internal medicine has, in some ways, served as a self-defined conscience for medicine. The history of internal medicine has consistently stressed certain themes: that absolutes in medicine are few, that technical skills are important but limited, and that judgment and perhaps the physician's character are paramount attributes of the good physician. It is no accident that it is the American Board of Internal Medicine, rather than other boards, that is now stressing the value of "humanism" as an intrinsic part of the practice of medicine.[32] Despite the leveling effects of the boards and the organization of the health care system, internal medicine still strives to see itself as qualitatively different from other fields. Its organizational persona is important to American medicine—as it has been for the past decades.

Second, and substantively, there is a compelling need for organizations in American medicine that can encompass all points of view, from primary to tertiary care. Pediatrics provides a similar opportunity. Indeed, the narrowing organizational domain of internal medicine sits oddly against the breadth and complexity of clinical problems in the field. The journals of internal medicine cover topics as diverse and wideranging as cardiac imaging, biofeedback, AIDS, chemical dependence, and the condition of the elderly in nursing homes. It may be that these are all different aspects of primary care, but here, too, there is an advantage in having structures that encompass primary and secondary care within one set of organizations, allowing for flexibility among their substances as the nature of medicine changes.

Third, acceptance of the notion of relative risk in chronic disease and in major surgery, by both doctor and patient, gives a new meaning to the internist as an arbitrator and negotiator between the patient and other physicians. Internal medicine is engaged in rethinking the relationship between medicine and surgery in areas ranging from the management of breast cancer to heart disease and gallstone removal. Rather than becoming a more limited field, it can be argued that "general medicine" is entering a new golden age. Moreover, while internal medicine has traditionally, over its history, responded to surgical leadership in medicine, it is the surgeons who are now under criticism. One interesting way of viewing the history of internal medicine would, indeed, be to examine the continuing dialogue, over time, within various fields, between medical and surgical approaches to disease and the relative power of internists and surgeons. That issue aside, if general internal medicine did not exist it would probably have to be reinvented—and might well blossom out into a new set of subspecialties.

A fourth reason for maintaining the present structure is that internists are past masters at dealing with uncertainty. Of all the specialties internal medicine has perhaps been the most openly willing to change: from a focus on consultant practice to clinical investigation in the medical schools in the early years of the century; to the establishment of a specialty board and a major base in clinical practice from the late 1930s; to the ability to encompass primary care after World War II. Its ideology has shifted in different periods, encompassing a mix of diagnostic medicine, university-based clinical research, subspecialty technique, and now an apparent shift to "humanistic" medicine. The location of the patient has shifted, too, from the home or private hospital room, to the clinical research unit of a major university, to huge hospital units focused on techniques of intensive care, and now (again) to a new focus on the ambulatory patient.

In addition, powerful systems extrinsic to the specialty per se have exerted widely varying effects over the years, from the era of university domination of medicine before World War II, to a hospital-dominated model, in turn replaced by the system-dominated medicine of the present. Even more fundamentally, over the life cycle of internal medicine, the primary cause of mortality and morbidity has shifted from infectious to chronic diseases. The professional organizations of internal medicine have survived all of these shifts, proving markedly adaptive as conditions have changed. Arguably, despite the early wish to keep internal medicine out of "medical politics," internal medicine has been the most successful specialty, politically, in all of American medicine.

Looking back over the past decades, one can only be struck by the continuous interweaving of the old themes—primary care versus consulting, generalism versus specialism, internal medicine as a democracy or an elite—through vast changes in the science, practice, and environments of medicine. The relative balance of these themes has been determined largely by forces external to internal medicine itself; for example, the ballooning development of the subspecialties following the availability of hospital reimbursement. However, internal medicine is too powerful and too central to medicine to be viewed as a passive or reactive discipline. The organizational success of internal medicine also makes it an important proactive force, which any move to carve up the field would lessen.

Political and economic issues in health care now dominate the agenda of professional organizations. The American College of Physicians has developed its own health policy initiative. The whole structure of graduate medical education is vulnerable to congressional legislation. Leaders of academic internal medicine are only too aware that the viability of their departments rests, at least in part, on the availability of research funding from NIH and other sources, on effective marketing of faculty practice plans in competition with other organizations, and on adequate reimbursement schemes for indigent patients in academic health centers.

Health care systems are becoming increasingly important in defining specialist roles and jobs and may become more important in the future in defining residency training programs (and in paying for them). As an increasing proportion of physicians becomes involved in large-scale practice organizations, the role of the "internist" will become defined by arrangements within specific organizations. Once again, internal medicine is faced by challenges and shifts. There is no reason to suppose that its organizations will respond any less adaptively or successfully than in earlier periods. Indeed, for those who see internal medicine as currently in a crisis, there may be some comfort in recognizing the history of internal medicine as one of constant crisis, ambiguity, conflict, and adaptability.

For historians, the development of internal medicine offers a window into fundamental questions in American medicine, suggesting new ways of defining several historical themes: the nature of scientific ideology; the connections between professional perceptions, practices, and organizations; the relationship between the specialty and external influences; the role of prestige structures within medicine (not forgetting the role of women and minorities); the relationship between the knowledge and skill base of a special field and its organizational arrangements; the nature of a "specialty" per se. In all of these areas, the cognitive and institutional aspects of internal medicine and its subspecialties have reinforced and reacted to each other in varying patterns over the years as variations on a set of central themes.

For internal medicine in the 1980s, as in earlier periods, the definitional and organizational questions intermesh. Questions of power, politics, and professionalism jostle uneasily for prominence as internal medicine struggles for consensus over purpose and mission in an environment dominated by health care systems. But in the 1980s, unlike the 1880s, internal medicine can address the issues of definition and organization from an established position of professional authority. No longer looking to German science or British models, internal medicine holds a pivotal position in American medicine. Because of the success of the organizations of internal medicine as a specialty, its leaders and institutions have power in the political and professional arenas far greater than those of early leaders. Thus internal medicine has a potentially large part to play in defining the future role of primary care and general medicine and in articulating, for the whole profession, the art of diagnosis and the nature of treatment. Looking back is a way of understanding internal medicine in the present—its inheritance, its environments, its cumulative stresses, and its changing opportunities.

My special thanks to Russell C. Maulitz and Charles E. Rosenberg for comments on an earlier draft of this paper. Background research was funded in part by a grant from the Commonwealth Fund for research on the history of hospitals and academic medical centers.

NOTES

1. Francis Delafield, first president of the Association of American Physicians, became widely quoted for defining that association as one in which "there will be no medical politics and no medical ethics." "Chronic Catarrhal Gastritis, with Opening Remarks by the President," *Trans Assoc Am Physicians* 1(1886):1. William Osler reinforced these aims in his presidential address nine years later, *Trans Assoc Am Physicians* 10(1895):xiii.

2. Cardiovascular diseases (first certificates granted in 1941), gastroenterology (1941), pulmonary diseases (1941), endocrinology and metabolism (1972), hematology (1972), infectious diseases (1972), nephrology (1972), rheumatology (1972), medical oncology (1973), diagnostic laboratory immunology (1986), and critical care (in development). American Board of Medical Specialties, *Annual Report and Reference Handbook, 1985* (Chicago: American Board, 1985), 60.

3. The ABIM granted 42,859 general certificates between 1975 and 1984, out of a total of 165,289 general certificates from all approved specialty boards. ABMS, *Annual Report*, 62.

4. Rosemary Stevens, *Medical Practice in Modern England* (New Haven: Yale University Press, 1966), 26–37.

5. Whitfield Bell's history of the College of Physicians of Philadelphia is in progress and should provide a much needed analysis of the eighteenth-century debates about a "College" and the role of a consultant elite.

6. The seven were Francis A. Delafield, William H. Draper, George L. Peabody, Robert T. Edes, William Pepper, James Tyson, and William Osler. See James Howard Means, *The Association of American Physicians: It First Seventy-Five Years* (New York: McGraw-Hill, 1961).

7. Samuel D. Gross, "Address of Welcome," *Trans Am Surg Assoc* 1(1883):xxii. The phrase "fast age" also comes from this source.

8. A vivid example is Maurice Richardson's Presidential Address to the American Surgical Association in 1903. For example: "Without exact demonstration of the truth, one diagnosis may be as good as another. Surgery affords a verification of

opinion, and is the control of diagnosis. No matter how painstaking the observer, how detailed his history, how educated his touch, how logical his deductions, no diagnosis—except by accurate operative demonstration—can be without possibilities of error. . . . Even if his deductions are good, his observations may be bad. Surgical explorations, I repeat, are establishing facts, and broadening experience is making deductions accurate; in a word, surgery is correcting premises and facilitating conclusions." "Address of the President," *Trans Am Surg Assoc* 21(1903):8–9.

9. William Osler, "Presidential Address," *Trans Assoc Am Physicians* 10(1895):xiii.

10. G. Baumgarten, "Presidential Address," 14(1899):xviii.

11. President Baumgarten of the AAP, for example, saw the association as standing both for specialization (that is, concentration of effort by the investigator and clinical observer) and as a counterbalance to overspecialization (a "one-sided devotion" to technique). The goal was to avoid both the "empty dogmatism" of generalism and the unthinking routine of specialization. Baumgarten, "Presidential Address," 14(1899):xviii.

12. In this respect, too, American internal medicine appears to have diverged from the British model of the consultant physician, whose prestige continued to be assured by hospital appointment rather than by a full-time medical school position. However, the relative roles, functions, and prestige of "internists" in the two countries in the early twentieth century await attention by historians.

13. The role of the university departments of medicine in this period, and later, also deserves special scrutiny. Obvious questions include, among others: (1) Where has the power in internal medicine actually resided, and how has power shifted over the years? (2) How far has policy been made by the professors, both in the university departments and through their influence in the American College of Physicians, on the specialty boards, and on the Residency Review Committee? (3) How far, in these respects, is internal medicine like or unlike other specialties? (4) How far has the medical school structure of departments and units dictated the board-examining structure of subspecialties, and vice versa? (5) What impact does the placing of fields, such as oncology, within internal medicine, the specialty, have on the cognitive skills and practice in the subspecialty field? If allergy and immunology are no longer organizationally part of internal medicine, why does hematology remain? How far do these reflect research interests in the universities? (6) Which have been, and are, the leading university centers in internal medicine development? How have they developed the field and how have they differed? (7) How have—and do—the university departments define "medicine" as distinct from "internal medicine"? Recent studies in the history of medicine and biomedical sciences provide a good base for specialized study of internal medicine and ask these and other questions; see especially: Kenneth Ludmerer, *Learning to Heal: The Development of Modern Medical Education* (New York: Basic Books, 1985); A. McGehee Harvey, *Science at the Bedside: Clinical Research in American Medicine 1905–1945* (Baltimore: Johns Hopkins Press, 1981); and Robert Kohler, *From Medical Chemistry to Biochemistry: The Making of a Biomedical Discipline* (Cambridge: Cambridge University Press, 1982).

14. William Osler, "The Coming of Age of Internal Medicine in America," *Int Clin* 4(1915):4.

15. Charles F. Martin, "My Recollections of the Period 1925–29," in *The*

American College of Physicians: Its First Quarter Century, W. G. Morgan, ed. (Philadelphia: American College of Physicians, 1940), 103.

16. See J. Harold Austin, "A Brief Sketch of the History of the American Society for Clinical Investigation," *J Clin Invest* 28(1949):404–6.

17. See "Graduate Education in the Specialties," *AMA Bulletin* 15(1921): 17–82.

18. See, for example, "Hospital Service in the United States," *JAMA* 96 (1931):1019–20; "Abstract of Minutes of the Board of Regents," *Ann Intern Med* 7(1934):1564–65; Editorial, *Ann Intern Med* 8(1935):1163–64; Editorial, "The American Board of Internal Medicine," *Ann Intern Med* 10(1936):411; and Walter L. Bierring, "The American Board of Internal Medicine," in *American College of Physicians,* W. G. Morgan, ed., 87–102.

19. "Hospital Services in the United States," *JAMA* 110(1938):975.

20. It would be interesting, in this context, to review dictionary and textbook definitions of internal medicine over the years. For example, *The American Illustrated Medical Dictionary,* ed. 22 (Philadelphia: W. B. Saunders, 1951), defines internal medicine as "that department of medicine which deals with diseases that cannot be treated surgically; medicine as distinguished from surgery." It assumes, in short, that internal medicine is general medicine. Examination of earlier editions and other texts would reveal how far this definition held, in general, and for earlier years.

21. See, for example, J. H. Means, "President's Address," *Trans Assoc Am Physicians* 57(1942):1–5.

22. A. H. Gordon, "President's Address," 61(1948):1–3.

23. See Rosemary Stevens, *American Medicine and the Public Interest* (New Haven: Yale University Press, 1971), 395.

24. C. L. Witten, A. N. Johnson, J. Michaelson, and W. Lotterhos, "The Core Content of Family Medicine: A Report of the Committee on Requirements for Certification," *GP* 34(1966):225–46.

25. See, for example, Paul S. Rhoads, editorial, "Internal Medicine and the Training of Internists," *Arch Intern Med* 102(1958):515–19; Arthur L. Bloomfield, editorial, "Origin of the Term 'Internal Medicine,'" *JAMA* 169(1959):1628–29; J. Lown Thompson, letter, "What is an 'Internist'?" *JAMA* 171(1959):1029–30; James V. Warren, "The Future of Internal Medicine," *Clin Res* 9(1961):111–13; Lowell A. Rantz, "The Image of an Internist," *Clin Res* 9(1961):218–20; Wright Adams, "Internal Medicine Under Stress," *JAMA* 186(1963):934–37; and Richard V. Ebert, "The Training of the Physician," *N Engl J Med* 271(1964):547–52.

26. James V. Warren, "The Training of the Internist: Today and Tomorrow," *JAMA* 195(1966):151–54.

27. Alvin R. Tarlov, editorial, "Academic General Internal Medicine," *Ann Intern Med* 96(1982):239.

28. Alvin R. Tarlov, Peter A. Weil, Mary Kay Schleiter, and the Association of Professors of Medicine Task Force on Manpower, "National Study of Internal Medicine Manpower: I. Residency Training 1976–77," *Ann Intern Med* 88(1978):413.

29. Robert H. Friedman, Janet T. Pozen, A. Lynn Rosencrans, et al., "General Internal Medicine Units in Academic Medical Centers: Their Emergence and Function," *Ann Intern Med* 96(1982):233–38.

30. John M. Eisenberg, "Sculpture of a New Academic Discipline: Four Faces of Academic Internal Medicine," *Am J Med* 78(1985):283–92. See also Eisenberg,

"The Internist as Gatekeeper: Preparing the General Internist for a New Role," *Ann Intern Med* 102(1985):537–43.

31. Robert H. Friedman and Janet T. Pozen, "The Academic Viability of General Internal Medicine," *Ann Intern Med* 103(1985):439–44.

32. See "Evaluation of Humanistic Qualities in the Internist, ABIM," *Ann Intern Med* 99(1983):720–24; Solomon Papper, "The Future of the General Internist," *Arch Intern Med* 143(1983):1601–2; and Richard Gorlin and Howard D. Zucker, "Physicians' Reactions to Patients: A Key to Teaching Humanistic Medicine," *N Engl J Med* 308(1983):1059–63.

CONTRIBUTORS

Paul B. Beeson, M.D., is Professor of Medicine Emeritus at Oxford University, where he held the Nuffield Chair, and the University of Washington. As medical author and editor of several editions of the influential *Cecil Textbook of Medicine*, he has put an indelible stamp on internal medicine as a medical specialty in the United States.

Thomas G. Benedek, M.D., is Professor in the Departments of Medicine and History at the University of Pittsburgh, as well as chief of ambulatory care and of rheumatology at the Pittsburgh Veterans Administration Medical Center. He is the author of several articles on the history and geography of the rheumatic diseases.

W. Bruce Fye, M.A., M.D., is chairman of the cardiology department at the Marshfield Clinic and Adjunct Associate Professor of the History of Medicine at the University of Wisconsin. Fye has published widely on historical topics, including a book titled *The Development of American Physiology: Scientific Medicine in the Nineteenth Century* (Johns Hopkins University Press, 1987).

Joel D. Howell, M.D., Ph.D., is Assistant Professor of Medicine at the University of Michigan. His major research interests are the history of cardiology and the use of medical technology in the United States and Britain during the late nineteenth and early twentieth centuries. He is currently studying the use of medical technology in hospitals as documented in patient case records.

Edward H. Kass, M.D., Ph.D., is William Ellery Channing Professor of Medicine and Director of the Channing Laboratory at Harvard Medical School. A long-standing leader in the Infectious Diseases Society of America, he has recently become its official historian. With Amalie Kass he is preparing a major biography of Thomas Hodgkin.

Joseph B. Kirsner, M.D., Ph.D., is Louis Block Distinguished Service Professor of Medicine and has been head of the gastroenterology service and Deputy Dean for Medical Affairs at the University of Chicago Pritzker School of Medicine. A pioneer in the study of gastroenterologic disorders in the United States, he has written over 650 articles in the field and is currently working on a longer history of this specialty.

Stephen J. Kunitz, M.D., Ph.D., is Associate Professor at the University of Rochester School of Medicine and Dentistry. His research interests extend beyond the history of medical specialization to several aspects of medical anthropology. His best known work examines health, health care, and cultural aspects of Amerindian populations and their medical systems, most recently *Disease Change and the Role of Medicine: The Navajo Experience* (University of California Press, 1983).

Diana E. Long, Ph.D., is Director of the Francis C. Wood Institute for the History of Medicine at the College of Physicians of Philadelphia. Her scholarship has centered on the history of endocrinology, sex research, women's studies, and physiology from the eighteenth century to the present. On this last subject, she has published a volume entitled *Why Do Animals Breathe: Physiological Problems and Iatromechanical Research in the Enlightenment* (Arno, 1981).

Harry M. Marks, Ph.D., does research on the contemporary history of social policy and medical care. He is presently a postdoctoral fellow at the Johns Hopkins Institute of the History of Medicine, where he is completing a book on the relation between therapeutic practice and medical experimentation in the United States during the twentieth century.

Russell C. Maulitz, M.D., Ph.D., is Lecturer in History and Sociology of Science in Medicine at the University of Pennsylvania School of Medicine. His most recent publication is a monograph on the history of pathology in the early nineteenth century entitled *Morbid Appearances: The Anatomy of Pathology in the Early Nineteenth Century* (Cambridge University Press, 1987). He practices internal medicine and directs the medical student program at Presbyterian-University of Pennsylvania Medical Center in Philadelphia.

Steven J. Peitzman, M.D., is Associate Professor of Medicine and of Community Medicine (Medical Humanities) at the Medical College of Pennsylvania, where his practice and teaching concern nephrology, internal medicine, physical diagnosis, and the history of medicine. His scholarly work in medical history has dealt with renal disease, medical education, and Philadelphia medical history and biography.

Rosemary A. Stevens, Ph.D., is Professor and Chair of the Department of History and Sociology of Science at the University of Pennsylvania. She has written numerous articles and books on health policy and the history of medical practice in England and the United States, including the landmark *American Medicine and the Public Interest* (Yale University Press, 1971). Her next major work will be a history of the twentieth-century American hospital (Basic Books, forthcoming, 1988).

INDEX